Biopsychosocial Perspectives on Arab Americans

Sylvia C. Nassar-McMillan • Kristine J. Ajrouch
Julie Hakim-Larson
Editors

Biopsychosocial Perspectives on Arab Americans

Culture, Development, and Health

Springer

Editors
Sylvia C. Nassar-McMillan
Department of Curriculum, Instruction, and Counselor Education
North Carolina State University
Raleigh, NC, USA

Kristine J. Ajrouch
Department of Sociology
Eastern Michigan University
Ypsilanti, MI, USA

Julie Hakim-Larson
Department of Psychology
University of Windsor
Windsor, ON, Canada

ISBN 978-1-4614-8237-6 (hardcover)
ISBN 978-1-4614-8238-3 (eBook)
ISBN 978-1-4899-7639-0 (softcover)
DOI 10.1007/978-1-4614-8238-3
Springer New York Heidelberg Dordrecht London

Library of Congress Control Number: 2013947471

Printed on acid-free paper

Springer is part of Springer Science+Business Media (www.springer.com)

We dedicate this book to the many current and future generations of individuals with Arab ancestry in the United States and worldwide.

Sylvia C. Nassar-McMillan
Kristine J. Ajrouch
Julie Hakim-Larson

Preface

From a perspective of ethnic identity, the process of my development as both a person and a professional has followed parallel paths. Due to ethnicities (and perceived ethnicities!) of the primary elders in my family of origin, coupled with the structure of my family of origin, I have grappled since childhood with the task of determining my own identity. Thus, despite over a decade of professional scholarship focused on Arab Americans, I continue to develop an identity and sense of place. Perhaps it is those developmental challenges that have continually led me into circumstances in which a broad range of possibilities and interactions is evident, albeit perhaps not always so clearly. For example, my scholarship spans multidisciplinary conceptual and empirical literature both within the counseling profession (with publications in journals across the American Counseling Association's primary divisions) as well as external to it (with publications across psychology, social work, cultural anthropology, and health care outlets). Within these publications, the overarching theme is the promotion of effective counseling research, practice, and more recently, policy-based interventions.

Perhaps the precursor of this particular vein of scholarship over the last decade can be attributed to a dual pivotal personal–professional experience that occurred just over a decade ago. In 1999, en route to Lebanon for the first time, I stopped off in Dearborn, Michigan (just outside my hometown) to attend the first inaugural International Conference on Health Issues in Arab Communities sponsored by the Arab Community Center for Economic and Social Services. During that conference, I participated in a breakout symposium with other mental health clinicians and scholars. It was at that time, as yet unbeknownst to me, that I was exposed to the criticality of culture within the biopsychosocial perspective on health care delivery. In hindsight it may have been my broad base of personal and professional experiences to date that allowed that concept to resonate within me. Subsequently visiting family in Lebanon, and the Arab Middle East for the first time, created an interactive synergy with that professional experience that I, only now, am realizing.

Within the subsequent decade, I had experiences in which I continually felt on the periphery—of my profession (i.e., counseling and counselor education); within the Arab American community nationally; within the community of interdisciplinary scholars; as a political entity. At the same time, I have had the extreme good fortune along the way to connect with interdisciplinary colleagues in fruitful personal and professional endeavors. I have come to believe that it was Kismet (Fate) that brought me the opportunity to put together this collective volume of works. When Janice Stern, Senior Editor for Health and Behavior publications at Springer, first approached me with the opportunity to create this book project, I was convinced there must be someone better suited, particularly because she clearly wanted a health focus for the project. Through her gentle urging and supportive negotiations, I realized that it was indeed the perfect opportunity to weave together key perspectives, across the multiple disciplines of which I had so long felt on the periphery! In so doing, I have had the opportunity to co-create, with my wise and wonderful coeditors, the synergy of these disciplines, taken together. I sincerely hope that this book will have the synergistic impact that our invaluable chapter authors, all of whom are top scholars and clinical experts focused on Arab American issues, along with my coeditors Kristine Ajrouch and Julie Hakim-Larson, to whom I owe a huge debt of gratitude, have envisioned.

Raleigh, NC, USA — Sylvia C. Nassar-McMillan

Preface

The study of Arab Americans has been my primary focus since I conducted my dissertation research in the mid 1990s. As a sociology graduate student aiming to work toward the promotion of cross-cultural understanding, the topic I examined was ethnic identity development. Convinced that we needed a deeper understanding of how people think about who they are relative to from where they come, I embarked on a project that included in-depth interviews with adolescent children of immigrants and their parents. That initial study laid the foundation of my future program of research. From there I expanded my interests to pursue the study of Arab American aging. In that quest, I developed a clear commitment to elaborating the Arab American experience over the life course, and most centrally the key role social relations play in health and well-being.

The decision I made to study Arab Americans stemmed from my personal experiences as the granddaughter of Lebanese immigrants. Growing up in an upper-middle class area of metro-Detroit in the 1970s and 1980s, where virtually no Arab Americans lived, I did not understand my heritage through the daily encounters of ethnic community living. Instead, my identity emerged through the stories that my maternal grandmother told. Yet my grandmother's stories of life in Lebanon, and her immigrant experience, clashed with media accounts of what it meant to be "Arab." Media portrayals of conflict in the Arab Middle East promoted an odious Arab culture that did not fit with the persona of my immediate family, extended relatives, or for that matter the Arab American community emerging during that time in Dearborn, Michigan. It was this dichotomy, between personal experience and larger social characterizations that first pulled me to the study of Arab Americans. Moreover, coming from an immigrant family kindled a fascination with the ways in which cultural world views inform relations between and among people.

The study of Arab Americans has developed over the last decades to include a wide array of disciplinary perspectives. The goal of promoting a biopsychosocial perspective to the study of Arab Americans has become possible due to the proliferation of scholars dedicated to discerning attributes of Arab Americans that are universally human, as well as culturally unique. The opportunity to work with Sylvia Nassar-McMillan and Julie Hakim-Larson, both established scholars in their own disciplines, to develop and coedit a volume intent on advancing a more rounded and multidisciplinary view of Arab Americans has been a distinct privilege and joy. Moreover, the opportunity to work with the leading Arab American scholars who contributed to our volume has provided an enriching academic and personal experience. It is my hope that this book provides a much needed resource to those interested in learning more about Arab Americans, especially for those who work directly with Arab Americans as well as those charged with policy directives that influence the lives of all Americans.

Ypsilanti, MI, USA Kristine J. Ajrouch

Preface

Like my coeditors, Sylvia C. Nassar-McMillan and Kristine Ajrouch, I too have a long and deeply felt history linking my sense of identity to my Arab American heritage. Like Kristine Ajrouch, I am the granddaughter of immigrants from Lebanon. My Lebanese-American parents, Simon David Hakim and Yvonne Mariam (Barrack) Hakim, were both born and raised in the United States; they nonetheless maintained strong cultural ties to the Arab community through Maronite Catholic church events, their love of Arabic music (especially the 'oud' that my maternal grandfather played), a large extended family network reaching from California to Detroit, and of course the preparation of traditional Lebanese foods. I am forever grateful to my parents for the rich ethnic legacy they provided in my background experiences. My childhood history is replete with stories of Arab Detroit family life in a working class neighborhood of not only Lebanese Americans but also of Syrian, Palestinian, Jordanian, and Iraqi Chaldean Americans. As a child clinical and developmental psychologist, my lifelong interest in Arab American families is both personal and professional, and is still quite entrenched in my everyday life as well as in my academic career.

My academic interest in Arab Americans began while I was a newly tenured faculty member at the University of Windsor, which is located just across the Detroit River in Ontario, Canada—easy commuting distance from southeastern Michigan. In 1997, as I planned my first research sabbatical, the American and Canadian Psychological Associations were encouraging researchers to include diverse ethnic groups in their studies. Because my parents taught me to have a sense of pride in my ethnic identity, I wholeheartedly embraced the idea and decided to plan research with Arab Americans. Thus, I took that opportunity during my first sabbatical over 15 years ago to proactively contact local southeastern Michigan Arab American community centers (ACCESS: Arab American Community Center for Economic and Social Services; ACC: Arab American and Chaldean Council). I am grateful to these centers for assisting me with my research. When I served on the Scientific Committees of Arab American health conferences sponsored by ACCESS, I met a number of Arab American scholars and began research collaborations involving

Arab Americans. Our connections and collaborations have endured now for over a decade. At these conferences, I was also fortunate enough to meet my two like-minded coeditors, Sylvia C. Nassar-McMillan and Kristine Ajrouch, at different times and under different circumstances. Our shared love for our heritage and our mutual understanding of the need for research with Arab Americans led to an immediate bond and a joint commitment between and among us to work together on this book as well as on other Arab American projects. I am delighted at our success and I look forward to our continued work together! It was also at the biopsychosocial health and refugee conferences sponsored by ACCESS that I met many of the excellent researchers and scholars who contributed chapters to this book. I am indebted to each of them for facilitating my understanding of the complex facets of Arab American life. They have been wonderful to work with throughout the process. Like my coeditors, I too have high hopes that this book will enhance the understanding of Arab Americans among health professionals, educators, research scholars, policy makers, and clinical practitioners. Future generations of Arab Americans will hopefully reap the rewards.

Windsor, ON, Canada — Julie Hakim-Larson

Acknowledgements

The editors would like to express deep appreciation and gratitude to the multiple chapter authors that joined us in this project. Without their shared knowledge and expertise, this edited text would not have come together as it did, nor would it make the contribution that it does to the literature, as the first of its kind geared toward enhancing the efficacy of research and practice relative to Arab American health and well-being. We are grateful to these authors for their patience and persistence in the developmental process of this text and their willingness to make *just one more* revision!

As in the development of any large-scale undertaking, there is a crew that provides the backbone and infrastructure to facilitate the creativity and communication flow among the writing team. For us that team was comprised first and foremost by Janice Stern, Senior Editor for Health and Behavior at Springer Science + Business, who provided consistent guidance and support throughout. Our project manager, Lynn Zagzebski Tovar, at North Carolina State University, also provided us with much needed administrative support.

Our respective universities, North Carolina State University, Eastern Michigan University, and University of Windsor, also deserve a note of recognition. By way of scholarly leave time and other in-kind contributions, these university structures provide the avenue for scholarship such as this text to be produced.

While there are many professionals that we would like to individually thank, this list would be too innumerable to mention here. Instead we would like to make mention of a few organizations that have made this current work possible. Throughout the text, organizations such as the Arab Community Center for Economic and Social Services (ACCESS) and the Arab American Institute (AAI) are cited and their work described. These organizations, among countless others, have been providing advocacy, health care, and other services critical to the health and well-being of individuals and families of Arab descent for decades, but more importantly they have been serving as the vehicles by which the Arab American community itself becomes healthier, stronger, and more vital with each year. They have also provided the avenue through which scholars, such as our editorial team members and chapter authors, can network and develop collaborative works and expertise.

We also thank the multitude of scholars, such as Nabeel Abraham, Nuha Abudabbeh, Alixa Naff, Margaret Nydell, Gregory Orafalea, and Andrew Shyrock among many others, whose work has paved the way for ours. In particular we wish to honor the memories of Drs. Edward Said, Evelyn Shakir, and Michael W. Suleiman. The profound contributions of these prominent scholars over the last few decades will always be remembered.

Finally, we thank our family members for the myriad of ways in which they have supported the development of this work.

The Editors

Contents

Contributors

Dalia Abdelhady is a Senior Researcher at the Center for Middle East Studies at Lund University in Sweden. She received a Ph.D. in Sociology from the State University of New York at Albany. The general theme in her work deals with the ways globalization shapes the lives of individuals in various ways. Primarily, she looks at Arab immigrants and their children in Europe and North America and investigates the complex ways they integrate to their new societies, maintain ties to their homelands, and construct global solidarities and cosmopolitan identities. She is the author of The Lebanese Diaspora: The Arab Immigrant Experience in Montreal, New York and Paris, NYU Press. A second line of Abdelhady's research investigates the impact of globalization on gender dynamics in the Arab World. Studying women's public roles, Abdelhady highlights the interplay of Islam, local traditions, and global cultural ideals in shaping women's experiences in the region.

Sawsan Abdulrahim is an Associate Professor of Health Promotion and Community Health at the Faculty of Health Sciences, American University of Beirut. She completed her Ph.D. from the School of Public Health at the University of Michigan, Ann Arbor, in 2005. Her doctoral dissertation research explored social identity formations and the subjective meanings of health among Arab Americans. Her work continues to center around the health impact of social inequities and immigration in the United States and the Arab region, with an emphasis on the well-being of immigrants across the lifespan. Dr. Abdulrahim's work on Arab Americans has been published in such international journals as Social Science & Medicine and Qualitative Health Research and in the form of book chapters. She is a member of the Kellogg Program in Health Policy Research and the Cross-National Network on Place, Migration, and Health.

Kristine J. Ajrouch, Ph.D. is Professor of Sociology at Eastern Michigan University and Adjunct Research Professor at the Institute for Social Research at the University of Michigan. She completed her doctoral studies in Sociology from Wayne State University in 1997, and postdoctoral training in the field of aging through the School of Social Work at the University of Michigan. Her research has focused, for over 15 years, on Arab-Americans in the United States and more recently in the Middle East. She was a Fulbright Scholar at Haigazian University in Beirut, Lebanon during 2008. Dr. Ajrouch has published in numerous national and international journals including the Journals of Gerontology, Social Science & Medicine, Ageing & Society, and is active in both national and international professional organizations. She currently serves as Executive Secretary/Treasurer of the Society for the Study of Human Development and works on projects that enhance global awareness and promote cross-cultural understanding.

Abdul Salam Al-Kassab, M.D. is an associate clinical professor in the Department of Medicine at Wayne State University in Detroit. He is also an Assistant Clinical Professor at Oakland University/William Beaumont Medical School. He is a practicing Endocrinologist and Diabetologist in Rochester Hills, Michigan which is a suburb of Detroit. He has been a founding member of the Arab American Diabetes Task force at the American Diabetes Association Michigan Chapter. His research work in the past involved Epidemiology of Diabetes in the Middle East. In his practice, he is involved in treating patients from all ethnic backgrounds including sizeable number of Arab American patients.

Mona M. Amer, Ph.D. is an Assistant Professor of Psychology at the American University in Cairo, Egypt. Her research interests are in minority mental health, with a specialization in the Arab American and Muslim American populations. She has examined sociocultural and acculturative factors associated with psychological well-being for Arab Americans, and identity development among Arab Muslim youth. Dr. Amer has developed cultural competence trainings for mental health providers serving Muslim and Arab clients, and is coeditor of *Counseling Muslims: Handbook of Mental Health Issues and Interventions*. She is the previous Editor-in-Chief of the *Journal of Muslim Mental Health*. Dr. Amer is a recipient of the American Psychological Association's (APA) Award for Distinguished Graduate Student in Professional Psychology and the APA Minority Fellowship Program's postdoctoral fellowship in mental health and substance abuse services, which she completed at Yale University School of Medicine.

Toni C. Antonucci, Ph.D. is the Douvan Collegiate Professor of Psychology, Program Director and Research Professor in the Life Course Development Program at the Institute for Social Research, both at the University of Michigan. Dr. Antonucci's research focuses on social relations and health including the family, life span and life course development, multigenerational relations, adult development and aging, and comparative studies in the United States, Europe, the Middle East and Japan. She is particularly interested in how social relations optimize or jeopardize an individual's ability to face life's challenges. She has numerous scientific publications; in 2010 she edited (with James S. Jackson) *Life Course Perspectives on Late Life Health Inequalities* and in 2011 edited (with Karen Fingerman, Cynthia Berg and Jacqui Smith) the *Handbook of Life Span Development*. She is currently series editor of the *Annual Review of Geriatrics and Gerontology* and is a member of the MacArthur Network on the Aging Society. She also serves on the Executive

Board of the International Society for the Study of Behavioral Development and holds the post of Secretary General-Elect of the International Association of Gerontology and Geriatrics.

Dr. Mireille Aprahamian is the Social Scientist at the Marine Corps Information Operations Center, responsible for socio-cultural and behavioral science research integration across various international analytic and planning efforts. She is also a Faculty Associate at George Mason University and Johns Hopkins University, teaching graduate courses in Human Growth and Development and Diversity and Social Justice within the Departments of Counseling and Human Services. Her expertise includes acculturation, identity development, diversity, and cross-cultural communication issues and their impact on mental health within Arab, Armenian, and Middle Eastern societies. Her most recent scholarship, published in the Journal of Mental Health Counseling, explored the relationship between the level of acculturation and mental health of Arab American adults in the United States, emphasizing the mediating effects of religion, age at migration, and discrimination experiences. Dr. Aprahamian has presented at several interdisciplinary conferences addressing cultural competency and multicultural issues. She has actively organized professional workshops that address counseling considerations when working with Arab American and minority populations. Prior to her current work, she was appointed as a research Faculty and Director of Evaluations at the Johns Hopkins Bloomberg School of Public Health, managing NIDA and NIH funded epidemiological research and evaluating school-based early childhood interventions in Baltimore City Public Schools.

Carolyn Archer, M.Sc. is an epidemiologist who works in research at Wayne State University. Ms. Archer has a strong record of public health research experience. She has 6 years of experience in public health research, with three of those years at the Wayne State University Department of Family Medicine, where she worked on an NIH-funded study of risk factors for preterm birth among African American women in Metro Detroit. Ms. Archer is currently working with the Arab American community in the Metropolitan Detroit Area to assess knowledge of vaccines and vaccine-preventable diseases among Hajj pilgrims. Ms. Archer's interests are primarily in conducting research within minority communities and maintaining ongoing relationships while furthering knowledge within these communities.

Cynthia L. Arfken, Ph.D. is Professor in the Department of Psychiatry and Behavioral Neurosciences at Wayne State University in Detroit Michigan (USA). Her research expertise is on alcohol and drug abuse epidemiology, and health service research, especially as it relates to health disparities. She has published over 100 peer-reviewed articles and been the principal investigator or investigator on multiple national and state grants. As part of a national sentinel system, she monitors and reports on drug trends for the Detroit metropolitan area, including use by different ethnic groups. From this work, she developed a focus on the alcohol and drug use patterns among Arab Americans and American Muslims. In addition to her publications and service on the editorial board of the *Journal of Muslim Mental Health*, she directs and collaborates on multiple research projects addressing mental health and substance abuse among Arab Americans and American Muslims.

Nicole Barakat, Psy.M. is a doctoral student in School Psychology at the Graduate School of Applied and Professional Psychology, Rutgers University of New Jersey. Her interests include understanding immigrants' experiences with the American school system, behavioral consultation with teachers, social-emotional program development in schools, and using mindfulness-based interventions with children and adolescents. She is currently working on her dissertation, "A program implementation evaluation of a behavior management program in a residential school for boys." Ms. Barakat also works as a behavior specialist for a suburban school district in New Jersey, where she consults with teachers and administrators to develop both individual and organizational-level programming in special education. She has published on the topic of evidence-based cognitive-behavioral therapy in the schools.

Ben K. Beitin, Ph.D., L.M.F.T. is Associate Professor and Program Director of the Marriage and Family Therapy Programs at Seton Hall University in South Orange, New Jersey. He has a doctorate in Marriage and Family Therapy from Virginia Polytechnic Institute and State University. He is first-generation Syrian American. His research has been in the areas of immigration experiences and acculturation of families in the Arab American community. Dr. Beitin has authored and presented nationally on Arab American families in the wake of September 11, 2001. He is also in private practice and has worked as an advocate for Arab American families in the New York/New Jersey areas.

Louise Cainkar is a sociologist in the Department of Social and Cultural Sciences at Marquette University and teaches courses in the social welfare and justice major. Her areas of expertise include Arab American studies, Muslims in the United States, and immigrant integration, fields in which she has published extensively. Her 2009 book, *Homeland Insecurity: The Arab American and Muslim American Experience after 9/11* (Russell Sage Foundation) was honored by the Arab American National Museum. In 2004 Dr. Cainkar won the prestigious Carnegie Scholar Award for her work on the reinvigoration of Islamic practices among second generation Muslim Americans. Cainkar has also conducted research in Palestine, Jordan, Iraq, Kuwait, and Yemen, studying, for example, the impact of economic sanctions on women and children and the forced migration of Palestinians and Jordanians from Kuwait. In addition to research for the academy, Cainkar has spent her career committed to public sociology, conducting community-based research and needs assessments in partnership with nonprofits and immigrant community organizations, serving on the boards of directors of various nonprofit agencies, and publishing in magazines that reach broad audiences. She is the treasurer of the Association for Middle East Women's Studies (AMEWS). Her current research is on second generation Arab American Muslim teenagers living transnational lives in Yemen, Palestine, and Jordan.

Florence J. Dallo, Ph.D., M.P.H. is an assistant professor in Wellness, Health Promotion, and Injury Prevention in the School of Health Sciences at Oakland University in Rochester, MI. As a Chaldean (Iraqi Catholic) immigrant growing up in a racially and ethnically diverse community, she was curious why some individuals led healthy lives, while others did not. After obtaining her M.P.H. and Ph.D., she completed a Kellogg Health Disparities Post-Doctoral Fellowship from 2004 to 2006. Since then, she has taught at the University of Texas, School of Public Health in Dallas from 2006 to 2009 and returned to Michigan in 2009. Her goal is to continue her research in better understanding and improving the health of Arab and Chaldean Americans in and outside of Michigan. Given that Arab and Chaldean Americans are categorized as "white" according to the federal government, one of her primary goals is to obtain an ethnic identifier on health forms and include them in the discourse on health.

Karen L. Haboush, Psy.D. is Visiting Associate Professor and School Psychology Internship Coordinator for the School Psychology program, at the Graduate School of Applied and Professional Psychology, Rutgers University. She also maintains a full-time private practice in Highland Park, NJ. Dr. Haboush's scholarly writing and publications have focused on culturally competent psychological practice with Arab American children and families. Her professional presentations both nationally and internationally have focused on training graduate students and mental health providers to work with this population in both clinical and school settings. Additional areas of professional practice and publication include clinical supervision and professional development of psychologists, treatment of trauma and child sexual abuse, psychological assessment, comprehensive mental-health program development for urban youth, integrating attachment theory with graduate student training, and international school psychology. Dr. Haboush is active in presenting at state and international professional groups aimed at promoting psychological services with traumatized and underserved youth.

Julie Hakim-Larson, Ph.D. received her doctoral degree in life span developmental psychology from Wayne State University in 1984 and obtained postdoctoral training in the field of Clinical Child Psychology. She has been on the faculty of the University of Windsor in Windsor, Ontario, Canada since 1991 where she is a Professor of Clinical Psychology. Her publications and research interests include culture and emotional development within a global perspective, emotion in families, Arab ethnic identity in North America, and the promotion of mental health in Arab immigrants and refugees. She has collaborated on projects that have resulted in peer-reviewed articles, book chapters, a training video, and conference presentations involving her work with individuals of Arab ethnicity. She is currently working on several books and organizing an international study group on Arab youth identity issues funded by the *Society for Research in Child Development*.

Adnan Hammad, Ph.D. is the founder and Senior Director of the ACCESS Community Health & Research Center, and Chairman of the National and International Health Research Initiative. Additionally, he serves as adjunct professor at both Wayne State University and Michigan State University. He holds numerous leadership roles on a number of regional, national, and international organizations including the American Cancer Society Board, the American Near East Refugee Aid Medical Committee Board, and the Advisory Committee on Health Research of the World Health Organization-Eastern Mediterranean Regional Office. He has been the principal investigator or coprincipal investigator on several research projects in the area of environmental health, diabetes, tobacco, cancer, and refugee health resulting in authoring over 100 articles focusing on Arab American health. To advance Arab American health research, he founded and is the Chairman of the Biennial International Conference on Health Issues in the Arab Community.

Linda A. Jaber, Pharm.D. is a Professor at Wayne State University. She has been extensively involved in the field of diabetes research. Her research program focuses on determining response differences in patients with type 2 diabetes to hypoglycemic agents. She has received the National American Diabetes Association Clinical Research Award to study the epidemiology and risk factors of diabetes and the metabolic syndrome among the Arab American population. She has also received NIH funding to examine the feasibility of diabetes prevention in the Arab American community. She has published numerous papers in the clinical pharmacology literature and has had numerous scientific presentations at local and national meetings. She is the recipient of the Excellence in Research Award from The Blue Cross Blue Shield of Michigan Foundation. Dr. Jaber is a member of the American Diabetes Association, and the American College of Clinical Pharmacy and is on the editorial board of *The Annals of Pharmacotherapy*.

Hikmet J. Jamil, M.D., D.V.D., D.I.H., M.Sc., Ph.D. is Professor, Director of OEM Graduate Courses at Division of Occupational & Environmental Health Department of Family Medicine & Public Health Sciences Wayne State University. He is the sole author of 18 books & first author of 2. He has 154 articles published in peer journals, 185 presentations at national and international conferences. He served as chief, deputy, secretary, and reviewer for several peer journals. He established the Diploma, Masters, and Ph.D. degrees in Occupational Medicine at Baghdad University. He has collaborated in research funded by: Karmonas, NIH, NIEHS, Pfizer, Roche, and NIMH. He founded "The International Society of Iraqi Scientists". His research interests fall in three areas: Iraqi refugees and immigrant health disorders, the impact of environmental exposure on health, and the impact of water-pipe (hookah) smoking on the health of smokers.

Ibrahim Aref Kira, Ph.D. is the director of the Center for Cumulative Trauma Studies, Stone Mountain, Georgia. His cross-cultural research is based on the new Development-Based Trauma Framework (DBTF). He served as the lead developer of the DBTF theoretical framework and its measurement tools. His primary interests include the effects of different trauma types and profiles of cumulative trauma on the health of refugees, torture survivors, minorities, and multiply traumatized children and adults. He is the past-director of the Center for Torture and Trauma Survivors, Decatur, Georgia, and past-supervisor of the Children Mental Health

Clinic, ACCESS community Health and Research Center, Dearborn, Michigan. Dr. Kira is the first author of over 30 peer-reviewed articles. He is a charter member of division 56 (Trauma Division) of the American Psychological Association (APA) and a consulting editor of the Journal of Psychological Trauma: Theory, Research, Practice and Policy (an APA Journal).

Dawn P. Misra, Ph.D. is Associate Professor and Associate Chair for Research in the Department of Family Medicine & Public Health Sciences at the Wayne State University School of Medicine in Detroit, Michigan. Dr. Misra received her B.A. and M.H.S. (Maternal and Child Health) from the Johns Hopkins University and a Ph.D. in Epidemiology from Columbia University. Dr. Misra has published more than 60 articles and book chapters and is the editor of the *Women's Health Data Book* (2nd edition, 2001). She serves on the editorial boards for the journals *Paediatric and Perinatal Epidemiology* and *Family Practice*. Much of her work focuses on racial and socioeconomic disparities in perinatal health. Dr. Misra has also led or collaborated on funded maternal and child health studies on a wide range of topics including racism, the placenta, infection, autism, and the effect of environment across the life course beginning in utero.

Sylvia C. Nassar-McMillan, Ph.D. is Professor and Program Coordinator of Counselor Education at North Carolina State University. Her professional background spans multicultural, gender, and career development issues, with a special focus on Arab Americans. She has published over 65 books, refereed articles, and other instructional materials. Dr. Nassar-McMillan currently serves on the CACREP Standards Revision Committee and has served as board member for the Census Information Center advisory board to the Arab American Institute, National Board for Certified Counselors, and North Carolina Board of Licensed Professional Counselors. She is past Associate Editor for Multicultural Issues for the *Journal of Counseling & Development*, for which she currently serves as Senior Associate Editor. Her recent NSF and NASA-funded projects have examined career stereotyping and evaluated curriculum tools. Dr. Nassar-McMillan's undergirding areas of scholarship and consulting include acculturation, advocacy, career development and underrepresentation issues, program evaluation, clinical supervision, and internationalization.

Kiumarss Nasseri, D.V.M., M.P.H., Ph.D. is an emeritus professor of epidemiology, is currently the lead scientific research advisor to Palm Tree Capital, a private equity firm actively investing in the health and health services industry. Dr. Nasseri has led a diverse and international career in academia and research. Some of his past work experience include collaboration with the World Health Organization on various public health issues, including cancer registration in the Middle East. His research interest is currently focused on ethnic variations in cancer incidence and mortality in the Arab and Middle Eastern immigrants in California and the United States. He has developed unique methods for identification of this ethnic population in cancer registry and other databases. He has authored over 40 peer-reviewed articles and monographs mostly on cancer epidemiology, 2 textbooks, and numerous scientific reports. He is currently on editorial boards of various journals, including: "Suicidology Online," and "International Scholarly Research Network (ISRN)."

Ashley Paterson, M.A. is currently a doctoral candidate in the child track of the Clinical Psychology program at the University of Windsor, Ontario, Canada. Her research focuses on identity development and acculturation within families of ethnically diverse backgrounds. Specifically, she has examined psychological outcomes as they relate to acculturation, enculturation, and social support among Arab youth living in Canada. Her doctoral research involves identity and the role of sibling conflict in an ethnically diverse sample of youth and emerging adults.

Jen'nan Ghazal Read is an associate professor of sociology and global health at Duke University and Associate Director for Special Initiatives at the Duke Islamic Studies Center. She is a Carnegie Scholar who has spent her career exploring the political, cultural, and economic experiences of Muslim and Arab communities in the west. She has published widely on this topic, including a book and numerous scholarly articles and her work has been featured in numerous media outlets, including the New York Times, Newsweek, and the Charlie Rose Show. Her current work focuses on Muslim integration in the United States and England, focusing specifically on the role of Islamic schools in the identity formation of Muslim youth. She is also beginning a project that will examine social determinants of obesity in several Middle Eastern countries.

Virginia Hill Rice, Ph.D., R.N., C.S., F.A.A.N. is a Professor in the Wayne State University College of Nursing with a joint appointment at the Karmanos Cancer Institute. She is a Clinical Nurse Specialist in Medical-Surgical Nursing and a Fellow in the American Academy of Nursing. Dr. Rice's research expertise and sustained contribution to nursing scholarship is evident in her teaching of students at both the graduate and undergraduate level and an almost continuous pattern of extramural research funding and refereed publications for more than 20 years. She has presented papers regionally, nationally, and internationally and conducted national and international research consultations on tobacco use. She currently serves on the ACCESS Scientific Committee, the Teen Health Committee, and the Health Disparities Reduction and Minority Health Capacity Building Grant Partners Committee. Dr. Rice has mentored more than 150 graduate student research projects (including those of students from Canada, China, Egypt, Jordan, & Thailand).

Manal Said, M.S.W., I.C.P.S., C.P.C.-R. is Programs Supervisor of the Health Promotion Section at the Arab Community Center for Economic and Social Services (ACCESS) Community Health Center. She is responsible for managing multiple publicly funded grant projects including Health Disparities Reduction and Minority Health Initiatives with a focus on reducing infant mortality, the Tobacco Prevention Program, Substance Abuse Prevention, and the Maternal & Infant Health Program. As an internationally certified prevention consultant, she works to eliminate health disparities among the Arab and Chaldean American population by pursuing health equity-related initiatives to build capacity, expand partnerships, and eliminate racial and ethnic disparities both within the local community and across the State. Additionally, she actively collaborates in research examining factors underlying disparities and risky behaviors among Arab Americans.

Helen Hatab Samhan, M.A. has spent 35 years in nonprofit advocacy, research and cultural outreach work about Arab Americans and US-Arab relations. She completed a Masters degree in Middle East Studies at the American University of Beirut, Lebanon in 1975. From 1985 to 2010 she served as a senior executive at the Arab American Institute (AAI) in Washington, DC where she led research programs including the first and only Census Information Center on the demographics of Americans of Arab ancestry. She publishes and lectures extensively in the field of Arab American studies: their immigrant experience in the United States, their identity and demographics, anti-Arab racism, political involvement and Arab American women. She currently is Senior Outreach Advisor to the Arab American National Museum (AANM).

Kendra Schwartz, M.D., M.S.P.H. is professor in department of Family Medicine and Public Health Sciences, Wayne State University School of Medicine, has research expertise in primary care and cancer epidemiology, with over 100 peer-reviewed publications. Dr. Schwartz focuses on the health disparities often experienced by vulnerable groups and the role of socioeconomic factors in those disparities. Because Detroit is home to the largest concentration of Arab and Chaldean Americans in the United States, Dr. Schwartz has worked with the community to develop a validated name list to determine the disease burden in this population group. She uses a name algorithm to identify Arabs/Chaldeans in registry and health statistics databases including the Metropolitan Detroit Cancer Surveillance System, which she co-directs, and is one of the founding members of the National Cancer Institute's Surveillance, Epidemiology, and End Results (SEER) program.

Emad Shehada, M.D. is an active clinician in critical and pulmonary care medicine at the Detroit Medical Center, where he is doing a fellowship, while at the same time completing a master's in public health through Wayne State University School of Medicine. Dr. Shehada is board-certified in internal medicine and certified by the Society of Critical Care Medicine. Dr. Shehada is dedicated to community efforts to inform Detroit-area citizens about healthy lifestyles and disease prevention. He has volunteered as a health screener and counselor at numerous community events, where he has provided individual advice on weight loss, and management of diabetes and hypertension.

Nancy Howells Wrobel, Ph.D. is Professor of Psychology and Chair of the Department of Behavioral Sciences at the University of Michigan—Dearborn. Her research addresses the validity of assessment and diagnostic practices across groups varying in gender, age, race, ethnicity, and cultural experiences. She has been engaged in research in collaboration with the Arab Community Center for Economic and Social Services in Dearborn, MI, with funded projects directed toward improving assessment and diagnosis of elderly Arab Americans through producing and validating Arabic versions of common screening instruments. Recent writings include work on the impact of acculturative stress on mental health. In addition to publications on multicultural issues, she has research interests and clinical expertise in child mental health and neuropsychological assessment. She has served on the Scientific Advisory Committees for the National Conference on Arab American Health and the ACCESS Annual Symposium on Refugees and Victims of Torture.

Chapter 1
Biopsychosocial Perspectives on Arab Americans: An Introduction

Sylvia C. Nassar-McMillan, Kristine J. Ajrouch, and Julie Hakim-Larson

For centuries, the mind–body connection has been debated. While perhaps associated more with an Eastern vs. Western worldview, the concept of the mind and body as intimately intertwined has waned in and out of popular discourse throughout human civilization. Arguably, corresponding with the World Health Organization's initiatives to define *integrated health services* (2008), efforts toward evidence-based treatments and practices have been reported with greater frequency over the past decade or so. These efforts have included scholarly inquiry into contemporary models of *integrated*, or *collaborative care*, wherein the focus is on the whole person, administered collaboratively between teams comprised of physicians and mental health counselors (Glueck, 2012; Miller, Mendenhall, & Malik, 2009).

The biopsychosocial model of care is one in particular that has been given attention in the scholarly and medical bodies of literature recently, including in the Arab world (e.g., Nasir & Abdul-Haq, 2008). Credited to Engel (1977), this approach suggests that while the biomedical model may explain the root causes of health issues, psychological variables, demands on life, and social and cultural conditions may just as likely impact the course of any disease progress, be it physical or mental.

S.C. Nassar-McMillan (✉)
Department of Curriculum, Instruction, and Counselor Education,
North Carolina State University, 2310 Stinson Drive, Poe Hall 520, Campus Box 7801,
Raleigh, NC 27695-7801, USA
e-mail: snassar@ncsu.edu

K.J. Ajrouch
Department of Sociology, Anthropology, Criminology, Eastern Michigan
University, 712 Pray-Harrold, Ypsilanti, MI 48198, USA
e-mail: kajrouch@emich.edu

J. Hakim-Larson
Department of Psychology, University of Windsor, 401 Sunset Avenue,
Windsor, ON, Canada N9B 3P4
e-mail: hakim@uwindsor.ca

S.C. Nassar-McMillan et al. (eds.), *Biopsychosocial Perspectives on Arab Americans: Culture, Development, and Health*, DOI 10.1007/978-1-4614-8238-3_1,

Center for Disease Control research on this topic at national levels in the USA has empirically validated this notion by showing that unhealthy lifestyles and behaviors lead to chronic illness and, conversely, that early intervention targeting such behaviors demonstrate improvements in a variety of health outcomes (Chiu & Wray, 2010; LaRowe, Wubben, Cronin, Vannatter, & Adams, 2007; Merrill et al., 2008).

Within the USA in particular, the medical model has been the predominant vehicle for delivery of health care for quite some time, despite the 1948 call for a more integrated approach to providing health care. The landmark legislation, in the form of the Affordable Health Care Act enacted in June 2012, is the first of its kind in the USA to mandate that prevention screenings and treatment for mental disorders, including substance abuse, be incorporated into medical care (Glueck, 2012; United States Department of Health and Human Services, 2011).

While perhaps more recently embraced by the medical field, mental health practitioners across a variety of settings and disciplines have employed the biopsychosocial model in their work for several decades. In addition to the presenting problem, typical clinical intake sessions include questions about developmental history over the lifespan, education and occupation, family of origin, social support, and religion. More comprehensive assessments may also consider historical and current substance abuse, mental health, and legal status in addition to medical issues. While categories such as family of origin and social support, among others, could certainly include cultural factors, culture itself is not typically articulated as a descriptor within this approach. Mental health clinicians, particularly those within rich ethnic communities and those otherwise more highly attuned to the potential impacts of culture on mental health, often talk about the importance of attention to this issue and may personally advocate for the inclusion of culture within initial client assessment as well as ongoing treatment. Including a "cultural lens" to a biopsychosocial approach to health was recently introduced (Jackson, Antonucci, & Brown, 2004), to suggest that cultural distinctiveness—that is, specific behaviors, attitudes, beliefs, and values—serve as resources and contribute in complex and significant ways to health and well-being. Associated with culture are matters of stratification that occur because of racial or ethnic affiliation, suggesting that attention be drawn to historical context and structural position as they relate to members of specific racial, religious, and ethnic groups. These issues are critical for health professionals to understand in the delivery of care. Recognition of culture in health care delivery appears to increase not only the effectiveness of such service in cost-effective ways but also contributes to a more complete understanding of the health status and health needs of persons more generally (Jackson et al., 2004). It is this stance that we attempt to convey in the present text. We weave together, through the book's major sections, salient factors of culture, development, and health, supporting the notion that these dimensions are inextricably related, particularly for Arab Americans. The full structure of the book and chapters are reviewed at the end of this Introduction, but first we will provide an overview of some of the more undergirding issues that will be found throughout the text. Beginning with immigration history as a backdrop, we will describe some basic information about the immigration of Arabs to the USA, define some key terms related to that immigration history, and identify critical incidents in the context of immigration and their implications for research, practice, and policy, along with their potential influences on assimilation and ethnic identity of Arab Americans. Finally, we will briefly overview the rationale and thematic undergirding for each of the three sections, as well as the chapter topics and their structure. As in any edited text, the richness of the material is enhanced by the diversity of authors and their respective perspectives. We hope you will find this even more to be the case in our holistic approach, vis-à-vis the biopsychosocial model, as well as the corresponding interdisciplinary nature of the overall text.

Immigration History

Several of the chapters, particularly those in Part I, will detail comprehensively the immigration waves of Arabs to the USA. As a reader, you may notice discrepancies among the various chapters in terms of the number of waves that are cited, as well as among countries of origin or time periods identified. Most scholars cite anywhere from two (e.g., Suleiman, 1999) to four (e.g., Nassar-McMillan, 2010) primary waves of immigration from the Arab world to the USA. The wide range of countries represented by this immigration also may serve to complicate this dynamic even more. For example, scholars focusing on immigration specifically from Lebanon, or Iraq, or any number of other countries (i.e., virtually any country in question), might identify a somewhat different wave based on the uniqueness of immigration from that country or region, often based on a country- or region-specific critical incident or incidents, such as the civil war in Lebanon in the 1970s or the Gulf War in Iraq in the early 1990s. Following are, generally stated, the various waves of immigration that have been cited in the literature over the past several decades:

- 1400s—Arabs accompanied Columbus and Spanish settlers to the New World (Arab American National, 2013).
- 1500s—millions of Arabs with origins in African countries were brought to the USA as part of the slave trade. Because their names were changed during that process, immigration and lineage for this group of immigrants is difficult to track (Arab American National, 2013).
- 1880s–1920s—the first waves are said to have come as part of the Great Migration, joining immigrants from countries worldwide in search of better economic opportunities. In many cases these Christian Arabs were fleeing the vast Ottoman (i.e., pan-Islamic) Empire (Orafalea, 2006).
- Post-World War II—often referred to as the Brain Drain, these Arab immigrants came to the USA to escape political tensions in their region. This group was primarily Muslim and well educated (Orafalea, 2006).
- 1960s—this group, like its immediate predecessors, was predominantly educated and Muslim; with reason for immigration to the USA being economic opportunities, opened up by loosened immigration restrictions; many were also unhappy with the continued political strife in the region (Orafalea, 2006).

- 1970s–1980s—Civil War and Israeli invasion of Lebanon prompted large numbers to leave Lebanon for the USA via chain migration (Samhan, 2014).
- 1990s—the Gulf War caused an Iraqi refugee crisis, with US President George W. Bush agreeing to allow refugees who had supported the USA to immigrate to the USA (Samhan, 2014).
- 1990s and beyond—refugees and immigrants from the Arab Middle East continue to immigrate to the USA for various reasons.
- September 11, 2001—the Twin Tower, New York City bombings and the subsequent *War on Terror* and its corresponding long-term occupation of Iraq by the United States, have provided a context for continued immigration from the Arab Middle East, most notably from Iraq (United States Citizenship and Immigration Services, 2012).

In many cases the USA is a key player in the political situations indirectly or directly leading up to the immigration. One example of this interaction is the Gulf War, as a result of which many Iraqis who fought on the side of the USA fled or otherwise immigrated to the USA and other countries for safety-related reasons (Jamil, Nassar-McMillan, & Lambert, 2007; Jamil, Nassar-McMillan, Lambert, & Hammad, 2007; Nassar-McMillan, Jamil, & Lambert, 2010). A second is the US-initiated War on Terror and the US occupation of Iraq mentioned above. It remains to be seen how the USA will become involved in the Arab Spring movements across the Arab Middle East and whether and how that involvement will interact with the US immigration policies and trends.

Key Definitions

The terms Middle Eastern and Arab American have historically been utilized interchangeably across various bodies of literature. A simple Internet search for maps of the *Middle East* yields vastly different portrayals of this region (e.g., Google, 2013; University of Texas Libraries, 2013; WorldAtlas, 2013), with many covering countries that do not define themselves as Arab (e.g., Turkey, Iran). Thus, *geographically*, the Middle Eastern region spans countries that are clearly non-Arab, such as Afghanistan, Pakistan, Turkey, Israel, among others. Other entities have defined Arab countries, or individuals of Arab descent, as being from Arab-speaking countries (e.g., de la Cruz & Brittingham, 2003). Still others, and this is by and large the perspective of the chapter authors in the present text, link the terms *Arab* or *Arab American* with origins from the countries belonging to the League of Arab States. These 22 countries are Algeria, Bahrain, Comoros, Djibouti, Egypt, Iraq, Jordan, Kuwait, Lebanon, Libya, Mauritania, Morocco, Oman, Palestine, Qatar, Saudi Arabia, Somalia, Sudan, Syria, Tunisia, United Arab Emirates, and Yemen. Despite the variety in defining Arab American, many scholars of multiculturalism agree that key in the distinction is the individual or groups' self-definition or identification (Samhan, 1999, 2014).

One additional point that needs to be noted here is the recent emergence of the term *Middle Eastern/North African* (*MENA*). While we applaud the domestic and global communities for their earnest efforts to understand and give credence to issues unique to these regions and those with ancestry from them, we have concerns that have not yet been fully explored related to this relatively recently emergent umbrella term. As can easily be interpreted, the regions inherently identified by MENA (i.e., Middle East and North Africa) or other relatively new synonymous terms such as WANA (West Asia/North Africa) or NAWA (North Africa/West Asia) exclude multiple Arab League States. While the World Bank's establishment of the MENA term might be fiscally appropriate on a global level, it falls short in its application of clarifying and defining a population that has, particularly in recent decades, striven hard to create a unifying self-definition. To that end, we avoid the term and caution readers not to conceptualize *Arab Americans* as being fully synonymous with those of MENA descent. In this text, the most likely terms to refer to our population of interest are *Arab American* or *individuals of Arab descent*.

A final distinction that needs to be made and will indeed be made further salient in the following chapters is the religious diversity among Arab Americans. As can be explicated from the key immigration points identified above, it is not accurate to assume *Arab* and *Muslim* as synonymous terms. In fact, because the late nineteenth-century wave of immigration was predominantly Christian, the majority of Arab Americans today are Christian, or at the very least, non-Muslim. Even today, the many refugees and immigrants from Iraq represent Iraqi Christians (called Chaldeans or Assyrians), along with their Iraqi Muslim (Shiite, Sunni) counterparts (Samhan, 2014).

Critical Incidents: 9-11, the Palestinian-Israeli Conflict, and the Arab Spring

Although the upcoming chapter on sociopolitical history will include all of the relevant critical incidents characterizing the relationships between the USA and various countries and regions within the Arab Middle East, one key incident is worthy of note here. The tragedy of the bombing of New York City's Twin Towers that occurred on September 11, 2001, caused a resounding impact, built upon already uneasy foundations. That fateful event set off a series of events that still strongly reverberate more than a decade later. As many Arab Americans will recount, any act of terror, whether on domestic or international soil, instills immediate fear and concern over retaliation toward Arab Americans or the Arab Middle East, regardless of the perpetrator's ethnicity. This emotional response clearly has the potential for impact upon an individual or groups' ethnic identity. In some cases, it may heighten ethnic identification, while in others may cause individuals to strive for invisibility within society at large.

In any case, the 9-11 bombing indirectly lead to a US-based invasion of Iraq, along with a subsequent decade-long occupation by the US military troops. Clearly, this is a salient issue among Arab Americans, as it is within the mainstream USA. Although these circumstances may have served to somewhat mask the decades-ongoing Israel-Palestine conflict, this issue also remains one of critical importance for Arab Americans (Arab American, 2013). Finally, the Arab Spring movements, ranging from minor civil unrest to major protests and governmental overthrows occurring across the Arab Middle East since December 2010, have clear implications for public relations between that region and the USA, with public opinion toward the USA in some countries there polling in at record lows (Zogby, 2010).

Present day empirical inquiry has only just begun to examine the tip of the iceberg represented by these issues and their impacts on individuals' ethnic identities. While various authors will discuss terms such as ethnic identity and assimilation (often-corresponding terms), it should be again noted that the interdisciplinary nature of the scholars across and even within book sections may serve to approach these terms from new or unique and sometimes seemingly disparate discipline-specific perspectives.

Thematic Undergirding and Chapter Structure

Although the present text is intended to provide a comprehensive biopsychosocial view of Arab Americans and their health care, each section can be influential in its own right as a stand-alone text of sorts. As previously mentioned, each section, and indeed chapters within each section, represent a diverse array of disciplinary backgrounds among chapter authors, as well as section-specific thematic undergirding. Each section examines the overall salience of assimilation and ethnic identity issues with different manifestation foci.

Part I provides societal context and examines outcomes from a corresponding social relations perspective. Chapters in this section, authored by prominent sociologists and scholars in closely related fields, include topics of sociopolitical history; intra-ethnic diversity and religion; gender; family traditions and values; the aging process; and culture, forgiveness, and social relations. Part II, with its prominent developmental focus, examines personal and developmental contexts and corresponding outcomes. Authors in this section span various clinical mental health fields and include both scholar and clinician perspectives. Part II chapters include topics of acculturation, ethnic identity, and gender; Arab refugees; mental health risks; education and employment; and environmental health. Finally, Part III blends together overall physical and behavioral contexts and examines epidemiological and mitigating factors within both context and outcome perspectives. This section's author teams include academic and clinical professionals. Part III includes topics of substance abuse, diabetes, maternal and childhood health, cancer, and advocacy needs for the Arab American community nationally. Finally, the book concludes with a synthesis chapter, clearly discussing implications concerning the need for prevention efforts at local, national, and international levels.

Across sections, readers will find the same, or similar, basic elements within each chapter. These include an introduction to the chapter topic; historical background and context, sometimes referring to historical regions of origin; relevant theoretical constructs; methodological approaches and their critiques; and implications for practice, research, and policy. Although the rationale for our biopsychosocial approach was introduced in this Introduction, along with our perspective of the need for culture to be more clearly articulated within the overall assessment across diverse client or patient settings, one final point of note in our perspective is the need for interdisciplinary professionals to impact policy change. While implications for research and policy might be inherently obvious within the sociological domains (and hence, Part I chapters) and implications for research and practice more clearly applicable within clinical domains (spanned by Parts II and III chapters), our view is that an *advocacy* role is inherently prescribed within an overall effective biopsychosocial approach. This relatively newly emergent role spans multiple health and mental health disciplines in its development as well as in the multidisciplinary perspective of its criticality and urgency.

In 2002 the American Psychological Association approved as policy a set of guidelines, namely, the *Guidelines on Multicultural Education, Training, Research, Practice, and Organizational Change for Psychologists*. This document details six domains relevant to culturally appropriate psychology practice, ranging from cultural knowledge of self and others coupled with multiculturally relevant responsiveness, to the importance of and need for employing constructs of culture across education, research, and clinical practice (American Psychological, 2002). Lastly, it cogently calls for scholar-practitioners to facilitate organizational change through culturally relevant policy development and practice. This latter component is embodied in the final Guideline and is particularly salient for work with Arab American populations (Nassar-McMillan, 2007).

Many clinicians and scholars alike may view themselves as apolitical. Implications for policy within the contemporary interdisciplinary literature at large, paralleling our own textbook's structure, are limited somewhat typically to the enhancement and efficacy of relevant research and corresponding evidence-based practice. These pleas represent critical precursors to the striven-for levels of recognition in the immediate domains (e.g., aging research, clinical interventions with refugees or diabetic patients) that likely impact clients' mental and physical health and well-being. At the same time, they are in and of themselves insufficient to change the ways in which society at large views the issues at hand. In other words, attention to the larger context within which people live includes political dynamics that influence the status, resources, and constraints experienced by various populations, including Arab Americans. Without appropriate legislation and policy change, the status of Arab Americans in terms of acculturation, mental health, and wellness is not likely to change (Nassar-McMillan, 2007). Thus, we make the case that broader, sweeping issues such as discrimination and violations of civil liberties have direct and indirect impacts upon the well-being of Arab Americans. And that, while our attempts in this text encompass a holistic and comprehensive perspective to assessment and treatment, true prevention must strive to eradicate the root causes of illness altogether. With that said, this edited volume challenges each and every scholar and clinician committed to the well-being of all people, to advocate for and support constructive changes at political levels beyond even the intuitively broad and comprehensive biopsychosocial approach whenever possible. In doing so, the resulting domestic and foreign policy changes will ultimately lead to a healthier and safer global context for all individuals.

References

American Psychological Association. (2002). *Guidelines on multicultural education, training, research, practice, and organizational change for psychologists*. Retrieved from http://www.apa.org/pi/oema/resources/policy/multicultural-guidelines.aspx

Arab American Institute. (2013). *Issues*. Retrieved from http://www.aaiusa.org/pages/issues/

Arab American National Museum. (2013). *Coming to America: Gallery one permanent exhibit*. Retrieved from http://arabamericanmuseum.org/Coming-to-America.id.18.htm

Chiu, C.-J., & Wray, L. A. (2010). Factors predicting glycemic control in middle-aged and older adults with type 2 diabetes. *Preventing Chronic Disease, 7*(1), A08. Retrieved from http://www.cdc.gov/pcd/issues/2010/jan/08_0250.htm

de la Cruz, G. P., & Brittingham, A. (2003). *The Arab population: 2000*. Washington, DC: US Census Bureau.

Engel, G. L. (1977). The need for a new medical model: A challenge for biomedicine. *Science, 196*, 129–136.

Glueck, B. P. (2012). *An interpretive phenomenological study of mental health counselors' experiences in integrated primary care settings*. Unpublished manuscript, Department of Curriculum and Instruction and Counselor Education, North Carolina State University, Raleigh, NC.

Google Maps. (2013). *Map of Middle East*. Retrieved from https://maps.google.com/maps?hl=en&q=map+of+middle+east&ie=UTF-8&hq=&hnear=0x157ec4658142ffb7:0xa5b8320215ea72c,Middle+East&gl=us&ei=hcTtUMydEvOv0AHZtYCwAw&sqi=2&ved=0CC8Q8gEwAA

Jackson, J. S., Antonucci, T. C., & Brown, E. (2004). A cultural lens on biopsychosocial models of aging. *Advances in Cell Aging and Gerontology, 15*, 221–241.

Jamil, H., Nassar-McMillan, S. C., & Lambert, R. G. (2007). Immigration and attendant psychological sequalae: A comparison of three waves of Iraqi immigrants. *Journal of Orthopsychiatry, 77*, 199–205.

Jamil, H., Nassar-McMillan, S. C., Lambert, R. G., & Hammad, A. (2007). Medical complaints of Iraqi American people before and after the 1991 Gulf War. *Ethnicity & Disease, 17*(Suppl. 3), S3-77–S3-78.

LaRowe, T. L., Wubben, D. P., Cronin, K. A., Vannatter, S. M., & Adams, K. (2007). Development of a culturally appropriate, home-based nutrition and physical activity curriculum for Wisconsin American Indian families. *Preventing Chronic Disease, 4*, 4. Retrieved from http://www.cdc.gov/pcd/issues/2007/oct/07_0018.htm

Merrill, R. M., Aldana, S. G., Greenlaw, R. L., Diehl, H. A., Salberg, A., & Englert, H. (2008). Can newly acquired healthy behaviors persist? An analysis of health behavior decay. *Preventing Chronic Disease,* 5, 1. Retrieved from http://www.cdc.gov/pcd/issues/2008/jan/07_0031.htm

Miller, B. F., Mendenhall, T. J., & Malik, A. D. (2009). Integrated primary care: An inclusive three-world view through process metrics and empirical discrimination. *Journal of Clinical Psychological Medical Settings, 16*, 21–30.

Nassar-McMillan, S. C. (2007). Arab American populations. In M. G. Constantine (Ed.), *Clinical practice with people of color: A guide to becoming multiculturally competent* (pp. 85–103). New York, NY: Teachers College Press.

Nassar-McMillan, S. C. (2010). *Counseling Arab Americans*. Belmont, CA: Brooks-Cole/Cengage.

Nassar-McMillan, S. C., Jamil, H., & Lambert, R. G. (2010). Chemical, environmental, and trauma exposures and corresponding health symptoms among Iraqi American women. *Journal of Applied Biobehavioral Research, 15*(2), 88–102.

Nasir, L. S., & Abdul-Haq, A. K. (Eds.). (2008). *Caring for Arab patients: A biopsychosocial approach*. Oxford, UK: Radcliffe Publishing.

Orafalea, G. (2006). *The Arab Americans: A history*. Ithaca, NY: Olive Branch Press.

Samhan, H. (1999). Not quite white: Race classification and the Arab American experience. In M. Suleiman (Ed.), *Arabs in America: Building a new future* (pp. 209–226). Philadelphia, PA: Temple University Press.

Samhan, H. H. (2014). Intra-ethnic diversity and religion. In S. C. Nassar-McMillan, K. A. Ajrouch, & J. Hakim-Larson (Eds.), *Biopsychosocial perspectives on Arab Americans: Culture, development, and health*. New York, NY: Springer.

Suleiman, M. (1999). Introduction: The Arab immigrant experience. In M. Suleiman (Ed.), *Arabs in America: Building a new future* (pp. 1–24). Philadelphia, PA: Temple University Press.

United States Citizenship and Immigration Services. (2012). *Iraqi Refugee Processing Fact Sheet*. Retrieved January 14, 2013, from http://www.uscis.gov/portal/site/uscis/menuitem.5af9bb959 19f35e66f614176543f6d1a/?vgnextchannel=68439c7755cb9010VgnVCM10000045f3d6a1R CRD&vgnextoid=df4c47c9de5ba110VgnVCM1000004718190aRCRD

United States Department of Health and Human Services. (2011, June 6). *News release: New Affordable Care Act support to improve care coordination for nearly 200,000 people with Medicare*. Retrieved January 4, 2013, from http://www.hhs.gov/news/press/2011pres/06/20110606a.html

University of Texas Libraries. (2013). *Northern Africa and the Middle East*. Retrieved January 9, 2013, from http://www.google.com/imgres?imgurl=http://www.lib.utexas.edu/maps/middle_east_and_asia/n_africa_mid_east_pol_95.jpg&imgrefurl=http://www.lib.utexas.edu/maps/middle_east.html&h=790&w=1264&sz=204&tbnid=bV-OS6jTGz5R-M:&tbnh=76&tbnw=121&zoom=1&usg=__sY8QBBSvLM5E0NExpb0Zeo-h4o0=&docid=bRIaCXk8GJ0XuM&hl=en&sa=X&ei=hcTtUMydEvOv0AHZtYCwAw&sqi=2&ved=0CDwQ9QEwBA&dur=11902

WorldAtlas. (2013). *Middle East Map*. Retrieved January 9, 2013, from http://www.worldatlas.com/webimage/countrys/me.htm

World Health Organization. (2008). *Integrated health services. What and why? Technical Brief No. 1*. Retrieved January 8, 2013, from http://www.who.int/healthsystems/technical_brief_final.pdf

Zogby, J. (2010). *Arab voices: What they are saying to us and why it matters*. New York: Palgrave Macmillan.

Part I
Arab American Culture

Kristine J. Ajrouch

But from the moment when it is recognized that above the individual there is society, and that this is not a nominal being created by reason, but a system of active forces, a new manner of explaining men (and women) becomes possible.
(E. Durkheim, 1915, The Elementary Forms of the Religious Life, p. 495-parentheses added).

Introduction

Society provides the foundation for specifying the cultural elements that shape Arab American life. To understand Arab American life, attention must be directed toward the underlying elements that drive their social reality. Social reality, "...is a matter of particular social actors, in particular social places, at particular social times" (Abbott, 1992, p. 428). Though it is now widely understood that culture patterns behavior in unique ways (Hall, 1966), it must also be recognized that culture is produced in the course of social interactions and relationships, through which meanings arise, persist, and change. Human actions occur within structures that provide opportunities as well as present constraints. Social relationships occupy a special place in the social sciences, serving as a critical foundation for the scientific study of culture, as well as for enhancing health and well-being. The chapters in this part present aspects of Arab American culture and their implications for health by

K.J. Ajrouch (✉)
Sociology, Anthropology, Criminology, Eastern Michigan University,
712 Pray-Harrold, Ypsilanti, MI 48197, USA
e-mail: kajrouch@emich.edu

focusing on social relations that range from the interpersonal up to the group level in the areas of social identity, family, gender, aging, and forgiveness.

The nature of social relations has preoccupied philosophers and social thinkers for centuries. Early theorists in the tradition of European and American sociology often described and sought to explain social change by highlighting the influence of various contexts on social relations or conversely by outlining how the nature of social relations, or repeated social interactions, ultimately extended to create society. Indeed, social relations have emerged as a key predictor of health and well-being (Antonucci & Jackson, 1987; Cohen & Syme, 1985; House, Landis, & Umberson, 1988). Social relations may involve close, interpersonal relationships, or relationships with groups and institutions. From the micro- to macro-level, the structure, type and quality of relationships hold enormous significance for daily life and overall well-being. Social relations hold an added layer of significance for understanding Arab American culture. The study of culture emphasizes a focus on meaning. Meaning is produced and reproduced through interactions that occur in social relationships (Blumer, 1969; Strauss, 1978). Hence, highlighting social relations as the core element to elucidating Arab American culture provides an important means by which to present issues of key importance in striving to present a biopsychosocial perspective on Arab American health.

The uniqueness of Arab Americans as a cultural group stems from the social conditions under which the group arose as a distinct, recognizable, and visible ethnicity. Contrary to the domestic policies (e.g., slavery, geographic expansion, industrialization) that brought about pan-ethnic groupings of Native Americans, Hispanics/Latinos, Asians, and African Americans, the impetus for carving Arab Americans out from the dominant white category into a distinct entity has involved US foreign policy directives in the Arab world (Cainkar, 2009). Indeed, political instabilities in the Arab world, beginning with the Arab-Israeli conflict (along with the United States' clear support for the state of Israel) are often cited as critical determinants of anti-Arab sentiment in the United States (Abraham, 1994; Salaita, 2006). Because the construction of Arab ethnicity is so intimately tied to events and political instabilities in the Arab world, Arab Americans incur a special situation, marginal in their status, "not quite white" (Samhan, 1999), yet not fully accepted as a legal minority (Cainkar, 2009), what Nadine Naber terms "ambiguous insiders" (Naber, 2000). Indeed, Arab Americans tend to adopt social identities that vary along national origin, age, and religious affiliations (Ajrouch & Jamal, 2007). Addressing the situation and needs of Arab Americans would benefit from a deeper understanding of culture.

This part addresses Arab American culture in a broad sense. Recognizing first, that similar to other pan-ethnic groupings (e.g., Hispanic/Latino), Arab American constitutes an umbrella term that essentially lumps a highly diverse group of people into one homogenous category, two chapters directly tackle the complexity of an Arab American social identity by examining the sociopolitical history of the Arab American experience as well as the ethnic and religious diversity found among those who fall within this category. Through these presentations, we gain insights into social relations between Arab Americans and others, as well as the nature of relations among diverse subgroups of Arab Americans. Second, the foundation of social relations for Arab Americans is the family. To understand gender dynamics, as well as the experience of aging among Arab Americans, references to family situations are critical. Moreover, gender and family issues overlap with the topic of forgiveness, which is presented within a framework that privileges social relations and culture as key to elucidating the conditions that shape the experience of hurtful social relations, or a sense of being wronged. As such, though each topic stands alone in importance, unavoidable overlap arises as this part seeks to clarify the importance of these issues for health and well-being. The six chapters in this part are summarized below.

In her chapter on the sociopolitical history of Arab Americans, Dalia Abdelhady traces the immigration history of Arab Americans by presenting multiple perspectives on the ways in which immigrants from Arab lands integrated. She challenges the traditional assimilation-pluralism framework as the only means to understand the social and political experiences of Arab immigrants and introduces the concepts of Transnationalism and Diaspora to reflect the complicated nature of the Arab American experience. Social relations are highlighted as the chapter illustrates the multiple ways that Arab Americans interact with the host society and home country. Through those interactions, the status and social identity of Arab Americans emerges.

In the chapter that follows, Helen Samhan outlines the intra-ethnic and religious diversity found within the pan-ethnic category of Arab American. In detailing underlying differences, Samhan elucidates the complexity of Arab ethnicity, illustrating why an *Arab identity* is not embraced by all. She provides valuable data on immigration from the multiple countries (22 total) that comprise the Arab world, identifies subgroups labeled as ethnic and cultural minorities in their country of origin (particularly Chaldeans, Assyrians, and Kurds), and furthermore describes religious diversity within the broader Christian and Muslim religions. The ways in which sectarian and national-origin boundaries facilitate or obscure acculturation are discussed. Indeed, social relations among Arab Americans as well as with others outside of the Arab American ethnicity again surface as a key element to the creation of identity. A poignant outcome arising from this chapter involves the difficulty inherent to identifying Arab Americans, raising questions about existing data and scholarship.

Ben Beitin and Mireille Aprahamian present a portrait of family. They first identify underlying values and traditions in the Arab world as a much needed context to the Arab American experience. They provide a thorough depiction of dominant values in the Arab world concerning the institution of family including large and extended family forms, and patrilineality, as well as the nature of the marital and parent–child relationship. By juxtapositioning traditional Arab values with US values, the authors offer important insights into potential tensions and conflicts members of Arab American families may face. For instance, the authors illustrate the challenges of collectivistic values in a self-reliant society and furthermore explain how gender roles are paramount to the structure of family relations and expectations. Social relations between men and women, young and old, therefore become a key site of negotiation in the US context. Beitin and Aprahamian conclude with a call for more research on the Arab American family to provide much needed insight into family change and continuity.

Louise Cainkar and Jen'nan Ghazal Read address the issue of gender. The dynamics of gender are discussed within a family context. The authors note that not all families are the same and gendered norms may be treated more flexibly in some families and more strictly in others depending on family resources (e.g., social class), the social capital (e.g., relationships and community) they build in the United States and their interpretations and management of interactions with the host society. The prominence of social relations in the articulation of gender dynamics provides an important lens. Noteworthy is the illustration of human agency, i.e., active decision-making, among Arab American women, and how decisions regarding gender norms facilitate social belonging. Noted is the paucity of data on the Arab American male experience.

In the chapter on aging, Sawsan Abdulrahim and Kristine Ajrouch focus on family relations and immigration as fundamental influences on well-being in later life. Four contemporary theoretical perspectives are discussed and applied to the Arab American experience. First, a life course perspective provides a lens by which to consider ways in which sociohistorical (e.g., war) and life events at various developmental stages (e.g., immigrating as a child or as an adult) shape outcomes in old age. Second, the Convoy Model of Social Relations draws attention to key relationships within (e.g., spouse, child, sibling) and outside (e.g., friends and neighbors) the family as key influences on health and well-being over the life course. Such relationships are thought to change in some respects, but remain the same in others. Third, intergenerational solidarity/ambivalence draws attention to relationship quality and provides a mechanism by which cultural ideals may be deconstructed to show pragmatic realities of social relations between older adults and adult children. Finally, the cultural assumptions behind the term successful aging are critiqued and applied to the Arab American experience.

In the final chapter, Kristine Ajrouch and Toni Antonucci discuss forgiveness in the context of culture and social relations. The concept of forgiveness is reviewed with cultural dimensions elaborated to suggest that in cultures tending toward collectivism the motivation to forgive may emanate from relationships with key others as opposed to a quest for inner peace. Data are then presented to illustrate how social relations influence the experience of forgiveness among Arab American college students in the metro-Detroit area. In particular, the authors consider how social relations influence within-group articulations of what it means to be Arab as well as shape explanations concerning strategies used when faced with difficult or hurtful situations.

Arab American culture involves multiple facets, the meanings of which are fruitfully guided by attention to the practice of social relations. In this part, the sociohistorical conditions of the Arab American experience and the diversity that marks the social identity of Arab Americans is illustrated. Both provide key insights into macro-level social relations. The interpersonal nature of social relations represents the key focus in the treatment of family, gender, and aging. Finally, both micro- and macro-level social relations emerge in discussions of forgiveness. Taken together, the chapters in this part provide key ideas to inform a more complete understanding of social aspects that shape the Arab American experience and ultimately their health and well-being.

References

Abbott, A. (1992). From causes to events: Notes on narrative positivism. *Sociological Methods & Research, 20*(4), 428–455.
Abraham, N. (1994). Anti-Arab racism and violence in the United States. In E. McCarus (Ed.), *The development of Arab-American identity* (pp. 155–180). Ann Arbor, MI: University of Michigan Press.
Ajrouch, K. J., & Jamal, A. (2007). Assimilating to a white identity: The case of Arab Americans. *International Migration Review, 41*(4), 860–879.
Antonucci, T. C., & Jackson, J. S. (1987). Social support, interpersonal efficacy and health. In L. L. Carstensen & B. A. Edelstein (Eds.), *Handbook of clinical gerontology* (pp. 291–311). New York: Pergamon Press.
Blumer, H. (1969). *Symbolic Interactionism*. Englewood Cliffs, NJ: Prentice-Hall.
Cainkar, L. (2009). *Homeland insecurity: The Arab American and Muslim American experience after 9/11*. New York: Russell Sage Publications.
Cohen, S., & Syme, S. L. (1985). *Social support and health*. New York: Academic.
Durkheim, E. (1915). *The elementary forms of religious life*. New York: The Free Press.
Hall, E. T. (1966). *The hidden dimension*. New York: Anchor Books.
House, J. S., Landis, K. R., & Umberson, D. (1988). Social relationships and health. *Science, 241*(4865), 540–545.
Naber, N. (2000). Ambiguous insiders: An investigation of Arab American invisibility. *Ethnic and Racial Studies, 23*(1), 37–61.
Salaita, S. (2006). *Anti-Arab racism in the USA: Where it comes from and what it means for politics today*. London: Pluto Press.
Samhan, H. H. (1999). Not quite white: Race classification and the Arab-American experience. In M. W. Suleiman (Ed.), *Arabs in America: Building a new future* (pp. 209–226). Philadelphia: Temple University Press.
Strauss, A. (1978). *Negotiations: Varieties, contexts and social order*. San Francisco: Jossey-Bass.

Chapter 2
The Sociopolitical History of Arabs in the United States: Assimilation, Ethnicity, and Global Citizenship

Dalia Abdelhady

Introduction

The Arab American population has been increasing rapidly during the last few decades. It grew by 42 % in the 1980s, reaching over one million in 1990 (Samhan, 2001). Despite the perceived underestimation of the size of the group, the 2000 census indicated that 1.2 million Americans report an Arab ancestry, making Arab Americans one out or 33 ancestry groups with a population over one million (De La Cruz & Brittingham, 2003). Like other ethnic identities in the United States, the formation of Arab American ethnicity took many years to crystallize, and there is much debate on the way it has been historically constructed. According to many scholars, the pan-ethnic identity "Arab American" is relatively new, dating to the early 1970s and resulting from a rise in political consciousness among people of Arab origin (whether immigrant or native to the United States). Orfalea (2006) finds the first appearance of the term "Arabic-speaking American" in the 1946 publication by Habib Katibah and Farhat Ziadeh under the same title and affirms that the term "Arab American" began to be used by the community itself around the same time. Suleiman (1999) traces the construction of the ethnic identity to the 1967 defeat of Arab forces and the Israeli occupation of the West Bank. Cainkar (2006) connects the rising political mobilization under the pan-ethnic identity to the US imperial aspirations in the Arab World around the middle of the twentieth century. Both Suleiman and Cainkar draw our attention to the political nature of Arab American identity and its relationship to global dynamics. Like other ethnic categories in the United States, being Arab American is fraught with diverse origins, religions, orientations, and dispositions. People originating in Arab countries are in no way homogeneous; they do not all

D. Abdelhady (✉)
Center for Middle East Studies, Lund University,
PO Box 201, SE 221 00 Lund, Sweden
e-mail: dalia.abdelhady@cme.lu.se

S.C. Nassar-McMillan et al. (eds.), *Biopsychosocial Perspectives on Arab Americans: Culture, Development, and Health*, DOI 10.1007/978-1-4614-8238-3_2,

consider themselves Arab (Ajrouch & Jamal, 2007). At the same time, similar to other ethnic labels, an Arab American identity and community are continuously and actively being constructed and reconstructed (Haddad, 2004). Identity formations take place through dynamics internal to the community itself, such as the activities of ethnic organizations, community centers, and political activists (Nagel & Staeheli, 2004), and external developments such as the foreign and domestic policies of the American government, the political environment in Arab countries, and the interactions members of the Arab American community have with other communities around them (Salaita, 2005; Suleiman, 1999). Scholarly works also contribute to the strengthening of such labels and render them meaningful.

In an attempt to depict the sociopolitical worldview of Arab Americans, this chapter traces the development of an ethnic political community among the different waves of immigrants by illustrating the global, transnational and national, social and political conditions shaping the context for the development of the community. The first part of the chapter summarizes the migratory patterns of the members of the community and highlights the dynamics that shaped their emigration, reception, and formation of identity and community. The second part explores the theoretical constructs that shape our understanding of the Arab American experience.

Traditionally, analyses of Arab American communities in the United States have been understood through the assimilation–multiculturalism paradigm. Assimilation refers to the ways members of an immigrant community became absorbed by the dominant society through various mechanisms such as language absorption, socioeconomic mobility, and intermarriage. Generally, assimilation is defined as a one-sided process of incorporating migrants into host societies. In the process of adapting to the new setting, migrants are expected to give up distinctive cultural and social attributes so as to become indistinguishable from members of the new society (see, for example Naff, 1985; Truzzi, 1997). On the other hand, multiculturalism refers to a more plural context of reception that allows immigrants to be incorporated into their new societies through multiple paths. Immigrant communities are accepted as ethnic minorities. Multiculturalism emphasizes that ethnic groups retain their distinguishable character (such as language, culture, social behavior, or public sphere) from the majority population within a larger multicultural society (see, for example, Basch, Glick Shiller, & Szanton Blanc, 1994; Castles, 1997; Glazer & Moynihan, 1970; Portes & Rumbaut, 1996).

This chapter highlights the ways analyses of the Arab American community have either stressed the various processes through which the group has assimilated into the American mainstream or traced the development of an ethnic identity and awareness of difference within the structure of American racial ethnic hierarchies. Next, this chapter extends such analyses by highlighting the growing global awareness that shapes contradictory forms of identification and are best understood through notions of transnationalism and diaspora. Transnationalism often reflects incomplete assimilation and the strengthening of ethnic pluralism in host societies (Morawska, 2008) by drawing attention to the ongoing connection with the immigrants' homeland and involvement in its political life. Diaspora provides a framework through which to understand immigrant integration that moves beyond traditional sociological models, such as assimilation and ethnic pluralism (Abdelhady, 2006). As an explanatory paradigm, diaspora possesses malleable qualities, such as the awareness of simultaneous inclusion and exclusion that complicates our understanding of immigrant communities and worldviews. The chapter concludes by underlining the contested nature of Arab American identity and the challenges faced by members of the community at present.

Historical Background and Migratory Patterns

The First Wave: 1880–1918

From the middle of the nineteenth century onwards, people from the Middle East have been moving in large numbers to North America. Most of these immigrants came from Mount Lebanon, which was then part of the Ottoman Empire, and the Syrian–Lebanese continue to make up the largest group of immigrants from the Middle East (De La Cruz & Brittingham, 2003; Hourani & Shehdi, 1992). Mount Lebanon was inhabited by heterogeneous groups of different ethnic and religious backgrounds, and a range of push–pull factors varied for each of the groups. Some were driven by push factors such as economic desperation, religious discrimination, or political oppression. Numerous accounts emphasize the importance of economic factors as the strongest in motivating early waves of emigration (see Karpat, 1985; Naff, 1985; Suleiman, 1999). The opening of the Suez Canal and the diversion of trade routes from Syria to Egypt, the inability of the Lebanese silk industry to compete with declining prices of Japanese silk, and rapid population growth which was unmatched by agricultural and industrial productivity are among the major economic factors behind Syro-Lebanese emigration (Suleiman, 1999).

According to Arab-American historian Naff (1994), the first waves of Arab immigrants to the United States were mostly Syrian–Lebanese Christians, farmers, or artisans, relatively poor, and poorly educated.[1] These immigrants were referred to as Syrians or Syrian–Lebanese and rarely Arab, which indicates a lack of a definite ethnic identity (Suleiman, 1999). These immigrants were emphatically sojourners, who have left voluntarily, as they wanted to improve their economic condition and to return home in a short time wealthier and prouder than when they left (Naff, 1994). Early settlers as well as missionaries played an important role in this respect. Both groups helped create the desire for improving material well-being by telling stories of the "entrepreneurial Eden" where "President Ulysses Grant was giving land away for free" (Younis, 1995, p. xiv).

[1] The religious origin of those emigrating from the Ottoman Empire is not a straightforward matter. According to Middle East Historian Karpart (1985) Muslim subjects were forbidden to emigrate, which may have led some to state that they were of Christian origin on official records. Fear of deportation if their true faith was discovered may have led them to conceal their Muslim origins after arrival.

In addition to the economic reasons for migration, sociopolitical factors played an important role as well. The beginning of the disintegration of feudalism brought about social and political instability to the region in form of communal clashes (which started in the 1840s and 1850s) and triggered large-scale migration from Mount Lebanon. Specifically, the granting of the special administrative status to Mount Lebanon in 1861, which meant relative autonomy from the Ottoman Empire, increased political and social instability and led to the isolation from the more prosperous regions of the Empire as well as more freedom for individuals to migrate (Karpat, 1985). Religious conflict, the imposition of conscription and the spread of foreign education were also contributing factors to migration from Greater Syria (Issawi, 1992; Orfalea, 2006).

Given their self-understanding as sojourners, early immigrants never felt that they belonged to American society (Suleiman, 1994). They mostly settled with co-ethnics and learned barely enough English to engage in back-peddling (McCarus, 1994). Since most early arrivals came with the idea of staying only long enough to accumulate a fortune and return home, they often started their economic activities in the new land as peddlers. With suitcases full of items such as needles, lace, and thread, Arab immigrants got on the road to sell their goods only a day or two after they arrived to the United States (Suleiman, 1999). Naff (1994) stresses that pack-peddling was the only activity Arab migrants had in mind as they had no interest in joining the American labor force or the isolated farm life. The Syro-Lebanese considered peddling as the most appropriate activity upon their arrival. Their lack of capital and limited knowledge of English constrained earning opportunities. Indeed, peddling, often supported by networks of friends and fellow countrymen, was seen as an activity compatible with quick financial rewards and a quick return home, as well as one being dependent almost entirely on individual effort (Truzzi, 1997). According to Suleiman (1999, p. 4), success in peddling required "thrift, hard-work, very long hours, the stamina to endure harsh travel conditions (mostly walking the countryside on unpaved roads), and not infrequently, the taunting and insults from children or disgruntled customers." These conditions were made tolerable for most early arrivals given their vision of a brighter economic future that would bring about social prestige for the immigrants and their families in the homeland. Suleiman notes that, as soon as they could afford to, early Arab immigrants switched to the "luxury" of a horse and buggy and later to a dry goods store.

Early Arab immigrants arrived in a country in which racial segregation was becoming increasingly institutionalized and nativist movements were pressuring immigrants to assimilate rapidly and to adopt American values and customs (Higham, 1955). Arab Americans were made aware of their racial difference and experienced opposition when using "White only" restaurants and restrooms (Conklin & Faires, 1987). In response to the racism of Jim Crow America and to court decisions labeling them as "Mongolian" or "Asiatic" and therefore not eligible for the US citizenship, Arab American leaders mounted a series of successful court cases between 1909 and 1915 seeking to be officially identified as "white." The judges who ruled in their favor were persuaded by a set of pseudo-scientific, legal, and religious arguments, including skin color, Christian identity, historic "contributions to civilization," Semitic identity, geographic proximity to Europe, and individual social and moral characteristics. While these characteristics do not apply to all Arab Americans and many of them faced resistance, the Syrian–Lebanese were officially included in the Caucasian racial category and were gradually characterized as belonging to the "white" race within American society (Truzzi, 1997, p. 21). Their incorporation within the privileged racial group allowed members of the Syrian–Lebanese community to utilize their "whiteness" and become legal citizens and more "Americanized."

Inter-War Isolation: 1918–1948

World War I and the restrictive quotas to immigration that followed isolated early Arab immigrants from the homelands and limited the growth of the immigrant community. The Immigration Restriction Act of 1921 and Johnson-Reed Act of 1924 set quotas on non-European immigration to the United States and limited the number of Arab immigrants permitted to enter the country. Nevertheless, immigration continued as families, mainly women and children continued to join their family members in this country (Naff, 1985). While immigrants were allowed to unite with their families, the replenishment of ethnicity by newcomers (Jimenez, 2009) was still limited resulting in a sense of isolation from the homeland. The sense of isolation had two effects on the Arab immigrant community (Suleiman, 1999). On the one hand, it led to enhancing the sense of solidarity among community members and more calls to end inter-sectarian conflicts that facilitated the emergence of an ethnic identity. The growth in self-help community organizations during the great depression can be viewed as a sign for the weakening of inter-sectarian conflict as they increasingly targeted all Syrian immigrants and their families (Orfalea, 2006). On the other hand, however, it also strengthened the assimilationist trend, especially for the American-born children of the early immigrants. For example, the early second-generation spoke only English and quickly moved away from ethnic churches (Suleiman, 1999) and is often characterized as being the most assimilated of all generations of Arab immigrants to the United States (Orfalea, 2006). The process of Americanization of the Syrian–Lebanese progressed with their incorporation, or rather acceptance, in the dominant white culture. In one example, Najeeb Halaby, who became the first chairman of NATO's Military Production and Supply Board described:

> The first generation of the immigrant Arabs really wanted to be 100 percent American and changed their names and their religions even. They wanted to arrive socially, politically, professionally. And so when you're raised in that kind of atmosphere, you want to be all-American. Yet… I've found in going back to Syria or Lebanon, though the food, the atmosphere, the air, the sights, sounds, you feel a root that just comes without logic or intellectual activity. It just is down inside you (Orfalea, 2006, p. 139)

Halaby is an example of successful assimilation trends that was experienced by early Arab immigrants and their children in the United States. Truzzi (1997) describes that success in business activities and professional occupations triggered the interest of Syrian–Lebanese immigrants in the United States to participate in politics and take on government positions. The author goes on to stress that "they entered not as Arab-Americans, but rather as assimilated Americans" (Truzzi, 1997, p. 13). Many analysts of early Arab experiences in the United States tend to conclude that members of the first wave of Arab immigrants were "Americanized to the point of extinction" (Kayal, 1995, p. 253).

While Arabic-speaking immigrants were reuniting with their families in their "new country," political changes were taking place in their homeland that affected the life in the diaspora. Following World War I, the Ottoman Empire crumbled and its rule over Arab communities was replaced by France and Britain (the two great powers at the time). In 1918, the French mandate for Syria and Lebanon was granted by the League of Nations and entailed the incorporation of diverse villages and cities and religious communities such as Christians, Muslims, and Druze into one entity. Under the French mandate, political tensions and religious divisions intensified and were only strengthened by its termination in 1946. The emergence of two separate nation-states from the mandate, first the Lebanese and later the Syrian, caused ethnic or national sentiments and attachments to surface which affected the immigrant community in the United States (Suleiman, 1999). Disturbances in Palestine with Zionist settlers and the British rulers motivated many Palestinians to escape the British mandate and migrate to the United States (Orfalea, 2006).

While most Arab immigrants had left before the creation of nation-states in their homeland and initially adhered to identities based on villages or families of origin, some of them started to encourage distinction from the larger Syrian identification to more nationalist terms such as Lebanese or even Syrian–Lebanese. Names of some social clubs also changed. During the period between the two World Wars, Arabs in America "functioned as a collective of communities whose bonds of solidarity beyond the family were mainly related to sect or country affiliation" (Suleiman, 1999, p. 7). While many of them could have returned to their homelands having fulfilled their dreams of economic success, many of them chose not to. They opted to maintain a transnational relationship with their places of origin instead and sent remittances to support families, villages, and nationalist struggles (Gualtieri, 2010).

At the same time, Arab Americans strived to remove their differences from the mainstream. They were eager to prove their worthiness to American society, which mostly took the form of shedding their cultural distinction and replacing it with an assimilated outlook (Kayyali, 2006). As a result, Arab immigrants almost lost their common language; with the exception of music and food, they became what Suleiman (1999, p. 9) describes, "an indistinguishable group from the host society." Their assimilation to white, middle class America was facilitated by their entry into the manufacturing of silk, dry food store ownership, and to a lesser extent intermarriage (Orfalea, 2006).

Arriving to the United States before the creation of modern nation-states, Arab immigrants at the time shared an understanding of difference that was mostly based on religious affiliation. Their encounters with institutions that shaped racial stratification and growing awareness of white privilege strengthened their desire to identify as white in order to reap such privilege and escape the stigma of otherness (Gualtieri, 2001; Samhan, 1997). Seeking whiteness, however, was often characterized by struggle and discrimination leading to a contradictory sense of identification and ambiguity about their inclusion in American society that lasts until the present (Gualtieri, 2010). Suleiman (1994) asserts that being sick of the outsiders' position, Arab Americans started to assimilate more into the American way of life during and after World War I when they started joining the army and fighting on behalf of the United States (see also Orfalea, 2006). Following the war and realizing that America was their permanent home, those immigrants started to develop a more inclusive community that was not divided along class and religious lines. For the first time, they also started to engage in campaigns to better inform the American citizens and others about their Arab heritage. Philip Hitti's 1924 book on *The Syrians in America* is considered the first attempt to introduce the community to American society. In the process, Hitti aimed to engender cohesion and unity to the community and the way it was perceived by others. Hitti's goals included the desire to establish an interest group that participated in American public life instead of accepting the community's invisibility. While the assimilation of the early wave of Arab Americans was often challenged and contested (see, for example Gualtieri, 2010), Americanization was still an important goal that was pursued by many ethnic organizations. The first wave of immigrants established a number of charitable societies that maintained group cohesion, ethnic ties, and fostered assimilation. Members of the small elite in the first wave started organizations to improve the conditions of other members of the community, such as clubs to learn English, and to promote American ideals and mutual understanding (Naff, 1985). Furthermore, there were societies based on family name and place of origin which were interested in modernizing their respective villages in the homeland and maintaining transnational ties (Naff, 1985).

The Second Wave: Emerging Nationalism (1948–1965)

According to the various accounts of Arab immigration to the United States following World War I, waves of immigrants were becoming more diverse and sophisticated. Yet, it was only after World War II that the second wave of Arab immigration became distinct (see Abraham & Abraham, 1983, for more information on historical trends of Arab migration). According to Suleiman (1994), by the end of World War II, the Arab American communities nearly assimilated fully and almost lost their Arab identity but this identity loss was reversed because of the Palestinian cause and the influx of new waves of immigrants. The establishment of the nation of Israel in 1948 in Palestine is considered a critical moment in the history of Arab American communities. The resulting expulsion of many Palestinians from their homeland brought many Palestinian refugees to the United States. The expulsion resulted in the allocation of Palestinians to different Arab countries, including but not limited to Lebanon, Syria, Algeria, Tunis, and Libya. With the passing of the Refugee Relief Act in 1953 and its extension in 1957, many of the Palestinian refugees settled in the United States (Alfaro-Velcamp, 2011), bringing the total number of Palestinians in the United States to an estimated 12.5 % of its total Arab population in 1980 (Seikaly, 1999). The Palestinian cause became a central concern in the ideological and identity questions of Arabs and Arab Americans.

Generally speaking, the post-World War II wave of Arab immigrants consisted of highly educated and politicized individuals and professionals. Unlike the early arrivals, the immigrants of the post-World War II wave were motivated by the desire to escape political deterioration and warfare as opposed to a search for better economic opportunities (Orfalea, 2006). In addition to Palestinians, the second wave of Arab immigrants included Egyptians, Iraqis, Yemenis, Syrians, and Lebanese. These new arrivals came at a time when the Arab countries started gaining, or at least fighting for, their independence from the colonial powers as western ideas of democracy and equality made their way into these countries. These ideas contributed to their political socialization before and after migration as they were fascinated by democratic opportunities and eager to participate in American political and public life (Seikaly, 1999; Suleiman, 1999). Unlike their forebears who came as temporary sojourners (but most of whom stayed), post-World War II Arabs came as immigrants who sought a new life in the United States (Haddad, 1994; Suleiman, 1994). Unlike the pioneer generation, those new arrivals had the education and skills to adapt more quickly to American society. However, they were more interested in homeland politics and possessed political views and religious beliefs that set them apart from other Americans. For many, their Palestinian origin (or pro-Palestinian orientation) and Muslim faith not only alienated them from the majority of American society but from early Syrian/Syrian–Lebanese immigrants who were already fully assimilated to the middle class white strata of American society (Orfalea, 2006).

Despite the divisions between the two waves of Arab immigrants, the creation of the State of Israel and the expulsion of Palestinians from their homeland motivated a growing unity among many Arab Americans, and to an extent a growing awareness of an Arab identity and community. The first attempt to establish a political interest group took place in 1951, when the Federation of Syrian–Lebanese Clubs managed to achieve ethnic unity and met with President Truman (Orfalea, 2006). For many historians of the Arab American community, it was not until after World War II that Arab Americans began to develop an Arab identity to counter the ignorance about the history of Arabs (see Naff, 1994). The emerging Arab American identity paralleled the development of Arab identity itself and reflected the emergence of Arab nationalism that resisted European colonization and political intervention in the region (Naber, 2008). This political identity found articulation in civil society organizations and political activities that aimed at not only educating Americans about Arabs, which was the popular strategy for members of the earlier wave of migrants, but forming a political interest group as well.

The Third Wave: Arab Defeat and Political Awakening (1965–2001)

Since the 1960s, the Arab American population has grown rapidly as a result of immigration policy changes. The loosening of the US immigration restrictions in 1965 allowed for larger and even more diverse numbers of Arab immigrants to move to the United States. Political and economic crises taking place in Arab countries motivated such increasing flows of Arab migrants to the United States. For example, Suleiman (1999) cites regional conflicts (e.g., Palestine-Israel, Iraq-Iran, Iraq-Kuwait) and civil wars (Lebanon, Yemen) as among the factors contributing to the increase of Arab migration. According to the author, the new immigrants were searching for democracy and freedom from their oppressive governments. Suleiman also adds the importance of improvements in transportation and communication as allowing immigrants to perceive of the world as a single unit and thus more accepting of the notion of migration especially to far away places in North America. According to Orfalea (2006), members of that third wave of immigrants are in many ways similar to those of the second: many of them came from Palestine, but others also came from Syria, Lebanon, and the Persian Gulf countries; the majority was highly educated and professional; and many of them left due to sociopolitical reasons. Unlike those of the second wave, however, members of the new wave of immigrants were fleeing their homeland due to intra-Arab warfare and an intensified US involvement in the region. While the Israeli aggression on Palestinians continued, the Lebanese civil war which started in 1975 and was intensified with Israel's invasion of Lebanon in 1982, Iraq's war with Iran and subsequent invasion of Kuwait that led to the imposition of harsh economic sanctions on the Iraqis, and the rise of religious fundamentalism in Egypt, Syria, and Iraq led many to flee such undesirable conditions and migrate to the United States. All these factors combine to make it less likely for members of the third wave of Arab immigrants to go back home (Orfalea, 2006). Given the political reasons motivating their migration and their dissatisfaction with the US policies in the region, members of the third wave are believed to be more likely to participate in American political life in an attempt to impact American policies in the Arab world (Orfalea, 2006).

While the creation of the state of Israel and the expulsion of Palestinians from their homeland motivated a growing interest in ethnic politics among Arabs in the United States, it was not until after the 1967 Arab–Israeli war that the Arab American community became visible in the United States (Abraham, 1994; Banks, 2003; Hooglund, 1987; Orfalea, 2006; Salaita, 2005; Seikaly, 1999; Shain, 1996; Suleiman, 1994, 1999). In an analysis of the political attitudes of Arab immigrants, Suleiman (1994) notes that the 1967 Arab–Israeli war marked Arab immigrants' political engagement in the United States based on their involvement with issues related to their ethnic community and homelands. Although Suleiman does not use transnationalism as a framework for his analysis, it seems that the 1967 defeat fostered transnational ties in the Arab American community more so than any other event.

Earlier waves of Arab immigrants may have assimilated to the US society by many measures (see, for example Kulczycki & Lobo, 2001; Naff, 1985). Yet, following the 1967 Arab defeat, Arab immigrants have expressed strong interest in maintaining ethnic attachments to their homeland as well as an ethnic community in the United States.[2]

The United States' strong support for Israel and partial media coverage of the conflict fostered Arab American unity and the emergence of an ethnic immigrant identity (see Haddad, 1991; Marshal & Read, 2003; Sandoval & Jendrysik, 1993). The 1967 war revived a nationalistic and ethnic identity among the Arab descendants and the newly immigrated Arabs in the United States. Sueliman (1999, p. 10) asserted that the "older and newer Arab-American communities… were dismayed and extremely disappointed to see how greatly one-sided and pro-Israeli the American communication media were in reporting on the Middle East." This assertion led Suleiman to stress that "members of the third generation of the early Arab immigrants had started to awaken to their own identity and to see that identity as Arab, not 'Syrian'" (Suleiman, 1999). For those who arrived in the third wave (post-1965), ethnic cohesion was sought after for political purposes as well (David & Ayouby, 2002).

According to Salaita (2005, p. 150) "nothing has been of more concern to Arab Americans since 1967 than the Israeli–Palestinian conflict, although Iraq has also been pivotal since 1990." Widespread American political and public support for Israel has infuriated Arab Americans and served to provide a rallying cause and a mobilizing political focus. Despite the diverse and sometimes opposing positions of Arab Americans, the issue of Palestine fostered the formation of Arab American racial identity and "transformed Arab Americans from a rapidly acculturated immigrant group into a radical, anti-mainstream community" (Salaita, 2005, p. 165, see also David, 2007). While Salaita and David's analyses may be accurate depictions of the public political lives of Arab Americans, it should be noted that among members of the Arab American community itself there is no agreement about the Israeli–Palestinian conflict, with many not having a position on the subject. In a study of Palestinian Americans conducted in the late 1980s, Barghouti (1989) found that American-born Palestinians were less politically engaged by the Arab–Israeli conflict than their foreign-born counterparts.[3] Analyzing Arab American political attitudes before 9/11, Wald and Williams (2005) find that members of the Arab American community are more attentive to the Middle East but without high levels of mobilization or unanimity. Suleiman's (1994) survey also supports this account

---

[2] Bawardi (2009) maintains that Arab immigrants' transnational activities can be traced back to independence movements which started at the turn of the nineteenth century but was accelerated following the second world war.

[3] A more substantial attitude variation was found by Sandoval and Jendrysik (1993) who surveyed Arab Americans about the Gulf War. The study found no difference between Arab Americans and other Americans about Iraq's guilt, the necessity of Iraq's withdrawal from Kuwait, and the desirability of disarming Saddam Hussein. However, the authors observe that younger, foreign-born, and Muslim Arab Americans have greater opposition to the U.S. policies relating to the Middle East. More recently, Salaita (2005) remarked that not all Arab Americans oppose the war in Iraq.

and adds that younger Arab Americans have stronger identification as Arabs (as opposed to American-only or based on their religion or national origin), but that such identification is mostly political since younger Arabs are not necessarily devoted to cultural traditions and ethnic practices. Nonetheless, unlike Arab Americans of the earlier waves, by the 1990, Arab immigrants and American-born Arabs alike shared a strong ethnic consciousness and were engaged in expressing their Arab consciousness intellectually and creatively (Salaita, 2005).

Arab Americans Today: 9/11/2001 and Beyond

In the aftermath of 9/11 attacks, Arab Americans became more visible actors politically, and the interest in political participation is believed to be pervasive among many members of the community (Abdelhady, 2006, 2011a). Most scholars consider the attacks as a turning point in the narrative of Arab Americans. While anti-Arab racism preceded the attacks and the systematic discrimination that followed, their impact on the daily lives of Arab Americans took on new forms and levels (see, for example Naber, 2008). Incidents of discrimination and anti-Arab violence were critical in their political mobilization, but government policies were at least equally significant. The passage of the USA Patriot Act and the broad investigative authorities it gave to government facilitated the detention of hundreds of Arab Americans. Cainkar (2003, p. 1) describes that "the US government's domestic legislative, administrative, and judicial measures implemented after September 11th have included mass arrests, secret and indefinite detentions, prolonged detention of 'material witnesses,' closed hearings and use of secret evidence, government eavesdropping on attorney client conversations, FBI home and work visits, wiretapping, seizures of property, removals of aliens with technical visa violations, and mandatory special registration." In addition to individual experiences, many philanthropic organizations were shut down by the FBI in fear of their support to terrorist groups. Muslim charities were especially scrutinized, and Arab or Muslim small businesses were threatened by the FBI.

Threat can be a source of mobilization and work to prompt ethnic consciousness engendering political capital (Ramakrishnane, 2005). Research on the 9/11 backlash (Bakalian & Bozorgmehr, 2009) has revealed that the mobilization of the targeted populations was one of the unexpected consequences. Unlike historical precedents (e.g., Japanese internment during World War II or the Iran hostage crisis), Middle Eastern and Muslim leaders across the country rallied their constituents to integrate into the civic and political institutions at the local and national levels. Almost immediately, they stood firm, claiming their rightful place in American society and protested the backlash by the government initiatives as well as the hate crimes and bias incidents. Instead of capitulating to exclusion, many Arab Americans distanced themselves from the terrorist attacks, and many organizations issued official statements condemning terrorist acts. One such attempt was portrayed in the candlelight vigil held in the heart of Arab New York on Atlantic Avenue. Others focused their efforts on educating the public about Arab cultural diversity. For example, following reports of police racial profiling of Arabs post-9/11, organizations such as the Arab American Association of New York and the American MidEast Leadership Network stepped in to provide cultural sensitivity training programs to officers of the New York Police Department (Millard, 2008). Many other groups organized voter registration, know-your-rights forums, and other activities that aimed at political integration. Bakalian and Bozorgmehr (2009) note the high levels of mobilization. They show that the increased racial profiling and stigmatization of Arabs in the US post-9/11, while remaining comparatively low, motivated many Arab Americans to reinterpret the multicultural structure of American society through participating in public life to shape the ways they wish to be portrayed by others. The mobilization of political capital resulting from the increased stigmatization reached out to many who may have been uninterested in establishing ethnic politics in the past. Rallying around specific issues affecting Arab Americans post-9/11, many have ended up with a stronger interest in addressing unjust policies that relate to the Arab world, and thus mobilized around transnational and sometimes global issues (Abdelhady, 2011a).

Transnational attachments of Arab Americans continue to be visible in post-9/11 political climate. However, as Howell and Shryock (2003, p. 459) note.

> In the post-9/11 era, transnational ties that connect the US to Arab and Muslim countries will be acceptable only insofar as they strengthen sites of belonging and social reproduction that are located in America (in the form of "ethnic communities") or are subject to US sovereignty (in the form of allied regimes).

This observation holds true in understanding the transnational involvement of Arab Americans today. Almost 10 years since 9/11, the pro-democracy movements sweeping many Arab countries today have garnered much support from Arab Americans who are pushing for a stronger support from the United States towards the political transformations taking place in their homelands (Abdelhady, 2011b). Seeing these transformations as threats to the political and economic stability in the region, and by association American interests that are protected by a number of dictators supported by the United States, the American government was slow to express its support to these transformations and in many instances ignored the mobilized efforts of Arab Americans who wished to alter the lukewarm support. Rallying in support for democratization movements in the Arab world, Arab Americans established new ethnic organizations but more importantly joined forces with others that have a more general commitment to peace and justice issues. Groups of Arab Americans that have previously disengaged from political activity in the United States (such as Yemenis, Libyans, and Syrians) partly as a result of the inhospitable climate for Arab Americans post-9/11 are expressing their transnational interests by attempting to impact the US policies towards the Arab world. Importantly, their transnational activities are taking place alongside a more inclusive strategy that aims at engaging with American (mainstream) organizations (such as political parties, colleges and universities, and civil rights organizations). To many Arab Americans, the pro-democracy movements in the Middle East are taken as significant events that can potentially alter the position of Arab Americans in American public life (Abdelhady, 2011b).

Theoretical Constructs in Understanding Arab American Experiences

Analyses of immigrant incorporation usually emphasize two contradictory trajectories that can be experienced by immigrant groups. On the one hand, assimilation—defined as incorporation into a middle class white majority through social mobility, language absorption and intermarriage—is considered the end goal of incorporation and is both desirable by the immigrant group and the host society. On the other hand, proponents of multiculturalism—who tend to emphasize the multiple paths to incorporation, minoritization, and discrimination—believe that immigrants are not likely to relinquish their ethnic identities and ways of life that add to enriching the fabric of host societies. To a large extent, the Arab American experience has been analyzed within these two frameworks. With very few exceptions, analysts of the Arab American pioneer generation often paint a picture of quick assimilation into a White middle class mainstream. Their Christian religion and desire for material gains, coupled with restrictions on ethnic replenishment are often cited as reasons facilitating their assimilation and adoption of American attitudes and lifestyles. Analyses of later generations often emphasize the ways immigrants from Arab countries gained or strengthened their identification as Arabs, and constructed and maintained an ethnic community in their new settings. Post-9/11 narratives tend to emphasize the nature of political and social exclusion faced by Arab American and in the process demonstrate the ways through which they are precluded from being considered full citizens. While the transnational aspect of the Arab American community (or the mutual strengthening of ties cross the boundaries of homeland and host society) has been traced to the pioneer generations and has been used to describe political participation in subsequent generations, the global effects of 9/11 lead us to draw more emphasis on the global context of reception that shapes the contemporary Arab American experience. The global context, best understood within the framework of diaspora (Abdelhady, 2011a) brings our attention to processes of simultaneous inclusion and exclusion that complicates our understanding of immigrants' communities and worldviews. Importantly, the framework of diaspora highlights forms of identification and community building that move beyond traditional groupings that may be based on ethnicity, nationality, or religion.

Treading Between Assimilation and Ethnicity

The assimilation of Arab Americans prior to 1967 is well documented in the literature. Suleiman (1999), Naff (1994), Hooglund (1987), Abraham (1994), and Naber (2000) all agree that early waves of Arab settlers in the United States were Christians who tended to assimilate to the predominantly white American middle class strata, even if at times retaining some distinctively Arab (also read Old World) characteristics such as food, religious behavior, family ties, and language. The newcomers exhibited a lack of ethno-political identity as their identities were rooted in family, regional, and religious affinities. Kayal (1995) explains that for many of the newcomers, "Arab" was a designation that referred to Ottoman Turks, and that Arab identification "marked them as backward, inferior, non-Christian and hostile to the United States," that they had little desire to preserve ties to their old world and its heritage (Kayal, 1995, p. 252).

The sojourning aspect of early Arab immigrants may have curtailed their assimilation to American society as it strengthened ethnic ties. For example, Suleiman (1999) notes that most newcomers relied on ethnic networks to start their peddling activities. Their interest in accumulating money quickly so that they can help their families and then return to their home villages made them uninterested in American life. Emphasis on the temporary nature of their life in the United States also meant that they were not interested in long-term investment such as buying homes, establishing families, or seeking different kinds of economic activities. Suleiman asserts that early arrivals only established connections with others who belonged to the same sects, town, or geographic region. They formed "residential colonies" especially in New York and Boston, and they strongly encouraged within-group marriage. More telling are the terms they used to distinguish between themselves and the larger American society. The Arab American community described itself as *Al-Nizala*, which means temporary settlement that is separate from and contrasted to "the Americans."

Despite its appeal to the sojourning aspect of Lebanese immigrants, a number of authors emphasize that pack-peddling was the fundamental factor in the assimilation of Syrian–Lebanese in America (see McCarus, 1994; Naff, 1985; Younis, 1995). According to Naff (1985), peddling forced the early arrivals to learn English quickly because learning English was critical to their success. Peddling further enabled them to see the country and experience its way of life firsthand. As such, it served as a window to new ideas and values and raised the immigrants' aspirations. Furthermore, Naff argues that peddling spared the early arrivals "a ghetto mentality" as it facilitated the acquisition of taste and manners of the larger society as well as the attainment of social acceptance. Thus, the success in trade and economic activities is emphasized as crucial in facilitating the assimilation of the Syrian–Lebanese to American society as it contributed to the continuous, multifaceted process of "becoming American" (Naff, 1985).

Traditionally the Arab American community has focused on assimilating into the United States mainstream instead of standing up and claiming their political power as a voting bloc. Perhaps the best evidence of this denial of identity is the long-term debate over whether members of the group should classify themselves as white or of Arab decent. Historically, many leaders in the community have campaigned for census surveys not to include an Arab-heritage checkmark, for fear of prejudice and exclusion from the mainstream (Samhan, 1997). For many immigrants being seen as indistinguishable from whites was a feat worthy of praise. To help accomplish this goal, a large portion of the group members even went as far as to make their names sound more American and less foreign (Goffe, 1999). It was common for Mahmoud to become Mike and Hussein, Sam. Ahmad Shebbani, the editor of the Arab community magazine Arabica, says that this pattern is because "People don't want to feel foreign. They want to imply 'we are part of you'" (Goffe, 1999). Truzzi (1997) describes that as a result of becoming successful in their business and professions, many Syrian–Lebanese in the United States entered politics and also did well in government, as governors, representatives, advisors to the President, and so on. Their descendants, having been socialized in communities that were not affected by new arrivals due to migratory restrictions, lacked political connections to the Arab world and the pan-Arab mobilization that swept their homelands in the 1950s and 1960s. As a result, they reacted to developments in the Arab world "primarily as Americans and only secondarily as Arabs" (Naff, 1985, p. 21).

According to many analysts, the manner in which immigrants understood their position in American society is an important difference between Arab immigrants of the first and the second wave. While first wave immigrants believed that they were sojourners who do not belong to American society, second wave immigrants were permanent settlers who came with well-defined ideas of democracy and citizenship (Suleiman, 1999). Higher levels of education and social status also motivated new immigrants to participate in American society. Members of the second and latter waves of Arab immigrants either came as university students or were members of the educated elite in their home countries and were more diverse in terms of religion and national origin. More importantly, while economic factors were the most significant behind the migration of the first wave, social and political reasons drove many Arab immigrants of the second wave to the United States.

Civil society organizations reflect the politicization of the Arab American community over the different waves. The first wave of immigrants established a number of charitable societies that maintained group cohesion and ethnic ties. Members of the small elite in the first wave started organizations to improve the conditions of other members of the community, such as clubs to learn English, and to promote American ideals and mutual understanding. For example, the Syrian Society was organized, in 1892, for the purpose of:

> Providing an educational and industrial institution for natives of that [Syrian–Lebanese] race, founded on Christian principles, by which they shall be taught the English language and such branches of learning and industry as may assist them to support themselves, and to become intelligent American citizens (Naff, 1985: 136).

The assimilatory mandate of the Syrian Society is clear. It was not until the second wave of migration, however, that community organizations started to promote participation in political or civic institutions, such as the Syrian Democratic and Syrian Republican clubs which were formed in the 1920s (Suleiman, 1999) which may be seen as strengthening political participation along ethnic terms.

Multiculturalism, Ethnic Politics, and Transnational Connections

While the first wave of Arab immigrants did not face major obstacles to their reception in American society partly due to their shared religious background with other settled ethnic groups, post-1965 immigrants were Muslims who arrived to a political climate that essentialized them as fundamentalist, patriarchal, extreme, and violent (Cainkar, 2006; Merskin, 2004). Marking Arab Americans an outsider Other is best analyzed through the framework of multiculturalism as it highlights the retention of ethnic identity in the new society and the associated discrimination and exclusion that often accompanies such processes. In the case of more recent waves of Arab immigrants, their distinguishable religious identity plays an important role in defining their ethnic identity and also their exclusion from the American mainstream. Research on Arabs in the United States refers to the post-1970 wave of immigrants as one that rejects secularism and Westernization while being more committed to ethno-religious culture and community than earlier cohorts of Arab immigrants (Haddad, 1983, 1994). According to Haddad (1983), this new cohort is mainly composed of Muslim Arab migrants who wished to transfer their strong religious traditions to their new Western environment. As a by-product of the post-1970 Islamic revival, religious identities (both Muslim and Christian) in the Arab World have prevailed over national and/or Pan-Arab identities. Thus, the new Arab migrants tended to assign a more devotional role to mosques and religious organizations, compared with their secular American-born ethno-religious peers of the second and third generation, whose implication in religious networks and mosques, if any, often assumed a social role of community binder (Haddad, 1983). The role of religious networks, especially among Muslim newcomers and their children is crucial in developing a sense of collectivity whose identity is clearly differentiated from the mainstream society (see, for example Jamal, 2005). Such collectivity is constructed through communal institutions that mark social boundaries between the minority group and the mainstream.

Beyond the internal dynamics of the community itself, a number of scholars stress that the racial formation of Arab Americans reflects American foreign policy interests in the region and thus political and economic events in the Middle East are important factors that we ought to take into account when investigating Arab American identity and political mobilization (see, for example Cainkar, 2006; David, 2007; Salaita, 2005). Cainkar (2006, p. 271) argues that "global events and the political agendas of powerful institutional actors" worked to increase the social distance and group distinctiveness for Arab Americans, and thus strengthening Arab American ethnic identities:

> Racial projects that moved Arabs into subordinate status began to clearly mark the Arab American experience in the last 1960s and provided momentum for the foundation of pan-Arab American activist organizations. In the 1990s, when Islamist challenges to American global hegemony became more powerful than Arab nationalism, these essentialized constructions were extended to Muslims and became grander; they became civilizational.

The "clash of civilizations" thesis has been used to justify racial profiling, mass detentions and deportations, and war against Muslim countries. The stigmatization of Arabs as the enemy/Other triggered the political mobilization of Arab Americans. Riemers (1992) notes, many Arab Americans felt victimized by negative media portrayals and social prejudice which motivated them to join or establish Arab Americans organizations. Stigmatized as a result of the political climate that demonized Arabs vis-à-vis Israel, Arab Americans tended to share the pan-Arabist identity politics of the Arab world at the time. The most notable Arab American organization that emerged in late 1967 is the Arab American University Graduates (AAUG). The transnational mandate of the organization was clear:

> There was special emphasis on the need to contribute the intellectual and professional skill of the Arab-American community to the fundamental transformation and development of the Arab world. The development of an accurate and scientific alternative literature, and an educational-informational program to challenge Zionist distortions and misinformation about the Middle East, were also seen as crucial. Furthermore, a viable national organization would leave the individual Arab-American less vulnerable, less isolated, and would promote cooperative efforts among the community (AAUG, 2001).

Similar to many other organizations that followed, the emphasis of the AAUG was to mobilize Arab Americans towards affecting change in the Arab world and defend against the negative portrayals of Arab Americans in the United States.

Ethnic organizations also reflect the strengthening of Arab American identity post-1967 as they started to develop as pressure groups. These organizations may have intended to reflect the strengthening of ethnic identification of the community and the growing transnational interest as well. Most prominent among these organizations are the Arab Anti-Discrimination Committee, which was formed to oppose media stereotypes and negative coverage of the Arab–Israeli conflict, the Arab American Institute, which focuses on affecting foreign policy through lobbying, and the Association of Arab American University Graduates, which was more interested in raising public awareness on Arab and Arab American communities and culture (see Majaj, 1999; Suleiman, 1994). Since these groups were more interested in educating the American public on Arab culture, they were fairly limited in their ability to provide a sense of cohesiveness that is important for maintaining an Arab American ethnic group. After 1967, however, the narrative of Arab American identification shifts. Many Arab immigrants arrived with an already politicized identity of Arab nationalism and political dispossession following the 6-day war. For many, their political identities also meant an opposition to the US foreign policy relating to the Middle East.

Many studies show that, for the descendants of the first wave of immigrants, political interests focus on civil rights and discrimination (Haddad, 2004; Howell, 2000; Nagel & Staeheli, 2004). More recent arrivals, however, focus on homeland issues related to the Arab–Israeli conflict (Howell, 2000; McCloud, 2003; Shain, 1996). Despite this analytical division, it is important to note that various studies point to the diversity in political attitudes among Arab Americans. While political exclusion and discriminatory US policies in the Middle East provide a source for ethnic pride for many Arab Americans, differences in migration experiences, national origins and religion inhabit a common political agenda and forestall collective action among Arab Americans (Wald, 2009). Nonetheless, the sparse empirical data reveal low levels of politicized ethnic identity among Arab Americans and continuing differences associated with religion and date of immigration (see, for example Barghouti, 1989 on political divisions related to the Palestinian–Israeli conflict and Sandoval & Jendrysik, 1993 on attitude variations related to the first Gulf War).

The transnational involvement of more recent Arab activists, however, continues to be seen. These transnational attachments signify that concerns with the Arab world and national integration in the United States are intertwined while simultaneously informing immigrants' political activism. Arab Americans maintain transnational ties with family and friends and may also engage in philanthropic and social activism that relates to the Arab World. At the same time, their transnational engagement does not preclude engaging in the US politics to address issues of discrimination, demand inclusion within the United States, and challenge the US governmental policies and attitudes of Americans towards Arabs and the Arab World (Nagel & Staeheli, 2004). For many Arab Americans, transnational involvement is important to their desire to be active members in their newly adopted country. Some focus their activities on ethnic organizations and politics as they wish to foster ethnic political mobilization for Arab-related issues. At the same time, many participate in mainstream organizations and cultural arenas as they wish to present Americans with positive role models of Arab Americans who are not threatening to the mainstream or challenge these organizations to be more inclusive and multicultural. While working for the benefit of their homelands, ethnic community, and mainstream society, Arab Americans also engage with universal issues of rights and freedoms with the intention to bring about global changes that may indirectly affect their various communities (Abdelhady, 2011a). Recent studies of Arab Americans question the utility of ethnicity as a framework for understanding the political dispositions and identity narratives of Arab Americans altogether. While highlighting transnational attachments, Nagel and Staeheli (2004) and Abdelhady (2011a) illustrate the ways immigrants move beyond traditional basis for membership and identification (national origin, ethnicity, or religion). Instead of navigating the contentious terrain of homeland and host society, Arab immigrants express cosmopolitan forms of identification and membership that also shape their desire to be involved with social and political issues in their current environment.

Political Exclusion, Global Politics, and Diaspora

Like other racial and ethnic groups in the United States, placing Arab Americans within the American ethnic/racial structure has been a source of debate. According to the 2000 census classification, individuals from North African and the Middle Eastern descent are classified as white/Caucasian, and 80 % of Arab Americans identified themselves as such in 2000 (De La Cruz & Brittingham, 2003). While this, together with their predominantly professional occupational status, English linguistic ability and overall socioeconomic success, may be seen as an indicator of successful assimilation into the white middle-class in American society, the process of Arab American identification and communal belonging is more complicated. It should not be seen within a simple linear, one-way process of assimilation framework. Despite their successful integration, the state and media racializes these same individuals as essentially other, which leads to a contradictory placement of Arabs in American culture (Naber, 2000). At one level, the conflation in the media of the categories Arab, Middle Eastern, and Muslim as mostly violent, backwards and irrational contributes to constructions of an inferior Arab/Muslim/Middle Eastern culture and the perception of Arabs as non-white Other. Thus, according to Naber (2000) the media representations emphasize the exclusion of Arabs from American society despite their inclusion among the majority white population. Despite the original debate within Arab American activist circles on the issue of classification and identity, the events of 9/11 marked a new historical juncture and a change in the racial formation of Arabs in the United States (for a report on discrimination against Arab Americans in the aftermath of 9/11, see Ibish, 2003). The new racial formation led many to realize that Arab Americans are undeniably people of color (Naber, 2002). Following the proclaimed war on terrorism, the political exclusion of Arab Americans continues to escalate.

Needless to say, forms of Arab American exclusion preceded the events of 9/11. According to Naber (2008, p. 31), discrimination against Arabs in the United States after World War II was shaped as a result of the interplay between the US military, political, and economic expansion in the Middle East, negative media representations, and institutionalized government policies targeting Arabs which "coincided with the increasing significance of oil as a commodity to the global economy and the United States' expanding interest in military and economic intervention in the Middle East." The last 3 decades of the twentieth century were ones of increasing anti-Arab sentiments and policies in the United States as they also brought about further political conflict in the Middle East. The oil embargo in 1973, the Iranian revolution in 1979, the US intervention in Lebanon in 1982, the two Gulf wars in the 1990s, the US bombing of Libya in 1986, and Sudan and Afghanistan in 1998 reflect the US political involvement in the region. These are also events that further strengthened anti-Arab sentiments in the United States and their exclusion from participating in American cultural politics.

Like any other racial and ethnic group in the United States, the political exclusion of Arab Americans took many negative forms. While specific policies, such as the 1996 Antiterrorism and Effective Death Penalty Act (commonly known as secret evidence law), highlight the legal discrimination that Arab Americans face, their political exclusion is harder to identify. For example, Arab American political analyst Zogby (1998) describes the negative lens through which Arab Americans are portrayed by political actors:

> Sometimes, Arab Americans found that their mere existence had become a campaign issue. A few weeks before the 1985 mayoral elections in Dearborn, Michigan, every household received a campaign mailer from one candidate announcing in thick, one-inch black lettering his solution to the "Arab problem," xenophobic concerns about the increase of Arab immigration into the city. Dearborn happens to be the city with the highest proportion of Arab Americans in its population—over 20 percent.

Furthermore, in the few incidents when Arab Americans managed to form a quasi-interest group, there groups were not well accepted, as evidenced by the rejection of campaign contributions from Arab Americans to Walter Mondale, Michael Dukakis and Hillary Clinton, all because of the politicians' fear of being connected to a "fringe" group (Hardy, Sentell, & Flores, 2001). This fear was perpetuated because the mainstream's view of Arab Americans was one of condemnation. Numerous accounts point to the ways the media and mainstream institutions stigmatize Arabs, which results in their exclusion from these institutions. Zogby (1998) cites an example:

> ABSCAM scandal of 1980 as a sting operation that netted five corrupt congressmen and one senator on charges of bribery and influence peddling. But to many Arab Americans, ABSCAM had an entirely different meaning. We were already acutely sensitive to the stereotypes of Arabs held by many Americans. The FBI surveillance footage—showing an agent dressed as an Arab Sheik corrupting American politicians—fed into the worst of these images. That the FBI would use and thereby propagate such stereotypes left us feeling vulnerable and angry. Unfortunately, the operation also exposed how little real political power we had, and made it even harder for us to gain access to the political process.

Generally speaking, Arab Americans were seen as "Others" who threatened the whole, largely because any success story of an Arab immigrant was kept hidden since that immigrant identified herself as white (Goffe, 1999); therefore, the only experiences with Arabs recognized by the white community were interactions with unsuccessful and often unmotivated immigrants.

The limited interaction between whites and Arabs drastically changed following the political backlash from the events of September 11. Almost immediately after the attacks, FBI agents, under the order of President George W. Bush, requested that anyone of Arab decent come forward to be interviewed about possible connections to terrorist groups (Taylor, 2006). According to Bush, it was "unlawful" for any Arab immigrant to not show himself or herself. This proclamation resulted in 4,793 Arab American legal immigrants being questioned by the Department of Justice in just 1 year after September 11 (Sachs, 2002). Coupled with this staggering figure is the fact that the Arab American community saw 1,200 Arab and South Asian Muslim men detained or arrested within just 2 months (Amnesty International, 2002). Hate crimes against the group increased dramatically, up to 500 % (Withrow, 2006), leading some to characterize Arab Americans as a community under siege (Yonge, 2004).

Increased awareness of exclusion, discrimination, and othering motivated many to mobilize politically and participate in combating existing stereotypes of Arab (and Muslim) Americans (see, for example Bakalian & Bozorgmehr, 2009; Millard, 2008). Such efforts often triggered alliances and political participation that extended beyond ethnic communities and included other immigrants and nonimmigrants who mobilized around issues of general appeal such as those relating to social justice, discrimination, and equality in general (Abdelhady, 2011a). Moving beyond identity politics, Arab Americans are building alliances no longer based on traditional understandings of identity and communal belonging, but now extend to issues of universal concern and broad global appeal. These forms of identifications and community alliances are best understood through the framework of diaspora, as it allows viewing identities and communities as flexible entities that are formed through processes of simultaneous inclusion and exclusion, rootedness and transitory realities, and local and global attachments. As processes of globalization intensify around the world, new forms of diasporic cosmopolitan identities also spread. Our understanding of the experiences of Arab Americans would benefit from incorporating these aspects of globalization in order to understand the ways in which ethnic belonging is changing in the contemporary world.

Contesting Singular Narratives

Like other groups in the United States, painting a picture of community life and history for Arab Americans is not an easy task. Historians provide contradictory analyses of early experiences as they tend to emphasize the aspects of community life that may resonate best with their ideological and political affiliations. Historical evidence may itself be incomplete, making it even harder to examine different aspects of incorporation and participation in American society. For example, Naff (1985, 1994) perceived of the early Arab immigrant experiences as one resulting in assimilation and integration into a white middle-class strata of American society. Bawardi (2009), on the other hand, perceived that experience as one of transnational connections centered around homeland politics and a rising political consciousness that was mostly concerned with homeland affairs. It is somewhat clear that Naff saw assimilation as a desirable process that prioritized Americanization over other aspects of community life. Gualtieri (2010) moved beyond such prioritization of Americanization and whiteness of Arab Americans to describe the ways the process of assimilation was never complete. She emphasized the ways assimilation was fraught with ethnic exclusion and discrimination from the early waves. The two dominant strands of immigration literature—namely assimilation and ethnic pluralism/multiculturalism—frame the specific questions and aspects of community life that scholars set to analyze and thus limit the kinds of analyses they provide.

In addition to historical and ideological limitations, diversity within the community itself further complicates any attempts to describe the experience of Arab Americans within singular narratives of either assimilation or ethnic identification. Among the many differences that shape the characterization of the Arab American community (see, for example Naber, 2000), generational differences shape identification, perceptions of assimilation and integration, levels of religiosity, and relationship to the homeland in many different ways. First-generation Arab Americans are likely to see themselves as immigrants who do not fully belong to their host society. Whether the same is true for the second and third generations is debatable at best. Furthermore, not all who fall within the objectively defined Arab American category agree on the meaning of the word Arab, and instead tend to define their ancestry in national terms (tracing it back to nation-states that indeed belong to the contemporary Arab World). Such differences and disagreements make it difficult to define the community under study, therefore instituting challenges for scholars to access respondents who likely portray the diversity of the community.

It has to be noted that such problems are not unique to the Arab American community, but reflect shared experiences of other ethnic groups when attempting to portray a community within singular narratives that stress only one aspect of community life and history. Since the goal is not to reach agreement among scholars of the Arab American experience concerning the "real" nature of the community, it remains important to highlight the diversity of experiences. There are often contradictory aspects that shape communal boundaries and identities. Focusing on diversity and internal contradictions or contestations would allow scholars to provide more comprehensive analyses as well as more nuanced descriptions of the dynamics of ethnicity and belonging in a changing context.

Conclusion

Transnational linkages, while not new, have taken on new meanings as a result of immigrants' ability to maintain strong economic, political, and social ties with their homelands as a result of inexpensive modes of communication and transport (Cohen & Vertovec, 1999). Castles and Davidson (2000, p. 127) hold that in the age of globalization "assimilation is no longer an option because of the rapidity and multidirectionality of mobility and communication." In understanding Arab American transnational social and political activism, it is important to note that early arrivals also formed transnational organizations that took issue with events in the homeland (such as Ottoman persecution, ethnic rivalries, and the development of the social infrastructure). These organizations were intended to address issues in the homeland while strengthening social bonds within the community. Importantly, these organizations also worked to strengthen integration in the United States as they dealt with issues relating to immigration, English language acquisition, and voting (see Al-Qazzaz, 1979; David, 2007; Naff, 1985). Successful assimilation weakened the need for such organizations that were replaced by ones more political in nature and reflected the interests of newer cohorts of Arab immigrants.

Post-1967 waves of immigrants displayed a pronounced Arab ethnic identity that was shaped by domestic interests and the international political climate. The organizations that formed reflected the political interests of these groups of immigrants as they focused on the political mobilization of Arab Americans towards impacting American policy towards the community and its homeland. These organizations, however, did not reflect the diversity of the Arab American community (based on national origin, religious affiliation, age, gender, or general political interests) and for the most part failed to form an Arab American political identity and interest group. During short-lived instances when Arab Americans managed to form a coherent political group, their stigmatization and exclusion by the general political climate worked to further disenfranchise them. The events of 9/11, however, represent an important disjuncture as it facilitated the mobilization of Arab Americans in face of mass detentions, deportations, and discrimination. Such large-scale mobilization facilitated the strengthening of transnational attachments that, while initially threatened, is on the rise given the major political transformations taking place in the region at present. The long-term implications of these transnational forms of involvement are yet to be determined.

While the identity of Arab Americans and their political involvement are shaped by a host of influences ranging from individual narratives, generational belonging, and involvement with homeland issues, it is rather difficult to arrive at a general understanding of how these individuals identify themselves or are identified by others. The theoretical perspectives discussed above shed light on the importance of accounting for waves of immigration, whether or not Arab Americans are immigrants, second or third generation, and how sociohistorical periods influence their identities and hence interactions with wider society and the institutions with which they interact. As such, understanding the relationship between membership to an Arab American community and health cannot take place without taking into consideration other factors such as age, class, and level of assimilation among other factors. Providing recommendations for mental health professional who provide services to Arab Americans, Erickson and Al-Timimi (2001) stress the importance of the providers' awareness of their own stereotypes of their clients and the need to interpret clients' behavior within the relevant cultural contexts in order to apply interventions that are most appropriate. Specifically, the authors call on mental health professionals who desire to work with Arab Americans successfully to gain awareness of their biases and assumptions about Arab Americans, identify their worldview and the cultural and socio-political factors that affect it, and determine the most relevant intervention strategies and techniques that suit their culture and experiences. The diversity in experiences and identity narratives among Arab Americans yield generalizing among members of the group an unfruitful and undesirable task for all those concerned about the well-being of the community members.

References

Abdelhady, D. (2006). Beyond home/host networks: Forms of solidarity among Lebanese immigrants in a global era. *Identities: Global Studies in Culture and Power, 13*(3), 427–453.

Abdelhady, D. (2011a). *The Lebanese diaspora: The Arab immigrant experience in Montreal, New York and Paris*. New York: New York University Press.

Abdelhady, D. (2011b). *The influence of Arab democratization movements on Arab American political activism*. Paper presented at the Contemporary Research in Arab American Studies: New Trends and Critical Perspectives: A Conference in Honor of Michael Suleiman, Detroit, Michigan.

Abraham, N. (1994). Anti-Arab racism and violence in the United States. In E. McCarus (Ed.), *The development of Arab-American identity* (pp. 155–214). Ann Arbor: The University of Michigan Press.

Abraham, S., & Abraham, N. (1983). Arabs in the world. In S. Abraham & N. Abraham (Eds.), *Arabs in the new world: Studies in Arab-American communities*. Detroit: Wayne State University.

Ajrouch, K., & Jamal, A. (2007). Assimilating to a white identity: The case of Arab Americans. *International Migration Review, 41*, 860–879.

Alfaro-Velcamp, T. (2011). Arab "Amirka": Exploring Arab diasporas in Mexico and the United States. *Comparative Studies of South Asia, Africa and the Middle East, 31*(2), 282–295.

Al-Qazzaz, A. (1979). *Transnational links between the Arab community in the U.S. and the Arab world*. Sacramento: California Central Press.

Amnesty International. (2002). *AI's concerns regarding post September 11 detentions in the USA*. Amnesty International. http://www.amnesty.org/en/library/asset/AMR51/044/2002/en/154256a9-d882-11dd-ad8c-f3d4445c118e/amr510442002en.pdf.

Arab American University Graduates. (2001). *Cited in David 2007*. http://www.aaug-asq.org

Bakalian, A., & Bozorgmehr, M. (2009). *Backlash 9/11: Middle eastern and Muslim Americans respond*. Berkeley: University of California Press.

Banks, R. R. (2003). Racial profiling and anti-terrorism efforts. *Cornell Law Review, 89*, 1201–1217.

Barghouti, I. (1989). *Palestinian Americans: Socio-political attitudes of Palestinian Americans towards the Arab-Israeli conflict. University of Durham occasional paper series*. Durham: Center for Middle East and Islamic Studies.

Basch, L., Glick Shiller, N., & Szanton Blanc, C. (1994). *Nations unbound: Transnational projects, postcolonial predicaments and deterritorialized nation-states*. Basel, Switzerland: Gordon and Breach.

Bawardi, H. (2009). *Arab American political organization from 1915–1951: Assessing transnational political consciousness and the development of Arab American identity*. PhD, Wayne State University, Detroit.

Cainkar, L. (2003). *Targeting Muslims, at Ashcroft's discretion. Middle east report online*. Retrieved from http://www.merip.org/mero/mero031403

Cainkar, L. (2006). The social construction of difference and the Arab American experience. *Journal of American Ethnic History, 25*(2–3), 243–278.

Castles, S. (1997). Multicultural citizenship: A response to the dilemma of globalization and national identity? *Journal of Intercultural Studies, 18*, 5–22.

Castles, S., & Davidson, A. (2000). *Citizenship and migration: Globalization and the politics of belonging*. New York: Routledge.

Cohen, R., & Vertovec, S. (1999). Introduction. In R. Cohen & S. Vertovec (Eds.), *Migration, diaspora and transnationalism* (pp. 12–17). Cheltenham: Edward Elgar.

Conklin, N. F., & Faires, N. (1987). Colored and catholic: The Lebanese in Birmingham, Alabama. In E. Hooglund (Ed.), *Crossing the waters: Arabic-speaking immigrants to the United States before 1940*. Washington, DC: Smithsonian Institution.

David, G. (2007). The creation of "Arab American": Political activism and ethnic dis(unity). *Critical Sociology, 33*, 833–862.

David, G., & Ayouby, K. (2002). Being Arab and becoming Americanized: Forms of mediated assimilation in metropolitan Detroit. In Y. Y. Haddad & J. I. Smith (Eds.), *Muslim minorities in the West: Visible and invisible* (pp. 125–142). Walnut Creek, CA: Altamira.

De La Cruz, P., & Brittingham, A. (2003). *The Arab population: 2000*. Washington, DC: US Census Bureau.

Erickson, C. D., & Al-Tamimi, N. R. (2001). Providing mental health services to Arab Americans: Recommendations and considerations. *Cultural Diversity and Ethnic Minority Psychology, 7*(4), 308–327.

Glazer, N., & Moynihan, D. (1970). *Beyond the melting pot*. Cambridge, MA: MIT Press.

Goffe, L. (1999). *Arab-Americans coming in from the cold: The growing political clout of the Arab-American community* (p. 22). The Middle East: Current Affairs.

Gualtieri, S. (2001). Becoming "White": Race, religion and the foundations of Syrian/Lebanese ethnicity in the U.S. *Journal of American Ethnic History, 20*(4), 29–58.
Gualtieri, S. (2010). *Between Arab and White: Race and ethnicity in the early Syrian American diaspora*. Berkeley: University of California Press.
Haddad, Y. Y. (1983). Arab Muslims and Islamic institutions in America: Adaptation and reform. In S. Abraham & N. Abraham (Eds.), *Arabs in the new world: Studies in Arab-American communities* (pp. 64–81). Detroit: Wayne State University, Center for Urban Studies.
Haddad, Y. Y. (1991). American foreign policy in the Middle East and its impact on the identity of Arab Muslims in the United States. In Y. Haddad (Ed.), *The Muslims of America* (pp. 217–235). New York: Oxford University Press.
Haddad, Y. Y. (1994). Maintaining the faith of the fathers: Dilemmas in the religious identity in the Christian and Muslim Arab-American communities. In E. McCarus (Ed.), *The development of Arab-American identity* (pp. 63–84). Ann Arbor: University of Michigan Press.
Haddad, Y. Y. (2004). *Not quite American? The shaping of Arab and Muslim identity in the US*. Waco, TX: Baylor University Press.
Hardy, K., Sentell, L., & Flores, V. (2001). *The Arab-Israeli conflict: Role profiles*. Retrieved from http://www.la.utexas.edu/chenry/aip/fall01/roles01/msg00007.html
Higham, J. (1955). *Strangers in the land: Patterns of American nativism 1860–1925*. New Brunswick: Rutgers University Press.
Hooglund, E. (Ed.). (1987). *Crossing the waters: Arabic-speaking immigrants to the United States before 1940*. Washington, DC: Smithsonian Institution Press.
Hourani, A., & Shehdi, N. (1992). Introduction. In A. Hourani & N. Shehdi (Eds.), *The Lebanese in the world: A century of emigration* (pp. 3–11). London: Centre for Lebanese Studies.
Howell, S. (2000). Cultural interventions: Arab American aesthetics between the transnational and the ethnic. *Diaspora, 9*(1), 39–59.
Howell, S., & Shryock, A. (2003). Cracking down on diaspora: Arab Detroit and America's "War on Terror". *Anthropological Quarterly, 76*(3), 443–462.
Ibish, H. (Ed.). (2003). *Report on hate crimes and discrimination against Arab-Americans: The post-September 11 Backlash, September 11, 2001-October 11, 2002*. Washington, DC: Arab-American Anti-Discrimination Committee.
Issawi, C. (1992). The historical background of Lebanese emigration, 1800–1914. In A. Hourani & N. Shehdi (Eds.), *The Lebanese in the world: A century of emigration* (pp. 13–39). London: Centre for Lebanese Studies.
Jamal, A. (2005). The political participation and engagement of Muslim Americans: Mosque involvement and group consciousness. *American Political Research, 33*(4), 521–544.
Jimenez, T. (2009). *Replenished ethnicity: Mexican Americans, immigration and identity*. Berkeley: University of California Press.
Karpat, K. (1985). The Ottoman emigration to America, 1860–1914. *International Journal of Middle East Studies, 17*(2), 175–209.
Kayal, P. (1995). Epilogue. In A. Younis (Ed.), *The coming of the Arabic speaking people to the United States* (pp. 249–265). Staten Island: Center for Migration Studies.
Kayyali, R. A. (2006). *The Arab Americans*. Westport, CT: Greenwood Press.
Kulczycki, A., & Lobo, A. P. (2001). Deepening the melting pot: Arab-Americans at the turn of the century. *The Middle East Journal, 55*(3), 459–475.
Majaj, L. S. (1999). Arab-American ethnicity: Location, coalition and cultural negotiations. In M. Suleiman (Ed.), *Arabs in America: Building a new future* (pp. 320–336). Philadelphia: Temple University Press.
Marshal, S., & Read, J. G. (2003). Identity politics among Arab-American women. *Social Science Quarterly, 84*(4), 875–891.
McCarus, E. (1994). Introduction. In E. McCarus (Ed.), *The development of Arab-American identity* (pp. 1–8). Ann Arbor: University of Michigan Press.
McCloud, A. B. (2003). Islam in America: The mosaic. In Y. Y. Haddad, J. I. Smith, & J. L. Esposito (Eds.), *Religion and immigration: The Christian, Jewish and Muslim experience in the United States* (pp. 159–174). Walnut Creek, CA: Alta Mira.

Merskin, D. (2004). The construction of Arabs as enemies: Post-September 11 discourse of George W. Bush. *Mass Communication and Society, 7*, 157–175.
Millard, R. (2008). *Seven years after 9/11: Arab Americans and the NYPD*. Retrieved from http://www.jjay.cuny.edu/cmcj/pdfs/NYPD%20Arab%20Americans_article.pdf
Morawska, E. (2008). Research on immigration/ethnicity in Europe and the United States: A comparison. *The Sociological Quarterly, 49*(3), 465–482.
Naber, N. (2000). Ambiguous insiders: An investigation of Arab American invisibility. *Ethnic and Racial Studies, 23*(1), 37–61.
Naber, N. (2002). *Arab San Francisco: On gender, cultural citizenship, and belonging*. PhD, University of California, Davis.
Naber, N. (2008). Introduction: Arab Americans and U.S. racial formations. In A. Jamal & N. Naber (Eds.), *Race and Arab Americans before and after 9/11: From invisible citizens to visible subjects* (pp. 1–45). Syracuse: Syracuse University Press.
Naff, A. (1985). *Becoming American: The early Arab immigrant experience*. Carbondale, IL: Southern Illinois University Press.
Naff, A. (1994). The early Arab immigrant experience. In E. McCarus (Ed.), *The development of Arab-American identity* (pp. 23–35). Ann Arbor: University of Michigan Press.
Nagel, C., & Staeheli, L. (2004). Citizenship, identity and transnational migration: Arab immigrants to the United States. *Space and Polity, 8*(1), 3–23.
Orfalea, G. (2006). *The Arab Americans: A history*. New York: Olive Branch Press.
Portes, A., & Rumbaut, R. (1996). *Ethnic America: A portrait*. Berkeley: University of California Press.
Ramakrishnane, S. K. (2005). *Democracy in immigrant America: Changing demographics and political participation*. Stanford: Stanford University Press.
Riemers, D. (1992). *Still the golden door: The third world comes to America*. New York: Columbia University Press.
Sachs, S. (2002, April 2). U.S. begins crackdown on Muslims who defy orders to leave country. *The New York Times*.
Salaita, S. (2005). Ethnic identity and imperative patriotism: Arab Americans before and after 9/11. *College Literature, 32*(2), 146–168.
Samhan, H. (1997, June 17, 2007). *Not quite white: Race classification and the Arab American experience*. Retrieved from http://www.aaiusa.org/foundation/355/not-quite-white.
Samhan, H. (2001). *Arab Americans. In Grolier's multimedia encyclopedia*. Available online from www.gme.grolier.com.
Sandoval, J. M., & Jendrysik, M. S. (1993). Convergence and divergence in Arab American public opinion. *International Journal of Public Opinion Research, 5*, 303–314.
Seikaly, M. (1999). Attachment and identity: The Palestinian community of Detroit. In M. Suleiman (Ed.), *Arabs in America: Building a new future* (pp. 25–38). Philadelphia: Temple University Press.
Shain, Y. (1996). Arab Americans at a crossroads. *Journal of Palestine Studies, 25*(3), 46–59.
Suleiman, M. (1994). Arab-Americans and the political process. In E. McCarus (Ed.), *The development of Arab-American identity* (pp. 37–60). Philadelphia: Temple University Press.
Suleiman, M. (1999). Introduction: The Arab immigrant experience. In M. Suleiman (Ed.), *Arabs in America: Building a new future* (pp. 1–24). Philadelphia: Temple University Press.
Taylor, M. (2006, November 23). FBI tactics put Muslims on edge. *The New and Observer.*
Truzzi, O. (1997). The right place at the right time: Syrians and Lebanese in Brazil and the United States, a comparative approach. *Journal of American Ethnic History, 16*(2), 3–34.
Wald, K. D. (2009). The diaspora project of Arab Americans: Assessing the magnitude and determinants of politicized ethnic identity. *Ethnic and Racial Studies, 32*(8), 1304–1324.
Wald, K. D., & Williams, B. (2005). *The diaspora consciousness of Arab Americans: The intersection of social identity and global politics working papers*. Middlebury: Middlebury College Rohatyn Center for International Affairs.
Withrow, B. (2006). *Racial profiling: From rhetoric to reason*. Upper Saddle River, NJ: Pearson Prentice Hall.

Yonge, G. (2004, October 16). *Under siege since 9/11, Arab voters turn to Kerry, the guardian.* Retrieved from http://www.guardian.co.uk/print/0,,5040778-111675,00.html

Younis, A. (1995). *The coming of the Arabic speaking people to the United States.* New York: Center for Migration Studies.

Zogby, J. (1998). The politics of exclusion. *Civil Rights Journal, 3*(1), 42.

Chapter 3
Intra-Ethnic Diversity and Religion

Helen Hatab Samhan

Understanding the population we call Arab Americans requires an appreciation of and respect for the many distinctions that define this ethnic community and shape its interactions within the American context. This chapter will explore the diversity of Arab Americans by national origin, religious affiliation, and ethnic descent and how competing and contrasting identities often determine where and if subgroups will be situated within the ethnic framework.

Information presented in this chapter addresses issues and experiences that are situated within theoretical constructs of minority status, assimilation, and identity. Minority status is often understood juxtaposed to dominant status in society, signifying not necessarily numerical differences, but instead differences in access to resources and power. Minorities from the Arab world have historically been identified as those communities that differ from the Sunni Muslim Arab majority in their religious affiliation and/or in their ethno-cultural identity (Hourani, 1947). Though a majority of the Arab world is Muslim, various sects of Islam as well as other religions and non-Arab subgroups make the diversity of the region quite complex.

Classic assimilation theory (Park & Burgess, 1921) implicitly operated from the assumption that immigrants slowly leave cultural attitudes and behaviors associated with the homeland to eventually assimilate into the economic and political fabric of the host society regardless of their cultural and ethnic background. Later iterations (Gordon, 1964) suggested that assimilation included both cultural and structural aspects, which do not necessarily follow one another. For instance, one may assimilate culturally in terms of language acquisition, but that did not necessarily guarantee one would attain full political or economic success. Moreover, the influx of non-European, post-1965 immigrants led to the notion that different patterns of assimilation processes depend on both individual-level factors (e.g., education,

H.H. Samhan (✉)
Arab American Institute Foundation, 6333 Lakewood Drive, Falls Church, VA 22041, USA
e-mail: hsamhan@verizon.net

S.C. Nassar-McMillan et al. (eds.), *Biopsychosocial Perspectives on Arab Americans: Culture, Development, and Health*, DOI 10.1007/978-1-4614-8238-3_3,

English language ability, national origin, age upon arrival, length of residence in the United States) and contextual/structural variables (e.g., racial status, family socio-economic status, school district as well as neighborhood characteristics). Some immigrants may assimilate into dominant American culture, while others assimilate less successfully into minority group culture (Ajrouch & Kusow, 2007; Portes & Zhou, 1993). Finally, identity represents a key aspect of group membership. Theoretical advancements concerning the study of identity now acknowledge that it is development (Erikson, 1985) situational (Stryker, 1980), and multi-dimensional (McCarus, 1994) Americans of Arab descent may identify along a myriad of dimensions, depending on the situation and developmental stage.

This chapter will seek to identify dominant and minority groups broadly represented in the Arab American category, highlight assimilation experiences of Arab Americans, and provide insight into how identities form and change. The theoretical constructs discussed above are interspersed throughout to provide a broad framework for understanding intra-ethnic diversity and religion in the lives of Arab Americans. The impact on identity development in the United States among members of minority communities from the Arab world will be examined, as will the differential social integration trends among Muslim and Christian immigrants. How time of immigration and socio-political conditions in the United States influenced the direction and strength of ethnic identity as part of, or distinct from, pan Arab American institutions and affinities will also be addressed. This chapter will hopefully challenge and deconstruct cultural assumptions and stereotypes about behavior and priorities of people with roots in the Arab world and provide an overview of the diverse and complex identities that have shaped their experience in the U.S.

Who Is an Arab?

Not surprisingly, the definition of who is an Arab American has been both dynamic and controversial. Change over time, immigrant experience, and the construction of pan-ethnic institutions to compete in the American political landscape have kept Arab American identity in flux. Political realities in the Arab world and the historical narratives of the region's minority populations have kept many subnational identities strongly independent of, and distinct from, their Arab neighbors.

Most scholars and ethnic practitioners accept the working definition of Arab Americans as a broad, regionally based affiliation with the Arabic-speaking countries of the Middle East and North Africa, which are internationally recognized as members of the League of Arab States: Algeria, Bahrain, Comoros, Djibouti, Egypt, Iraq, Jordan, Kuwait, Lebanon, Libya, Mauritania, Morocco, Oman, Palestine, Qatar, Saudi Arabia, Somalia, Sudan, Syria, Tunisia, United Arab Emirates, and Yemen (Kayyali, 2006; Suleiman, 1999). The diversity present in the Arab world, by religion, by phenotype, by regional variation, is fully reflected by emigrants from this region and their descendents in the United States. What binds Arabs together in their societies and with each other is their shared history, Arabic language, music, literature, cuisine, and customs that are their common legacy. The experience of Americans of Arab descent has reflected both the solidarity and the divisions within Arab society. This chapter will address groups living in America with roots in the Arabic-speaking world, even though some of the subgroups, particularly religious or indigenous ethnic minorities, may not self-identify as Arab or Arab American.

While later in this chapter the politics of identity formation among subgroups of Arab Americans will be explored, certain trends in immigration history and acculturation patterns have influenced how Arabic-speaking immigrants have related to an Arab identity. The first wave of pioneer emigrants to arrive in the United States prior to World War I from the Ottoman provinces of greater Syria identified primarily with their village or town and religious sect and adopted the concept of being "Syrian" as ethnic shorthand in their new home (Kayal, 1974). These early immigrants and their descendants are less familiar and comfortable with identifying as Arabs. Subsequent waves of immigration after World War II corresponded with newly independent nation states in the Middle East and a popular Arab nationalist movement. Many second-wave immigrants arrived in America with a distinct pride in their Arab origins and the institutions they formed in the 1960s and 1970s reflected this affinity to the ideals of Arab cultural and political solidarity. While current references to the Arab American population embrace the broadest definition of those with any roots in the Arab world, there are many subgroups, as will be discussed below, who have "opted out" of the whole.

Major Regions of Arab Immigration to the United States

Most Americans with roots in the Arab world trace their origins to six countries (Lebanon, Syria, Egypt, Palestine, Iraq, and Jordan), with the remainder of Arab states (e.g., Morocco, Saudi Arabia, Yemen, among others) having a shorter and smaller immigration experience. Measuring country of origin is challenging as the American-born generations increase, and mixed heritage families become more common. One tool available to track sub-ethnic affiliation over time is the US Census which is one of the only national surveys to measure ancestry of nonminority populations. Ancestry responses can be of national origin (Lebanese, Iraqi, etc.) or generic (Arab or Arabic) so the data are imprecise but still provide a longitudinal view of how a national sample of Arab Americans self-identify since 1980. It is from these survey responses that proportional representation in the U.S. can be tracked and analyzed. The following overview of national origin groups is organized by the relative size of the population group and also clustered by geographical proximity.

Lebanese and Syrians: Since the majority of pre-World War I wave of Arab immigrants came from what is present-day Lebanon and Syria, these national origins claim the largest population group in the United States. Until the 1930s, these immigrants and their descendants referred to themselves collectively, and their institutions, as "Syrian" and once Lebanon received its independence, there was a propensity to identify distinctly as Lebanese-Americans (Suleiman, 1999). The pioneer wave of immigration from greater Syria lasted until the 1920s when US quotas restricted the number of new arrivals permitted from areas outside of Northern Europe (Samhan, 1999). These immigrants were mostly semi- or unskilled village and townspeople, predominantly Christian by religion, and settled in major port cities like New York and Boston but soon migrated across the country as peddlers, shopkeepers, and merchants (Naff, 1994).

In a second major immigration wave that began with the open-immigration policies of the 1960s, graduate students, young professionals, and entrepreneurs from the newly independent states of Lebanon and Syria formed part of the region-wide brain drain of that postwar era. More educated and politicized than the first wave, this generation of immigrants reflected an array of nationalistic experiences about the modern Arab world as well as the role of the United States in the politics of the region (Samhan, 1999). The devastating and destabilizing civil war in Lebanon from the 1970s until 1990 resulted in a new wave of emigrants escaping that conflict—arrivals that included Christians as well as many Shi'a from South Lebanon who were disproportionately impacted by conflict and disruption throughout the 1980s and sought refuge in the United States.

It is estimated that more than two in five Americans of Arab origin trace their ancestry to Lebanon and Syria (United States Census Bureau, Decennial Census, 2000). The Lebanese-Americans are the single largest subgroup and represent about one third of all those who identify an Arab ancestry in the US Census. Persons of Syrian descent represent an additional 10 %. As the oldest subgroup of Arab Americans, Lebanese and Syrians are also the most dispersed geographically throughout the states, with concentrations in Michigan, California, New York, Texas, Ohio, and New England. Older Syrian settlements in Pennsylvania and Rhode Island have resulted in concentrations in these states; the community in Allentown, PA in particular has cultivated a strong ethnic pride in the city and is one of the few places where Syrian national day is recognized by local government officials.

Palestinians and Jordanians: The first immigrants from Palestine arrived with the wave of Christians from Greater Syria, representing about 10 % of that cohort of pioneer arrivals until the 1920s. The unrest and dispossession affecting Palestinian society during the 1930s and 1940s resulted in spurts of immigration to the West, particularly after the 1948 war. The US Congress allowed limited numbers of Palestinians to enter America as refugees throughout the 1950s, in spite of prevailing quotas on non-European immigration (Ameri & Ramey, 1999). The Arab-Israeli war of 1967, creating a new cadre of refugees and dislocation, resulted in an increase in Palestinian immigration, both Christians and Muslims, seeking education, economic opportunity, and refuge from the upheaval at home.

A large portion of those emigrating to the United States with Jordanian passports since the 1950s are of Palestinian origin (since Jordan administered the West Bank after the 1948 war), but Jordanians from the "East Bank" have also come to America with other Arab immigrants, mostly in the post-1965 period. Jordanian and Palestinian migration has frequently been by nuclear families, with many opening up small businesses or working in a professional field. Palestinians in particular have placed a high premium on education and have been well represented in medicine, higher education, and engineering fields. Palestinian communities have concentrated in metropolitan areas like Chicago, San Francisco, Washington, DC, New York, and Jacksonville, FL (United States Census Bureau, Decennial Census, 2000). Jordanian Americans also have settled in Chicago as well as Yonkers, NY, and other communities. According to ancestry identification in US Census surveys, Arabs of Jordanian or Palestinian descent make up at least 10 % of the total ethnic population, but probably more given the inclination for Palestinians to self-identify generically as Arabs.

Iraqis: Immigrants from Iraq first came to the United States in the early 1900s, with small numbers of Christians from the region of Telkaif, near Mosul, who formed a small enclave in the greater Detroit area (Sengstock, 1974). Iraqi immigration increased considerably in the post-1965 wave of broader Arab world immigration, when more Iraqi families, students, merchants, and professionals, both Christian and Muslim, came to America in search of stability and opportunity outside the confines of the political and economic upheaval in the newly independent nation states of the region. Forming part of the brain drain since the 1960s, educated Iraqis arrived in the United States for continued study and training and often chose to remain in America and continue professional careers in medicine and education, among other fields.

As will be discussed below, the Christians from Iraq are known as Chaldeans and Assyrians who are descendents of the Aramaic tribes who created the Second Babylonian Empire in the sixth century BCE (Kayyali, 2006). A distinct religious minority, Chaldeans, formed successful networks of grocery and other retail stores, especially in southeast Michigan. Iraqi Americans also include refugees from the Gulf Wars of the 1980s and 1990s, particularly Shi'a from the south of Iraq who were escaping government repression and violence (Ameri & Ramey, 1999). Iraqi refugees who arrived after the US-led attack on Iraq following its invasion of Kuwait in 1991 were more likely to have less education, English proficiency, or resources than earlier immigrants and needed more support in their absorption into American society. A new wave of refugees in the years following the US-led invasion of Iraq in 2003 has been comprised of mostly Christian families escaping sectarian violence as well as those Iraqis who worked with coalition forces and were targeted by the ongoing insurgency.

Iraqi Americans are geographically concentrated in Michigan, California, Illinois, Arizona, and Nevada (United States Census Bureau, Decennial Census, 2000). Immigrants from Iraq and their descendents, of all religious denominations, represent about 10 % of the population in America from Arabic-speaking countries. The Chaldean/Assyrian communities in Michigan and California in particular have constructed religious institutions and strong economic cooperatives that have facilitated the integration of new immigrants and the social cohesion of their offspring (Sengstock, 1974). While the Christian immigrants earned a reputation for success in business, immigrants from Iraq's ruling classes were well represented in the professions and in the development of professional ethnic organizations, both pan Arab and Iraqi-specific.

North Africa: Immigrants from Egypt and their descendents form one of the fastest growing populations among Arab Americans and have dominated emigration from North African countries. Egyptian immigration to the United States began in the 1950s and grew steadily in the following decades. Unlike chain migration, where single men arrived first and brought family members later, from other Arab countries, Egyptians tend to immigrate in nuclear families and retain a close relationship with extended families by taking frequent trips back to the homeland (Keck, 1989). Prominently represented among Egyptian immigrants are Copts, members of an ancient church dating to the earliest centuries of Christianity and now comprising about 10 % of Egypt's population (Kayyali, 2006), as well as Protestants. Muslims also immigrated in considerable numbers, particularly in search of higher education and advanced degrees. Egyptian-American men and women claim the highest percentage of educated and professional members of all Arab American populations (Ameri & Ramey, 1999).

Egyptian Americans, especially Copts, are likely to identify strongly as Egyptians, and Middle Easterners, and with their Pharaonic heritage before their Arab one. While there are exceptions where individual Egyptians have taken leadership positions in pan Arab American institutions, this population maintains an Egyptian-centered social network driven by sectarian and professional affiliations (Keck, 1989). Based on data from US Census surveys since 1980, there has been a threefold increase in the Egyptian-American population in the past 3 decades, with this subgroup comprising about 13 % of those who identify an Arab ancestry. Geographic concentrations include the New York/New Jersey metropolitan area, Southern California, greater Washington, DC, and Chicago (United States Census Bureau, Decennial Census, 2000).

After Egypt, Moroccan immigration to the United States has increased, particularly in the past few decades. While there was some post-World War II immigration to America by Moroccan Jews (Ameri & Ramey, 1999), most Moroccans chose France, Spain, and other European states as their destination of choice for economic improvement and higher education. Migration to America in recent years has been facilitated by preferential visa programs and greater exposure in Morocco to American institutions through cultural outreach programs and other bilateral initiatives, including a pavilion dedicated to Moroccan culture at Disney World in Florida. Moroccan immigrants to the United States generally have better job skills and education than their counterparts in Europe, with a propensity towards business-ownership for those with capital or jobs in the hospitality industry, including hotel and restaurant work.

It is estimated that the number of Moroccan Americans has at least doubled since 1990, with the largest communities located along the eastern seaboard from Boston to Florida (with the largest community found in greater New York City), in California, and in Texas (United States Census Bureau, Decennial Census, 2000). A network of social, cultural, and professional associations has emerged to serve this population and a number of national conferences are sponsored to solidify communication and collaboration among Moroccan American institutions. Like their Egyptian neighbors, Moroccans in the United States tend to visit their homeland frequently, maintain close ties with extended families, and according to a survey of expatriates (Association of Moroccan Professionals in America, 2005), fully two thirds reported their desire to retire in Morocco.

Among the remaining countries of North Africa, known in Arabic as *al-Maghreb*, Tunisia and Libya have relatively small numbers of immigrants who have chosen to settle in America. Immigrants from these less populous countries tend to have a connection to the United States through study, professional training, or diplomatic service. According to data collected on the foreign-born population, persons of Tunisian and Libyan origin are likely to be concentrated in the same major metropolitan areas as other Arab immigrants (United States Census Bureau, Decennial Census, 2000).

Gulf States: Like parts of North Africa, the Arabian Peninsula has experienced less emigration to the United States. The number of Americans with origins in the Gulf States, with the exception of Yemen, is relatively small. While the foreign student population from Saudi Arabia, Kuwait, and the United Arab Emirates continues to grow, these students tend to return home both to remain with their families and fulfill the terms of their scholarships to study in America.

Unlike its Gulf neighbors, Yemen has a considerable portion of its population living and working in the United States. Yemeni immigration to America began as early as the nineteenth century when young men from the port city of Aden, under British control, worked on ships and made their way to the United States where they found factory jobs in cities like Buffalo and Detroit, or as workers in the farmlands of California (Bisharat, 1975). Yemeni migration to the United States has been predominantly from the rural areas, transient and economically driven, with males living in group quarters to send remittances back to families in Yemen, where land ownership and social relationships were kept intact (Abraham, 1983). Yemeni chain migration was facilitated by a network of agents who facilitated passage to the United States, paperwork, loans, and remittance transmissions to Yemen. While some migrants brought wives to America, raised children here and became citizens, the majority of Yemenis in America have retained close ties to their extended families, with frequent visits to keep their children connected to their ancestral culture. The challenges for immigrant families to reconcile the aspirations of their American-born children, especially girls, with the traditional cultural expectations of Yemeni-born parents are exposed and explored by Sarrouf (2005) who helps shed light on the experience and frustrations of this second generation.

The sheer number of Yemenis living in America, with concentrations in upstate New York, Michigan, and California, has encouraged the creation of ethnic organizations to serve the needs of the immigrants and their families. Institutions include expatriate political organizations reflecting partisan affiliations inside Yemen, benevolent associations to offer charity to needy families and to causes in Yemen, and most recently civic institutions like the Yemeni-American Political Action Committee, based in Hamtramck, Michigan, and led mostly by US-born children of Yemeni migrants, which promotes voter engagement and other civic integration practices.

Other Arab Africans: The majority of immigrants from Arabic-speaking countries in Africa outside the Maghreb, especially Somalia and Sudan, are in America seeking refuge and political asylum from civil conflict at home. Somalis began coming to the United States in the 1980s but peaked in 2004–2006 when at least 35,000 refugees were admitted to the United States (Office of Refugee Resettlement, 2009). With the assistance of federal refugee resettlement programs, Somalis laid down roots in a number of states including Minnesota, where nearly one third of the population currently resides, Ohio, New York, Washington state, and Maryland. A number of social service and economic organizations have emerged to cater to this population, particularly in the mother colony of Minneapolis/St. Paul where Somali American activists work closely with other community advocates and local government to mediate the cultural integration, employment, and other economic needs of the community. Recent comparative studies point to the barriers that the double minority identities of Black race and Muslim religion create for Somalis as they negotiate their status in a White majority culture (Ajrouch & Kusow, 2007).

In smaller numbers, refugees from southern Sudan have taken root in the United States, with a significant number of children displaced by the civil conflict, victims of extreme poverty and often abuse. In 2001, 3,800 "Lost Boys of Sudan" were settled in American cities, a resettlement program that peaked in 2004 and resulted in Sudanese communities emerging in Omaha, New York, Des Moines, Alexandria, VA and San Diego, CA (United States Department of Health and Human Services/ Administration for Families and Children, Office of Refugee Resettlement, Refugee Arrival Data, 2002–2009). By the 2011 referendum on independence for Southern Sudan, it is estimated that up to 50,000 Sudanese citizens, migrants, or refugees residing in the United States were eligible to vote remotely (Malagon, 2010).

Ethnic and Cultural Minorities from the Arab World

There are immigrants in America representing communities that have historically lived in the Arabic-speaking world, but which have maintained cultural and linguistic traditions that have kept them distinct from the Arabic-speaking majorities. The most prominent of these ethnic minorities are Chaldeans and Assyrians, who are Christian, and Kurds, who are Muslim, both of which share ancestral connection to areas of present-day Iraq, Syria, Iran, and Turkey. While Armenians are another ethnic and religious minority with ties to a number of Arab countries, particularly Lebanon, Syria, Egypt, and Palestine, the experience of Armenian immigrants in the United States is distinct and not generally studied as part of the Arab world diaspora and therefore is not covered in this chapter.

There are religious and historical roots that tie the Chaldean and Assyrian communities together, and these alliances have created institutional solidarity and ethnic cooperation in the United States. They are descendents of the Nestorian sect which in the fifth century was censured by Rome and then in the 1830s was reunited as a recognized eastern rite affiliate. The majority of Christians living in northern Iraq became Chaldean at that time and preserved the heritage and practice of their sect through the ancient Aramaic language, a version of which is spoken by Chaldeans and Assyrians and serves as the basis of their liturgy (Sengstock, 1974).

The earliest Chaldean immigrants to the United States settled in Michigan in the early decades of the twentieth century and continued into the 1960s. The majority of refugees being admitted by the United States as a direct result of sectarian violence in Iraq after the toppling of Saddam Hussein in 2003 have been Chaldeans and Assyrians, with international attention drawn dramatically to terrorist attacks on their churches and leadership.

Most Chaldeans in America live in three states: Michigan, California, and Illinois (United States Census Bureau, Decennial Census, 2000). The community estimates their population to be about 260,000, with the Detroit metropolitan area representing the oldest and largest community—"the promised land of the Chaldeans" (Oasis Center, 2009, p. 1). Chaldeans have earned a reputation for strong economic cooperation, building family businesses, facilitating economic integration of new arrivals, and endogamous marriages (Sengstock, 1974). The cornerstone of their institutional foundation is a network of churches organized into two eparchies (like archdioceses) in Michigan and California. Complementing this active religious network are business organizations and chambers of commerce, cultural institutes and, more recently, advocates for civic and political representation like the Chaldean Federation of America.

Like other immigrant groups, Chaldeans organize to teach their children Aramaic, to highlight their culture and history, and to promote cultural preservation outside their ancestral home. And like other expatriate communities with political grievances and concerns in their home countries, Chaldean and Assyrian American organizations are active members of international umbrella groups like the Assyrian Universal Alliance, which is a coalition of organizations and political parties that most recently met in Irbil, Iraq in December 2010 (Oasis, 2009). Some Assyrian religious leaders have found alliance also with Lebanese Maronites whose liturgical use of the ancient Syriac language has created common ground and also nurtured the common cause of distinctions from what they see as Muslim-majority Arab culture. In 2007, the Chaldean Assyrian Syriac Council of America (CASCA) was organized to coordinate the expatriate political and religious concerns of these communities. Some scholars have observed more willingness to accept associations with Arab identity among Chaldeans who have immigrated more recently to the United States, and collaborations between Arab and Chaldean institutions exist in the greater Detroit region where both communities are well represented (Sengstock, 2005).

The Kurdish experience in the United States is another example where exile politics and historical grievances have driven their identity as a distinct ethnic community. The first Kurds to arrive in America came in the immediate aftermath of World War I, but the biggest influx occurred in the 1990s following the failed uprising against Saddam Hussein. It is estimated that about 100,000 persons of Kurdish origin live in the United States, with the largest concentration (about 15,000) living in Tennessee (Ahmed, 2009), with other communities located in Dallas, TX, and

Southern California. But Tennessee is the undisputed mother colony, with Nashville known as "Little Kurdistan" and serving as one of five voting locations organized across the country by the State Department for Iraqi citizens to participate remotely in that country's 2005 national elections. Like the tenor and agenda of the Chaldeans and Assyrian community organizations, Kurdish institutional life in America centers on exile politics. The Kurdish National Congress in North America was founded in 1988, shortly after the massacres by Iraqi forces of civilians in Halabja. There are, however, hints of an emerging civic awareness of their domestic role as US citizens: in 2008, a group of Kurdish Democrats formed a "Kurds for Obama" presidential campaign support committee.

Religious Diversity of Arab Americans

A surprising demographic reality of the Arab American experience is that the majority of this population is affiliated with a Christian denomination, due to the disproportionate number of Christian Arabs who emigrated over a longer period of time compared with their Muslim counterparts. According to private surveys conducted among Americans of Arab descent (Arab American Institute Foundation, 2002), 63 % of Arab Americans report Christian roots (35 % Roman/Eastern rite Catholic; 18 % Eastern Orthodox rites; 10 % Protestant) with 24 % reporting as Muslims and 13 % as other or no religious affiliation. A small number of Jews from Arab countries, or Sephardim, emigrated to the United States, mostly from Morocco, Syria, Iraq, and Lebanon.

Among Arab Christians, those affiliated with the Catholic Church originate from several Eastern rite sects: Maronites predominantly come from towns and villages in present-day Lebanon and form a large core of the Lebanese-American Christian community. Melkites or Greek Catholics are also from Lebanon as well as present-day Syria and Palestine and have a liturgy closer to the Byzantine rites practiced in the Orthodox tradition. More recent immigrants from Iraq who belong to the Chaldean church are also affiliated with the Roman Catholic Church, but like their Maronite and Melkite co-religious maintain the Syriac/Aramaic language in their worship services.

Arab Christians of Orthodox traditions are another well-established religious community which is represented by the Antiochian Orthodox Christian Archdiocese of North America, the Syrian Orthodox Church, and the Coptic Orthodox which follows the rite of Alexandria, Egypt, and traces its roots to St. Mark the Evangelist. Like the Latin rite Eastern churches, Orthodox churches began being established in immigrant communities over a century ago and now number an estimated 200 (Antiochian Orthodox Christian Archdiocese of North America, 2010). Arab Orthodox communities were at times affiliated with the larger Russian and Greek Orthodox patriarchies in the United States, but those in large Arab population centers—like New York, New Jersey, the New England states, Michigan, Ohio, Pennsylvania, Florida, Texas and California—have kept their Arab ethnic character and membership. Eastern rite churches founded by the first wave of Syrian and Lebanese immigrants before and after the First World War found new congregants among the Arab Christians who immigrated in the second wave, especially Palestinian families from Ramallah and other Christian towns and villages in the West Bank.

The churches and affiliated social clubs and charities founded by the Arab Christians became a lifeline to their heritage and culture and in many ways served as their primary ethnic identity in America. As will be explored later, the experience of the first wave of mostly Christian immigrants was dominated by allegiance to their extended family, to their sectarian denomination, and to their village or town of origin. The strength of their sectarian affinity is largely due to the practice of Ottoman rule over the subjects in their empire which designated minority communities to be administered by a magisterial system run by clerics of each recognized religious denomination. In the Ottoman *millet* framework, each denomination was "organized into a nationality" (Kayal, 1974, p. 120). This church-based culture for Arab Christians was intensified by how their civic obligations and rights differed from those affecting the majority Muslim population, and that sense of separateness, if not discrimination, accompanied them to their new life in the United States.

Arab Christian immigrants who affiliated with the Uniate churches, or those affiliated with Rome, were often the fastest to assimilate into the "Latinized" culture of American Catholicism. According to Kayal, the material and social appeal of Latin Christianity overwhelmed the immigrant Maronite and Melkite infrastructure, which was lacking the priests and seminaries needed to serve their congregations which were already dispersed broadly across the country and rapidly achieving economic success and American middle class values (Kayal, 1974). Among Arab Christians, assimilation has been most prominently accelerated by high rates of intermarriage with non-Arab Christians. By the 1980s, with the grandchildren of the first wave immigrants fully come of age, the estimate of exogamy among Arab Christians was as high as 80 % (Kayal, 1974).

The Eastern rite churches remain, however, important cultural lifelines for Arab Christian families, especially those in major metropolitan areas which benefit from the infusion of new immigrants into their memberships. Most Eastern liturgies have adapted to English to accommodate the native-born members and even non-Arab converts, but the churches and related activities provide a forum for social interaction and ethnic preservation, as the locus for wedding celebrations, youth clubs, Arabic classes, community picnics and *haflaat* (parties), wakes, and charitable events. Eastern religious traditions, such as elaborate Palm Sunday processions, Lenten fasts, celebrating Easter according to the Gregorian calendar, memorial masses after 40 days of mourning, wedding ceremonies, and the celebration of Christmas on the Feast of the Epiphany, are still followed and serve to preserve and perpetuate important links to these ancestral churches and associated ethnic relationships.

For the majority Muslim populations of the Arab world, immigration to the United States was less attractive or facilitated than for their Christian counterparts. It is estimated that no more than 10 % of the first wave of Arab immigrants were

Muslims, and most of these arrived from the Ottoman provinces of Greater Syria. Unlike for the Arab Christian immigrants of that pioneer generation who were eager to relocate to a predominantly Christian country, Muslim Arabs who came to the United States in the early 1900s were seeking economic relief only and not permanent displacement (Haddad, 1983). Those Muslims who did emigrate early gravitated to the Midwest cities where auto and other industrial jobs were available. The first mosque in the United States was established in Cedar Rapids Iowa in 1934.

Rapid economic and political transformations during the postcolonial period in the Arab world coupled with new, open US immigration policies in the 1960s created a larger wave of Arab Muslims seeking opportunity in America. A number of middle and upper class families escaping nationalization policies in Egypt, Syria, and Iraq, for example, chose to relocate in Europe and the United States. Arab nationals from across the newly independent states of the Middle East and North Africa were attracted to the United States to pursue their higher education and professional careers. It is estimated that in the decade prior to 1967 alone, over 50,000 Arab Muslim intellectuals and professionals entered the United States (Haddad, 1983). While Christian Arabs continued to emigrate to the United States in this second major wave, Muslims from Yemen, Egypt, Iraq, south Lebanon, Palestine, Jordan, Syria, and more recently Morocco and Somalia have dominated the demographics of new immigration and helped to diversify the religious makeup of the Arab American experience.

There are a number of factors that shape the acculturation and integration of Arab Muslims in America and the institutions they have built here to preserve their religious traditions and social cohesion. While Arab Christians may have encountered some difficulty in being fully accepted by the host society, their Christian affiliations and high rates of marriage outside the ethnic community helped to speed up their assimilation across the generations. For Muslim Arab immigrants, especially those who practiced their faith, America was largely unfamiliar with and culturally prejudicial against Islam, which for most of the twentieth century remained in the popular American imagination a symbol of otherness and exoticism, if not barbarism and oppression (Samhan, 1987). This negative predisposition was of course exacerbated by the political discourse since mid-century surrounding the Arab-Israeli conflict, the Cold War alliances between some Arab states and the Soviet Union, and the oil embargo of the 1970s, which spawned an image of Arabs and Muslims as anti-American, anti-Semitic, and ultimately dangerous. It is noteworthy that charges of anti-Semitism against Arabs of any religion have been particularly jarring since Arabs and Jews share a Semitic historical and linguistic heritage. It was into this challenging political and cultural environment that Muslim immigrants were left to navigate their identity and acceptance as new Americans, without sacrificing their strong affinity to their Arab culture and Muslim religious traditions.

Efforts to organize Muslim institutions to facilitate this acculturation challenge began in the 1950s when the Cedar Rapids community took the lead in convincing the United States Army to recognize and accommodate the needs of Muslims in military service. By the 1960s organizing goals expanded to the needs of Muslim students (the Muslim Student Association was founded in 1963), and the 1970s witnessed a surge in national consolidation through bodies like the Federation of Islamic Associations and the first convening in 1977 of the Islamic Conference of North America when the goals of the Muslim leadership expanded to focus on producing and discussing Islamic knowledge (Haddad, 1983). In the 1980s and 1990s, Arab Muslim organizing grew even further to encompass the civil rights, civic integration and legal advocacy needs of Muslims living in the United States.

It is the impressive network of mosques, Islamic cultural centers, and schools that has emerged in the past 2 decades that serves as the primary ethnic lifeline for Arab American Muslims today. Haddad observes that the role of the American mosque is much closer to that of a Western church than to mosques in the Arab world; the US mosque is the locus for weddings, funerals, charitable events, religious instruction, Arabic classes, and cultural celebrations. Likewise, the function of the Imam has been transformed from a prayer leader to that of an administrator, program manager, family counselor, spokesperson, and representative at interfaith events (Haddad, 1983).

While intra-Muslim distinctions are less emphasized than among Eastern Christian denominations, Arab Americans reflect the religious demographics of Islam in their home societies. The majority of Arab Muslims in the United States are Sunni, the dominant strain of Islam which reflects the historic acceptance of the Prophet Mohammed's successors in the seventh century as Abu Bakr, the Prophet's close friend and early believer. Shi'a Muslims are those who believe the rightful successors to the Prophet were his son-in-law Ali and grandson Hussein. Many aspects of Islamic practice and tradition are common to both sects, with Shi'a interpretation more dependent on rituals and on direct religious instruction than Sunni in general. Arab American Muslims who follow the Shi'a tradition include those who migrated from South Lebanon where they constitute Lebanon's fastest growing population group and were directly impacted by the Israeli incursions into Lebanon since the early 1980s, prompting considerable chain migration to places like Michigan in search of refuge and economic opportunity. Another sizable community of Shi'a left Southern Iraq as of the early 1990s following a failed rebellion against Saddam Hussein and to escape discriminatory treatment by that regime.

Iraqi Shi'a are more isolated in the United States than those from Lebanon, although they often worship at the same mosques. Institutions and leadership of Shi'a immigrants tend to reflect closely the ideological and political struggles of their home societies, whereas Sunni organizing seems to have a broader focus on scholarship, outreach, and religious accommodations in the United States (Walbridge, 1999). Another branch of Islam represented in the United States are the Druze, who descend from an eleventh century reform movement and follow the five pillars of Islam but also adhere to additional commandments and moral obligations (Ameri & Ramey, 1999). Druze immigrants are mostly from Lebanon and Syria and began coming to the United States before World War I.

The basic tenets of the faith practiced by most Arab Muslims form the core of their religious observances in America. While the level of religious adherence varies broadly, Muslim practice can include daily prayer and ablution (at five proscribed times), communal prayer on Fridays, dietary restrictions against pork, alcohol, lard, and non-*Halal* meat, modest dress codes for women (loose fitting clothing and covering the hair), and for some men, beards and prayer caps. In very observant families, social interaction between the sexes, including sports, dating, or unsupervised events, is avoided. Many Muslims observe the sunrise to sunset fast during the holy month of Ramadan and celebrate two main feast days: *Eid al Fitr* which marks the end of Ramadan, and *Eid al Adha* which observes the end of the annual *Hajj*, the pilgrimage to Mecca where Muslims renew their dedication as a community (*umma*) to worship God. These feasts are occasions for festive meals, visits among family and friends, gifts for children, and services at the mosque.

The fact that Arab Muslims make up only one fifth of the world's Muslim population, and the same proportion of the American Muslim population, has not prevented a stubborn conflation that "Arab = Muslim" in American popular culture, in political discourse, and even in the media. As will be discussed in the last section of this chapter, this conflation has been amplified in the period following the 9/11 attacks, but has been constructed over decades of political rhetoric that has associated Islam as a faith system of believers with the headline-grabbing terror attacks by violent extremists. This rapidly expanding association in public discourse of Muslims with suspicion of terrorist connections has deeply affected how Arab American Muslims feel about their sense of belonging or security in this country.

The Politics and Demographics of Identity

How Americans of Arab origin identify their ethnicity has been impacted by a variety of cultural and political factors both in the ancestral and host countries, and, like many ethnic realities, has changed over time. When the mostly Christian immigrants from Ottoman-ruled Syria arrived in the United States, they were unfamiliar with the concepts of nationalism or even citizenship, so they tended to accept readily the ideals of American civic identity. They held strong attachments to their cultural, religious, and village traditions and adopted a "Syrian" identity as the collective term easiest to self-describe in the American context (Kayal, 1974). These early immigrants may have referred to each other privately as *awlad Arab* (children of Arabs), but in no way did they identify as "Arabs" which in their mind, according to Kayal, meant Moslem and hence oppressor (1974).

The onset of French mandatory rule over greater Syria after World War I and the creation of borders delineating an independent Lebanon in the 1920s caused a new identity controversy among immigrants in the United States from this region, especially Maronites who began to form Phoenician clubs to distinguish themselves from Arab Syria and the larger Muslim world (Naff, 1994) and to insert Lebanese into existing institutional names. Regional federations of local Syrian and Lebanese American Clubs (SLAC) were formed in the 1930s, some of which remain active today, and when Lebanese-American Danny Thomas founded St. Jude Children's Research Hospital in Memphis in the 1960s, it was and remains funded by the

Associated Lebanese and Syrian American Charities (ALSAC). The churches and their national institutions continued to impart a strong sectarian identity on the children of the pioneer immigrant wave as they expanded and adapted to the needs of the assimilated, American-born generation.

Major events of the 1960s ushered in a new era of Arab immigration, the ideology of secular Arab nationalism, the Arab-Israeli war of 1967, and the civil rights movement in the United States—all of which had a direct impact on the way Arab Americans viewed themselves and projected their ethnic concerns publicly. American-born Arabs witnessed not only a new influx of educated, politicized, Arab immigrants who helped form new institutions, but experienced with them the anti-Arab prejudice that the 1967 war engendered in US popular and political culture (Kayal, 1983). The concepts of pan-Arabism, and particularly the injustice experienced by Palestinians after 1967, empowered a new generation of organizations, many with roots on US university campuses, which in turn helped foster Arab American as an accepted and purposeful identity in America. Unlike the country-centric identities of earlier institutions, Arab American as a designation "provided common ground as well as a common bond that made their national, religious and cultural differences seem anachronistic in the modern world" (Haddad, 1994, p. 8).

Organizing across many countries of origin was also a necessity in order to be heard in the crowded field of American ethnic politics. Arab American institutions that were founded in the 1970s and 1980s recognized the successful models of other ethnic communities in presenting political or policy positions, like US Jews, or in unifying around common cultural or regional bonds, like ethnic umbrella organizations created by US Latino and Asian communities. The Arab American identity was cultivated through the creation of these ethnic institutions that developed missions that addressed the needs and interests of their constituents—from anti-defamation and civil rights protections to political empowerment, social services, and professional associations—and could caste a wide net across the generations and geography of Arab America.

Just as there remains a vibrant network of country-based institutions alongside pan Arab ones, the ethnic identity of Americans of Arab origin can be strongly rooted in their ancestral homeland. Many Arab Americans have coexisting identities: their countries of origin may influence their choices in travel, social interaction, marriage choices, or where they worship, yet their civic, cultural, and political ethnic involvement may be Arab in focus. Surveys conducted by the US Census indicate that roughly one in six persons of Arab ancestry chooses Arab/Arabic as their primary ethnic identity. In more nuanced survey research, roughly two thirds of respondents to a national telephone opinion survey reported that they describe themselves as Arab American alone or alongside their country of origin. One-fifth reported self-description by only country of origin, and one-fifth by no ethnic identifier. Of this last cohort, respondents who are US-born, Christian, and older are most likely to eschew ethnic identifiers. Muslims, foreign-born, and youth are more heavily represented in those with strong ethnic identification (Arab American Institute Foundation, 2010). Another factor in ethnic identity formation is affiliation with White race classification, which Ajrouch and Jamal found to differ by religious affiliation, nativity, and country of origin (Ajrouch & Jamal, 2007).

Intra-Ethnic Diversity and Identity After 9/11

More than a decade has passed since the tragic events of September 11, 2001, but its impact on how Americans of Arab heritage relate to both their American and ethnic identities remains decisive. Prior to 9/11 one could observe a pattern that shaped each major immigrant wave's attitude towards Americanization. According to Haddad, the early, mostly Christian Arab immigrants were "eager to belong and in the process interpreted American culture as compatible with Arab concepts of virtue and honor" (Haddad, 2002, p. 116). For the largely Muslim, politicized post-World War II immigrants, their process of Americanization has been "impeded by a profound feeling of an American double standard that dismisses Arab sentiments and rights" and they are more likely to feel they are surviving in a hostile environment (Haddad, 2002, p. 116).

After 9/11, ethnic leaders spent considerable time making the case for compatibility of Arab/Muslim values with American ones in reaction to the scrutiny and suspicion levied against their community, where Arab ethnicity and Muslim affiliation became politicized in public discourse and questioned culturally at the American grassroots. In the immediate wake of the attacks, some permanent residents strengthened their civic attachments by applying for US citizenship, a step seen as "protection" against new detention and/or deportation policies. When federal agencies began to recruit Arabic-speakers as linguists and analysts in the 9 counter-terrorism efforts, immigrants were more likely to set aside their historical mistrust of these agencies for the "greater good" of helping their country through a crisis. In one response to the public aspersions on the patriotism or loyalty of the Arab community, the Association of Patriotic Arab Americans in the Military (APAAM) was founded by a Yemeni-American Marine to underscore present and historic contributions of Arab Americans enlisted in the armed forces. And attention by ethnic organizations to civic integration, voter registration, and "know your rights" meetings intensified in the post-9/11 period as a way to bolster the civic participation of Arab immigrants and protect their rights.

If there were measurable shifts in immigrant attitudes about American civic identity after 9/11, there were equally pronounced developments in how ethnic subgroups associated with Arab American efforts and identification. There is evidence that organizing as Arab Americans has expanded in the past decade: a National Network for Arab American Communities was set up in 2004 to support and increase the capacity of the growing number of local social service and cultural agencies that cater to Arab immigrants. There are, however, competing trends where religious affiliation may increasingly conflict with—or trump—secular Arab ethnicity.

The sensitivities of certain subgroups (e.g., Assyrians, Maronites, Copts) about their distinct identities and resistance to being aggregated with Arab American efforts have deep roots, but the unprecedented exposure to Arab and Muslim Americans in the wake of the 9/11 tragedy has sharpened these distinctions and taken them public, well beyond the boundaries of intra-ethnic discourse. Examples immediately preceding 9/11 include the request by advocates of Assyrian and Maronite identities to create a "Syriac" category in the US census and to discourage government officials from attending Arab American events. Since 9/11, the Arab American Institute (AAI) was challenged on its reports that include Christian minorities in overall statistics on Arab Americans. The Assyrian International News Agency initiated in 2002 an online campaign against AAI's demographics with the simple but forceful message "Assyrians are not Arabs!"

On the other end of the ethnic religious spectrum, the post 9/11 conflation of Arab and Muslim identities and the rapid growth of activist Muslim organizations with broader agendas have led not only to confusion in the media and within government agencies, but to pressures on Arab Muslims in America to identify as Muslims "first." The sheer weight of anti-Muslim rhetoric and Islamophobia that permeate current media, political, and even academic discourse itself is an incentive for some secular Arab Muslims to embrace their Islamic roots. It can be seen as a gesture of political defiance and self-respect, where their identity as Muslims confirms their stance against racism and western hegemony. And the fact that Islam is a universal religion offers Muslim Arabs the automatic solidarity of non-Arab co-religious in their political and cultural efforts.

Methodology: A Career Perspective on Identifying Arab Americans in the US Census

A particular challenge for researchers and practitioners serving Arab American populations is the lack of consistent and comparable data from government sources. Because persons from the Middle East and North Africa are considered "Caucasian" by federal standards defining race and ethnicity, there are few demographic sources to distinguish Arab Americans from the majority White population of European descent. The US Census question on "ancestry" since 1980 has provided limited demographic profiles on populations of Arab descent.

Attention by national organizations, most notably the Arab American Institute (AAI), to Census policies, data collection, and analysis began in earnest in the mid-1980s, and since the 1990s the Decennial Census Advisory Committee which provides advice, feedback, and expertise to the Census Bureau staff has included an Arab American representative. National bilingual outreach campaigns to inform Arab Americans about the importance and confidentiality of Census responses were launched by AAI in 1990 and each decade since. Advocacy efforts at the national level resulted in the inclusion of Arabic language paid media advertising in the communication budgets of the 2000 and 2010 Censuses and a national profile on "Americans of Arab Ancestry," a rare initiative on a nonminority population group, was published by the Census Bureau in 2004 based on data from the 2000 Census responses. What are strengths and shortcomings of this approach?

Among the strengths of data derived from the US Census question on Ancestry is that they are considered "official" in that they are collected by the US government, they allow for some longitudinal analysis (at least since 1980) and, unlike earlier Census questions on "birthplace of parents," ancestry data are multi-generational and measure up to two ancestries per respondent, thereby accounting in part for intra-ethnic marriages and their offspring. Another benefit of Census ancestry data is that they are available to the public on both large and small geographies, allowing agencies, service, and civic organizations the information they need to study educational, language achievement, income, and employment trends even at the local level. And the ancestry question is open-ended, allowing respondents to choose their own primary identities.

Census ancestry data are not without shortcomings. One challenge is that ancestry measurement is not treated like race or Hispanic origin: it appears only on sample surveys (not the basic form that is sent to all households in the United States) and may be considered by respondents as "optional." Unlike race and Hispanic origin, missing ancestry is not imputed, even within households. And nonresponse in the Arab American population can be more acute at both ends of the immigration/assimilation spectrum: recent immigrants with limited English proficiency may misunderstand the importance of the Census itself, or be wary of providing personal information to the government, and the descendents of the first wave of Arab immigrants often have several competing ancestries, and the form only allows 2. The Census Bureau also defines Arab more narrowly when it publishes ancestry data, excluding Arabic-speaking countries bordering North Africa like Sudan, Somalia, Mauritania, etc.

In spite of these shortcomings, the Census ancestry question is still a valuable tool for research on Arab integration, acculturation, and socio-economic mobility. While some advocates have recommended an "Arab American" ethnic category for US Census forms, it runs the risk of alienating the many religious and ethnic minorities from Arabic-speaking countries who do not identify primarily as "Arabs" yet who share many common experiences, social, and service needs with other Arab Americans. A more inclusive and flexible solution to measuring ethnicity of people who originate in the Middle East and North Africa is to change short-form Census to include a 3-part question on race, Hispanic origin, and ancestry, thereby allowing for self-identification in the place that makes most sense. Currently the Census Bureau is studying the extent to which people of Middle Eastern and North African (MENA) ancestries chose not to identify solely as "Caucasian" in the 2010 Census, but wrote in their ancestry as "Some Other Race." This conflation and confusion of racial and ethnic identities among MENA ancestries is attracting more attention at the federal level and is currently the subject of internal research at the Census Bureau.

Implications for Practice, Research, and Policy

Perhaps the greatest challenge to practitioners serving clients from Arabic-speaking countries is to avoid the cultural and political assumptions most Americans have formed about people from this region. The experiences that shape identity and feelings of acceptance among Arab Americans vary widely based on generational, historical, religious, and geographic factors. Understanding the complexities of how homeland politics, US policy, cultural stereotypes held by Americans and intra-group relations affect individuals and families profoundly but also differently is an important ingredient to culturally competent care.

Recognizing the diversity and nuances of the Arab immigrant experience is equally important in the formulation of policies that impact the welfare of this population and its future integration into American society. One size fits all strategies are rarely effective in addressing the needs of immigrants or refugees from distinct political, religious, educational, and religious backgrounds. The persistence of conflict and instability in the region will shape the attitudes and apprehensions of immigrant families who live here. Recent events affecting Christian minorities in Iraq and Egypt, for example, where churches and clergy have been attacked, will no doubt renew the sense of fear and vulnerability among Arab Christian immigrants from those communities. Arab Muslims continue to bear the brunt of political posturing where American Muslims are portrayed as a threat to national security and the object of suspicion and surveillance. Political instability anywhere in the Arab world will influence the way immigrants from those countries negotiate their status in America, at times provoking fear and isolation among subgroups, at times promoting solidarity and communication across national origin and even religious boundaries.

Intra-group diversity, the dynamics of identity, and why subgroups resist or embrace integration into American society are among the many topics that merit future research. A number of research tools, including public data sources from the US Census Bureau and private opinion research, like that sponsored by the Arab American Institute Foundation, merit closer attention in the tracking of ethnic identity and assimilation, recognizing that such tools are limited in addressing nuances among generations and within subgroups. The prevalence or dominance of religious identities among Arab Christians and Muslims deserves special attention, to track how sectarian affiliations may become substitutes for secular, pan Arab American identities and relationships. An important focus of future research should be to track the attitudes and ethnic habits of US-born children of the post-1960 cohorts of Arab immigrants. It will be useful to explore how this generation is coping with emotional and political ties to their parents' homeland, if they are breaking through sectarian and national origin boundaries in their ethnic behavior, and how strong is ethnicity among this generation as they consolidate political, social, economic, and family aspirations.

References

Abraham, N. (1983). The Yemeni immigrant community in Detroit: Background, emigration and community life. In S. Y. Abraham & N. Abraham (Eds.), *Arabs in the new world: Studies on Arab-American communities* (pp. 109–134). Detroit, MI: Wayne State University.

Ahmed, A. K. (2009, February 9). *Kurds in Nashville*. Retrieved from http://journeyintoamerica.wordpress.com/2009/02/09/kurds-in-nashville/

Ajrouch, K. J., & Jamal, A. (2007). Assimilating to a white identity: The case of Arab Americans. *International Migration Review, 41*(4), 860–880.

Ajrouch, K. J., & Kusow, A. (2007). Racial and religious contexts: Situational identities among Lebanese and Somali Muslim immigrants. *Ethnic and Racial Studies, 30*(1), 72–94.

Ameri, A., & Ramey, D. (Eds.). (1999). *Arab American encyclopedia*. Detroit, MI: The Gale Group.

Antiochian Orthodox Christian Archdiocese of North America. (2010). Retrieved from http://www.antiochian.org/about

Arab American Institute Foundation. (2002). *Religious affiliations of Arab Americans*. Retrieved from http://www.aaiusa.org/demographics

Arab American Institute Foundation. (2010). *Arab American voters in 2010: Their identity and attitudes towards Obama and the mid-terms*. Washington, DC: Arab American Institute.

Association of Moroccan Professionals in America. (2005, June). *Jaridati*. Retrieved from http://www.amp-usa.org

Bisharat, M. (1975). Yemeni migrant workers in California. In B. Abu-Laban & F. T. Zeady (Eds.), *Arabs in America: Myths and realities* (pp. 202–209). Wilmette, ILL: The Medina University Press International.

Erikson, E. (1985). *Childhood and society*. New York: W.W. Norton and Company.

Gordon, M. (1964). *Assimilation in American life: The role of race, religion, and national origins*. New York: Oxford University Press.

Haddad, Y. (1983). Arab Muslims and Islamic institutions in America: Adaptation and reform. In S. Y. Abraham & N. Abraham (Eds.), *Arabs in the new world: Studies on Arab-American communities* (pp. 64–83). Detroit, MI: Wayne State University.

Haddad, Y. (1994). Maintaining the faith of the fathers: Dilemmas of religious identity in the Christian and Muslim Arab American communities. In E. McCarus (Ed.), *The development of Arab-American identity* (pp. 61–84). Ann Arbor, MI: The University of Michigan Press.

Haddad, Y. (2002). Inventing and re-inventing the Arab American identity. In K. Benson & P. M. Kayal (Eds.), *A community of many worlds: Arab Americans in New York City* (pp. 109–123). New York, NY: Museum of the City of New York/Syracuse University Press.

Hourani, A. H. (1947). *Minorities in the Arab world*. London: Oxford University Press.

Kayal, P. M. (1974). Religion in the Christian "Syrian-American" community. In B. C. Aswad (Ed.), *Arabic-speaking communities in American cities* (pp. 111–136). New York, NY: The Center for Migration Studies.

Kayal, P. M. (1983). Arab Christians in the United States. In S. Y. Abraham & N. Abraham (Eds.), *Arabs in the new world: Studies on Arab-American communities* (pp. 44–63). Detroit, MI: Wayne State University.

Kayyali, R. A. (2006). *The Arab Americans*. Westport, CT: Greenwood Press.

Keck, L. T. (1989). Egyptian Americans in the Washington, DC area. In B. Abu-Laban & M. W. Suleiman (Eds.), *Arab Americans: Continuity and change* (pp. 103–126). Belmont, MA: The Association of Arab-American University Graduates.

Malagon, E. (2010, December 16). *Sudanese in America prepare to vote in January referendum*. Retrieved from Scripps Howard Foundation Newswire, http://www.shfwire.com

McCarus, E. (Ed.). (1994). *The development of Arab-American identity*. Ann Arbor, MI: The University of Michigan Press.

Naff, A. (1994). The early Arab immigrant experience. In E. McCarus (Ed.), *The development of Arab-American identity* (pp. 23–35). Ann Arbor, MI: The University of Michigan Press.

Oasis Center. (2009, April 19). *That corner of Iraq in Detroit*. Retrieved from http://www.oasiscenter.ebl
Park, R. E., & Burgess, E. W. (1921). *Introduction to the science of sociology*. Chicago, IL: University of Chicago Press.
Portes, A., & Zhou, M. (1993). The new second generation: Segmented assimilation and its variants. *The Annals of the American Academy of Political and Social Science, 530*, 74–96.
Samhan, H. H. (1987). Politics and exclusion: The Arab American experience. *Journal of Palestine Studies, 16*(2), 11–28.
Samhan, H. H. (1999). Not quite white: Race classification and the Arab-American experience. In M. W. Suleiman (Ed.), *Arabs in America: Building a new future* (pp. 209–226). Philadelphia, PA: Temple University Press.
Sarrouf, L. K. (2005). *All American Yemeni girls: Being Muslim in a public school*. Philadelphia, PA: University of Pennsylvania Press.
Sengstock, M. C. (1974). Iraqi Christians in Detroit: An analysis of ethnic occupation. In B. C. Aswad (Ed.), *Arabic-speaking communities in American cities* (pp. 21–38). New York, NY: The Center for Migration Studies.
Sengstock, M. C. (2005). *Chaldeans in Detroit*. East Lansing, MI: Michigan State University Press.
Stryker, S. (1980). *Symbolic interactionism: A social structural version*. Menlo Park, CA: Benjamin/Cummings Publishers.
Suleiman, M. W. (1999). Introduction: The Arab American experience. In M. W. Suleiman (Ed.), *Arabs in America: Building a new future* (pp. 1–21). Philadelphia, PA: Temple University Press.
United States Census Bureau, Decennial Census. (2000). Retrieved from http://factfinder.census.gov/home/saff/main.html?_lang=en
United States Department of Health and Human Services/Administration for Families and Children, Office of Refugee Resettlement, Refugee Arrival Data. (2002–2009). Retrieved from http://www.acf.hhs.gov/programs/orr/data/refugee_arrival_data.htm
Walbridge, L. S. (1999). A look at differing ideologies among Shi'a Muslims in the United States. In M. W. Suleiman (Ed.), *Arabs in America: Building a new future* (pp. 53–65). Philadelphia, PA: Temple University Press.

Chapter 4
Family Values and Traditions

Ben K. Beitin and Mireille Aprahamian

Introduction

Family values and traditions are central organizing parts of Arab culture. Family relationships have been well established as defining connections for Arab individuals (Barakat, 1993; Haj-Yahia, 2000; Joseph, 1999). Values and traditions are important, especially for immigrants, as sometimes they serve as the only connection between the immigrant and his/her country and culture of origin. Maintaining meaningful aspects of culture provides feelings of safety and connectedness to others (Lijtmaer, 2001). A sense of cultural loss may result in feelings of denial of or clinging excessively to one's culture of origin. Such potential outcomes underscore the need to help people remain connected to their culture. Identifying family values prevalent in the Arab world and their evolvement over time provide an important context for a better understanding of Arab American family patterns.

Families living in the United States who identify with Arab descent are diverse in many ways, such as religion, gender, country of origin, immigration narrative, generation, acculturation, and family structure. Immigration to the United States began during the late nineteenth century and early twentieth century. Arab families came predominantly from areas of Lebanon in what was then named the Syrian Province of the Ottoman Empire, and were predominantly Christian (Aswad, 1997). After World War II, families traveled from more areas of the Arab World such as Iraq, Egypt, and Yemen. They brought strong educational backgrounds. As the

B.K. Beitin, Ph.D. (✉)
Seton Hall University, 312 Jubilee Hall, 400 South Orange Avenue,
South Orange, NJ 07079, USA
e-mail: ben.beitin@shu.edu

M. Aprahamian, Ed.D.
Counseling and Human Services, Johns Hopkins University, MCC, A&R Building,
9601 Medical Center Drive, Rockville, MD 20850, USA
e-mail: mapraham@gmu.edu

S.C. Nassar-McMillan et al. (eds.), *Biopsychosocial Perspectives on Arab Americans: Culture, Development, and Health*, DOI 10.1007/978-1-4614-8238-3_4,

twentieth century progressed, Muslim families grew in number. Early families created communities which later waves of immigrant families often joined. Though successful in creating large communities, many families also dispersed geographically upon arrival. Early in their immigration history, members of Arab families had difficulty finding employment but ultimately found success as entrepreneurs and businesspeople. As of 2009, Arab American families showed prominent presence at both the high and low ends of the socioeconomic ladder. While 27 % reported a higher average salary than the national average, 13.7 % lived below the poverty line (Arab American Institute Foundation, 2011).

This chapter will present nuances and complexities of Arab American families whenever possible, recognizing the diversity of Arab Americans, but also drawing from the notion of an overarching Arab culture. When writing about a group of people, writers often risk making inappropriate generalizations and stereotyping. As such, this chapter begins with a presentation of the historical background of Arab American families, identifying terminology often used when referencing the Arab American family experience. A presentation of theoretical constructs follows, with a focus on acculturation, collectivism, patrilineality, violence, and resilience. These broad frameworks facilitate understanding key aspects of Arab American families. Finally, methodological approaches will be considered, as well as implications and recommendations for policymakers and professionals working with Arab Americans families.

Historical Background

Family Terminology

Definitions of family change as rapidly as family structures and demographic trends. In the middle of the twentieth century, Western researchers equated the concept of family with nuclear structures and constructed family as two or more people who shared a household and were connected by birth or marriage (Burgess & Locke, 1945). Some theorists added economic and reproductive functions to the definition. As family composition changes, the definition is more accurately reflected by "two or more persons related by birth, marriage, adoption, or choice … by socioemotional ties and enduring responsibilities, particularly in terms of one or more members' dependence on others for support and nurturance" (Allen, Fine, & Demo, 2000, p. 1). This recent definition of families in Western literature is more relevant for Arab families than definition by structure because it is congruent with Arab values of collectivism, patrilineality, and relational development. Large, extended, patrilineal, clearly delineated expectations of gender roles, religion, parenting, socialization of children, and marital dynamics are family values commonly identified in the literature specific to Arabs in the Middle East and North Africa (Beitin, Allen, & Bekheet, 2010). Identifying family values in Arab culture provides context for Arab American family patterns.

The word "family" does not permit a full understanding of the complexity surrounding Arab family dynamics. The term kinship provides a more meaningful way to describe Arab family values. Kinship represents ideas of an extended family that provide connection, security, and identity for Arab men and women. For instance, marriage represents more than a union of two people; it ensures a union between two families and connections among many people. Abraham and Shryock (2000) wrote:

> The strength [of Arab families] is not a by-product of family values or the idea that "kinship is important," vague notions to which Americans subscribe ... but the extent to which Arab immigrants use kinship to accomplish things and the extent to which things cannot be accomplished without resort to kinship ties (p. 574).

The complexity and multifaceted function of Arab families may be better described through a consideration of their traditionally large and extended nature.

Large and Extended

Traditional Arab families have many members who live in close proximity and depend upon each other for many reasons such as social needs, economic support, and cultural and religious maintenance (Cohen & Savaya, 2003). Obeid, Chang, and Ginges (2010) surveyed students at a university in Lebanon and reported participants having an average of four to five members in their family, with a small minority reporting extended family members living in the household. Reasons for large families are identified as due to religious beliefs, need for economic support, and a belief that there is strength in numbers (Khalifa, 1988). In 1960, an average of six members lived in a household in the Arab world. Significantly, this statistic indicates only members living in the same dwelling, and is not indicative of family size. By 2001, the childbirth rate dropped to 3.6, however, down from approximately seven in 1960. Improvements in access and quality of educational systems as well as more opportunities for women particularly have been documented over the last 4 decades (Amin & Al-Bassusi, 2004). Scholars point to these gains as key factors contributing to decreasing birthrates.

During the second half of the twentieth century, several social forces, many happening on a global level, have influenced change across the world including values and traditions practiced by Arab families. Disagreement lingers regarding the source most influential in family change. Until recently, it was thought that modernity, education, and technology were three factors that spurred change in Arab families as they grew in influence, and challenged traditional family rituals and beliefs. Family planning became a focus of government in Arab societies which previously depended on large family sizes for economic security. Women and children felt more empowered by increasing access to education, while technology led to more isolation and an increasing desire for privacy (Al-Haj, 1995).

Recent challenges to this line of thinking suggest that it was not structural components (i.e., governments), but instead, the dissemination of actual ideas that were responsible for family changes (Thornton, 2005). The influential factor was the Western value systems and associated beliefs, both of which were connected to structural changes in education and technological development. For example, women's growing desire to have equality and all its benefits was propagated through education. Whether or not changing family patterns stem from government policies or instead are lodged in ideological shifts, it is clear that families have been changing in the Arab world, from large and extended to smaller and quasi-co-residential (Ajrouch, Yount, Sibai, & Roman, 2013).

Gender Roles

Relationships in traditional Arab families are based on a patrilineal structure, which entitles males to determine descent, kinship, and title through their family lineage. The development of this social system is believed to have grown out of the desire to protect families from outside threats such as regional tribes competing for resources or foreign nations seeking domination and wealth (Tillion, 1983). Since increasing family size improved chances for survival, women held an elevated status because only they could assure the continuation of family lineage by their willingness and ability to give birth.

Patrilineality influenced and in some instances was responsible for the development of Arab family values. For example, an extended family structure ensured protection and survival of family members as well as preserved the authority and privileges held by male kin. Child development also links to the practice of patrilineality; it becomes a foundational aspect in the promulgation and continuation of family lineage. The parent–child relationships take on a specific meaning in this context. Building from a patrilineal understanding of the Arab family, Joseph (1993) addresses the role of patriarchy. She argued that patriarchy is more complex than male domination and female subjugation. She described traditional Arab patriarchal societies as hierarchical systems based on gender expressions, social connectedness, and age rather than gender alone. Using the term patriarchal connectivity, she suggested that patriarchy enables cultural and structural relations that foster self-development through connectedness in family relationships. Men and elders direct the lives of youth and women, but in a way that fosters interdependence between family members. Moreover, couples differ in their expression of gender and power from home to home. These variations are influenced by the age of women in the family as well as degree to which men express masculinity. These complexities challenge the tendency in the literature to label a whole society as patriarchal and as a result ignore the complexities and nuances of relationships in Arab families.

As found in most societies around the world, oppressive practices toward women in the name of patriarchy exist. Discussion about the influence of a patriarchal system on domestic violence, female genital mutilation, and honor killing in some

Arab societies persist. One point of agreement is that Arab societies vary in their support and enforcement of patriarchal beliefs and behaviors. Indeed, empirical research supports a connection between traditional patriarchal attitudes and violence against women (Dhaher, Mikolajeczyk, Maxwell, & Krämer, 2010; Haj-Yahia, 2011). As a point of comparison, research has not supported a relationship between Western men who endorse patriarchal attitudes and marital violence and aggression (Sugarman & Frankel, 1996). This contrast suggests that in both cultures a better understanding of patriarchal assumptions and processes is in need of attention.

The influence of patriarchy on gender roles in the Arab world extend to parent–child relations. Fronk, Huntington, and Chadwick (1999) studied Palestinian adolescents regarding family roles and discovered that the strongest predictor of gender role expectations was the employment of their mothers. Adolescents, whose mothers worked outside the home, had stronger egalitarian gender role expectations than adolescents whose mothers stayed at home. Scholars connect patriarchal structures in Arab families with the high rate and acceptance of domestic violence (Shalhoub-Kevorkian, 1997). Yet, recent challenges to traditional gender roles have been spurred largely by an increase in education of women (Moghadam, 2004).

Shalhoub-Kavorkian (1997) acknowledged great variation in sociocultural characteristics and practices across Arab cultures, including religion, history, language, and socioeconomics; however, despite these differences, she indicated that violence against women seemed to be a pervasive power dynamic that is mostly associated with gender role expectations and cultural values of women's role in society. Abuse of women is connected to a specific cultural belief that women's behavior brings honor or shame to a family. Expected behaviors include no sexual activity until marriage, caring for her husband's needs, and raising the children to follow cultural rules and norms. In addition, values of honor and shame are related to women's tolerance of violence against them. For example, women often tolerate abuse to protect family privacy and cohesion, which is a gender role expectation. Although women often increase their influence within the family as they age (Aswad, 1997; Olmsted, 2005), it is within the confines of the patriarchal bargain (Kandiyoti, 1988). In other words, a woman's power and influence in later life emanates from her role in perpetuating the patriarchal structure (Smith, 1990).

In sum, patriarchy is often a framework applied to understanding the Arab family. Though it undoubtedly permeates the experiences of many, it is not uniformly prominent and takes many forms. Additionally, patriarchy and the accompanying oppression tend to structure the lives of women all over the world. For instance, domestic violence continues to be an enormous concern for many women living in the United States, regardless of ethnicity. In other words, it is not exclusive to Arabs. Patrilineality, on the other hand, provides an insightful framework for better understanding gender roles and family relations in the Arab world. Patrilineality points to arrangements where descent, family responsibility, and personal security are guaranteed through relations to male family members, and, as such, illuminates unique attributes of the Arab family.

Couples and Marriage

The coming together of two people in a marriage is often a family affair. Decision making in Arab societies traditionally occurred with extended family involvement (Barakat, 1993). For example, couples typically meet and marry through family negotiations. If families are not drawing up the terms of the marriage, they are in close consultation with the bride and groom about major decisions. This influence is connected to family honor. The choice of marital partner is discussed by the larger community as a positive or negative reflection of one's parents and family legacy.

Values about love and marriage in Arab societies have historically been distinct from the West. For example, extended family approval, more than romantic love, often becomes the basis upon which the decision to marry is made (Lev-Wiesel & Al-Krenawi, 1999). Recent research shows the impact of modernization and globalization on family influence in marital partner selection, however. Raz and Atar (2004) surveyed young Bedouins in Israel and found a higher rate of resistance to parental intervention in the partner selection as well as a desire for romantic love. These results are congruent with reports of increasing rates of young adults, particularly women, who are marrying at a later age or not at all (United Nations, 2007). The increases are occurring at the same time as changes in social and legal reforms to women's roles and rights as well as higher levels of education in the Arab world are taking place.

Other values include the tendency to marry consanguineous. Arab marriages may occur between those who share a close ancestor, estimated at 20–50 % of the Middle East (Alwan & Modell, 1997). The reasons for this preference are many, but usually function to keep wealth in the family and preserve the family legacy. Additionally, the importance of marital satisfaction pales in comparison to the primacy given to raising children and expanding a family. In sum, marriage is traditionally practiced as part of a larger family relationship, with focus rarely on the couple dyad (Shah, 2004).

Parent and Child Relationships

Parent–child relationships in Arab society are extremely important to well-being across the life course. A child's identity is very much influenced by the parent–child relationship, and this remains the case into adulthood. For example, Joseph (1999) illustrates the intense closeness between a parent and child in the Arab family, which is achieved through interactions that communicate to the child that he/she is an extension of the parent. It is common for a mother or father to refer to the child as *mama* or *baba*. This approach, which begins at birth, communicates to the child that he/she is one and the same with his/her parent, facilitating high levels of emotional closeness that continues into adulthood.

Some characterize the parent–child relationship in Arab societies as authoritarian, interdependent, and controlled (Dwairy, 2008). Research is mixed on the effects of authoritarian parenting and punishment on Arab children. Contrary to Western literature, some scholars have reported that Arab children do not suffer in their mental health under authoritarian parenting and parental inconsistency was a stronger predictor of poor mental health (Dwairy, 2004). It is important to note that the relationship between the effects of authoritarian parenting on children's mental health is fairly complex and other compounding factors have to be accounted for in order to better understand parent–child dynamics within Arab families. Rudy and Grusec (2006) conducted a comparative study between individualistic and collectivistic families, to include Arab societies, and found that in contrast to individualistic (Western) societies, children who came from collectivistic families are not impacted negatively by authoritarian parenting. However, the study found an association between maternal negative feelings, cognition, and children's low self-esteem in both societies, indicating authoritarianism should not be used as a standalone factor in determining mental health in children.

Individuation for Arab adolescents in the Arab World is experienced differently than Arab adolescents raised in the United States. Adolescents living in the United States are expected to become individuals who enter the world as self-reliant. Arab adolescents in Arab countries grow as individuals in close relation to their families. They remain in a pattern of mutual interaction with their families throughout their lives. Hatab and Makki (1978), in their survey of Arab adolescents in Lebanon, found that a majority reported following their parents' direction regarding behavior with others, relationships, marriage, occupation, and political beliefs. This family dynamic is consistent across Arab countries. Egyptian college students generally favor "absolute submission" to parents (Al-Khawaja, 1999). When the interaction between location, gender, and connectedness was examined in Arabs living in Israel, urban adolescents were more connected than nonurban and girls felt a higher level of connectedness to their families than boys (Dwairy, 2003).

Gender affects the experience of individuation—which refers to the process of becoming an individual and having distinct characteristics from others—in traditional Arab families. Generally speaking, stricter rules apply toward females than males and they are given less choices and options (Shabib, 2001). Daughters are under more control and supervision by their parents than sons and this is often contextualized as supporting the value of protecting family honor through clearly delineated gender roles. For example, in some families, females are more likely to have stricter dating rules and dress codes applied to them than are males (Ajrouch, 2000). In addition, sons are often expected to take on the role of provider and are seen as a source of security for parents in old age, or even during the absence of an adult male figure in the family. As a result, men are allowed more flexibility to socialize given the key role they play as provider and protector of the family. Through a Western lens, high control and supervision would be expected to result in adolescent rebellion; however, Azaiza (2005) found that not only did female adolescents report a more positive attitude toward their parents they also felt more connected to them than did males. Parent–child attachment and children's positive response toward their parents are often reinforced by Arab family values of respecting elders, including parents and grandparents. Indeed, the caregiving relationship between parents and children is developmental and bidirectional. As children become adults, they expect to begin to care for their aging parents. This tradition is valued by both parents and children as parents can access more resources and support and children can repay the sacrifice of their parents (Khalaila, 2010).

The literature on living arrangements systematically shows that the number of surviving children does influence where an elderly parent resides in Arab societies (Sibai, Beydoun, & Tohme, 2009). Elderly parents with a larger number of children are less likely to live alone compared to those without children or with one to two. Parents are more likely to live with married sons compared to married daughters or unmarried children. In terms of gender, studies show it is a significant predictor of living arrangements, and that women are more likely to live alone because of longer life expectancy, widowhood, and a lower likelihood of remarriage (Tohme, Yount, Yassine, & Sibai, 2011). We turn next to a presentation of theoretical constructs that provide insight into the growing literature that investigates the area of Arab American families.

Theoretical Constructs

Several theoretical constructs have been discussed in the literature relating to Arab Americans' family values. This chapter highlights the constructs of collectivism, patrilineality, acculturation, violence, and resilience. Each appears in the literature to inform practitioners about Arab family values in the United States. More importantly, the focus of most writers is the negotiation between Arab American families and the dominant culture with a focus on how greatly these constructs impact Arab family values and traditions. The constructs trickle down into multiple facets of families.

Collectivism in a Self-reliant Society

Arab families are rooted in collective, extended family support systems (Ben-Ari & Pines, 2002). The collective takes precedence over the individual and the nuclear family is not primary as it is in the United States. Arab families in the United States feel the strain as their primary support network becomes smaller (May, 1992). As a result, families experience increases in stress and decreases in support. As Arab American families shift away from relying on extended family support, there has been a change in traditions.

Large families, many with five or more children, are valued by Arabs in the United States, yet size declines as socioeconomic level increases (Aswad, 1994). In line with gender role expectations, young men and their wives will attempt to live near their fathers and brothers to access support, guidance, and remain close to their culture. This proves difficult, however, as reported by a study indicating only 15 % of men lived near their fathers (Aswad, 1991). Immigration and assimilation are significant factors in the separation of men from their fathers. Tension between immigrant fathers and their American born sons have been reported in Arab American communities in which sons become highly assimilated and lose connection with their cultural traditions. Arab immigrants, who came to the United States for college education in the last half of the twentieth century, married out of their culture at a high rate. This lessened the chances of retaining Arab cultural values and traditions.

Though extended family support is often touted as ideal, research suggests that spousal support is highly valued. After the attacks on September 11, 2001, couples were dependent on each other to cope in a social climate that made them feel more targeted and isolated (Beitin & Allen, 2005). This was further supported by Aroian, Templin, and Ramaswamy (2010), who studied social support in 539 Arab immigrant women and found husbands to be a larger source of support than family and friends. Yet, a potential negative impact of losing the collective, extended family support system and having increased spousal dependence is domestic violence. Financial dependence is the biggest barrier to Arab American women leaving abusive relationships (Kulwicki & Miller, 1999). Often, immigrant women are unable to achieve financial independence because their husbands are their sponsors and use their status to threaten them if they attempt to leave the marriage.

Parent–child relationships are greatly affected by culture in the United States. Part of this is the inherent conflict in wanting their children to succeed in the United States as well as remain connected to their ethnic community. Adolescents sense that accessing the privilege that comes from being a member of United States society comes at the cost of losing connection to their ethnic group. A collectivistic outlook, however, encourages children to privilege family over friends. Indeed, Ramaswamy, Aroian, and Templin (2009) reported Arab Muslim adolescents were more likely to seek social support from their family than their peers. Further, when adolescents felt strong family support, particularly that they could take their problems to their parents, they were less likely to experience emotional and behavioral problems. Eisenlohr (1996) interviewed Yemeni adolescent females about the experiences of the home and host cultures. Females described a delicate line between the desire to fit into teen culture and wish to maintain respect for their parents. Benefits of social support within the family context, especially the parent–child relationship, were not only found to benefit adolescents but also extend to later life. Ajrouch (2007) found that aging parents, who have less education and are more vulnerable, report better health when they perceive high quality support from their children.

In sum, a collectivistic outlook remains important. Even though the large extended family form has begun to fade, the primacy of family relationships continues to mark the experience of Arab Americans.

Patrilineality

Patrilineality, a structure in which males pass on their title and kinship through family lineage, underscores the importance of gender relations in traditions and values found among Arab American families. The impact of patrilineality and strong women's rights has received the most scholarly discussion regarding how Arab family values are affected by US culture. This tension affects the spousal relationship as well as the parent–child relationship. In a survey of 60 family crisis cases at the Arab Community Center for Economic and Social Services, Aswad and Gray (1996) found that half of the problems related to husbands not paying the bills and restricting their wives' employment. A large number of crisis cases initiated requests for separation or divorce. The availability of work and welfare to women challenged the traditional patrilineal structure of the family. Additionally, to protect the system of patrilineality, families are especially watchful of their daughters (Aswad, 1997). If girls tarnish the reputation of their family, the patrilineal structure is threatened, and so reprimand provides a means of control. A daughter or sister may be cut off from her family as a result of dishonoring her family by marrying outside the culture or having sexual relations outside of marriage. Sons have more freedom to date outside the culture but are expected to ultimately marry within culture. These practices vary by country of origin. Lebanese men and women are less likely to have their marriages arranged than Yemeni individuals (Aswad, 1991).

Researchers have also focused on transitions in gender roles, and how those shifts impact family life. Faragallah, Schumm, and Webb (1997) found that more egalitarian gender roles were associated with reduced marital and family satisfaction, partly due to more conflicts in gender role expectations, religious values, and traditionalism. Meleis (1991) argued that Arab American women need to negotiate between American and Arab cultures while carrying primary role responsibilities at home. The accumulation of stressors results in physical and mental health problems. Jordanian immigrant women reported loneliness, sadness, emotional distress, anxiety, and social isolation related to acculturation stressors such as societal prejudice, financial instability, household management, protection of children from perceived disapproved Western behaviors, and maintenance of ethnic identity (Hattar-Pollara & Meleis, 1995). In contrast, however, Amer and Hovey (2007) studied immigrant and second generation Arab Americans finding that men and women did not differ in their levels of acculturative stress, family dysfunction, or depression. These results indicate that gender role transitions have varying impacts on men and women. Moreover, related acculturative stress can be mediated by a number of cultural and environmental characteristics to influence degree of connectedness to traditional values.

Another factor that influences the impact of gender role transition is religion. Read (e.g., Read, 2003, 2004) has focused on religion with a specific emphasis on gender and power. Though she does not address the impact of patrilineality, Read's findings suggest that Arab culture rooted in traditional gender roles is more responsible than religion for gender inequality in Arab American families.

Gender and religion are interconnected in that religion and religious facilities often serve to connect men and women to their communities and culture. This is particularly true for Arab American Muslims. Muslim women are significant in the transmission of Islamic belief, ritual, and history to younger generations (Abu-Laban, 1991). Men and women are informed about behaviors in marriage, parenting, filial ties, and responsibilities by Islamic teachings. When they transition to the United States, they face a societal structure that threatens to undermine their family values because of high divorce rates, child abuse, out of wedlock births, and isolation of elders (Waugh, Abu-Laban, & Qureshi, 1991). These experiences are also true for Christian Arab Americans who often share similar cultural values, despite religious differences.

Acculturation

Acculturation is a dominant theoretical construct in Arab American family studies. Researchers examine how acculturation affects values, traditions, and relationships within Arab American families as they adjust to life in the United States. Berry (1997) has a widely accepted model of acculturation which measures individual preference for their heritage as well as the dominant culture in society. Based on these preferences, individuals fall on a continuum of four acculturation strategies: assimilation, integration, separation, and marginalization.

Acculturation involves adaptation to various elements in the host society, including identity, as well as the traditions and cultural norms surrounding family. Ajrouch and Jamal (2007) found that Arab Americans show different patterns of acculturation with regard to a "racial" identity. Some individuals identify as both white and Arab American, while others prefer a white identity and reject the Arab American category, and still others reject a white identity in favor of an Arab American identity. Identity choices may vary within families as well, with younger members rejecting a white identity and older members more likely to embrace whiteness (Ajrouch, 2004; Ajrouch & Jamal, 2007). The expectations associated with acculturation may induce high levels of stress on families. Indeed, the impact of acculturative stress on families can be a strain if resources are not available. On one hand, Arab American families can act as a buffer against the effects of acculturative stressors on individuals (Ajrouch, 2000; Hattar-Pollara & Meleis, 1995). On the other hand, acculturative stress may be associated with reduced Arab American family satisfaction (Faragallah et al., 1997; Kulwicki & Miller, 1999). Laffrey, Meleis, Lipson, Solomon, and Omidian (1989) surveyed 47 Arab American men and women about their most prevalent health care problems. The most frequently reported problems included: family stress, adjusting to life in the United States, managing acute illness, coping with adolescents, and marital stress. Three out of the five directly inform Arab American family values and traditions, posing a potential threat to family stability.

Acculturation also involves possible encounters with discrimination. Muslim Arab Americans report greater experiences of discrimination than Christian Arab

Americans, partially explained by Christianity being the dominant religion in the United States (Awad, 2010). However, ongoing political tensions in the Arab world and media's negative portrayal of Arab Muslims often generate misunderstanding among the public and contribute to the discrimination differences experienced by Muslim Arab Americans (Cainkar, 1996; Orfalea, 1988). Muslim Arab Americans also differ in their experience of integration into US culture, reporting higher acculturative stress as they integrate (Amer & Hovey, 2005). These struggles compel some Arab families to return to their countries of origin. Others face persistent adversity, yet many find political, economic, and religious security in a beloved new country.

Arab American marital relationships are identified as a source of resilience in the process of acculturation. Further, marriage has remained an important value. Endogamy is less likely among Arab American men and women with higher levels of acculturation, who are likely to marry a partner not of Arab descent (Kulczycki & Lobo, 2002), yet Arab Americans are more likely to be married and less likely to be divorced, separated, or widowed than the overall US population (Abi-Hashem, 2008). With the nuclear family as a dominant US societal value, couples often report isolation as they find themselves increasingly needing to rely on their spouse for support.

Relationships between parents and adolescent children have been widely studied in Arab American families. Arab American parents struggle with their child's desire to fit into US culture. Ajrouch (2000) found that tensions existed for many adolescents between feelings of support and belonging and feelings of frustration from a limited amount of privacy in the Arab ethnic community. Differences in levels of acculturation between parents and children are also indicators of parent–child conflicts and increase in rebellious behavior. Many studies indicate that children of immigrants experience higher levels of mental health problems because of conflicts with parental views and those of the host country (Phinney, Horenczyk, Liebkind, & Vedder, 2001). Significant gaps in values between parents and children pose a struggle in disciplining children and enforcing cultural expectations. Aswad and Gray (1996) reported that difficulty disciplining children and even children running away were frequent problems that lead Arab American parents to seek professional services. Cultural and religious differences between traditional Arab families and dominant values exercised in the United States may cause some Arab parents to limit their children's societal interactions, fearing it would negatively impact their Arab upbringing. Hattar-Pollara and Meleis (1995) reported that Jordanian American mothers felt anxiety and fear that their children might assimilate and lose their Arab cultural values. They worried that their children might adopt values of the United States, such as engaging in dating, arguing about their "rights," becoming self-centered, and seeking independence, rather than Arabic traditions that emphasize collectivity. Because children were often acculturating faster than their parents, the traditional hierarchy was challenged, which then posed a direct confrontation with traditional family structure. In an effort to compensate for the potential negative impact of US culture on their children, Arab American parents often send their children to Islamic schools or Christian Arab congregations to learn Arabic and religion as a means to expose children to traditional social expectations (Abu-Baker, 2006; Beitin & Allen, 2005).

The unwavering support of family members to one another has also been shown to help second generation Arab Americans in their development of ethnic identity. Some Arab immigrant youth see value both in their heritage and in mainstream US culture. Ajrouch (2000) suggested that second generation Arab Americans use selective Americanization or selective acculturation. They have a strong ethnic identity but they also desire social interaction with mainstream culture. Hakim-Larson, Kamoo, Nassar-McMillan, and Porcerelli (2007) discussed the idea that first and second generation Arab American adolescents can create a sense of self that incorporates a mainstream identity and a private identity. In their study, Hattar-Pollara and Meleis (1995) discovered that Jordanian Arab American mothers make a point of providing their adolescents with support, praise, and nurturance to prevent assimilation.

In sum, Arab Americans experience various patterns of acculturation and identity development in the United States. The acculturation process may expose Arab Americans to face family conflict, discrimination, and acculturative stress, as well as opportunity to capitalize on resources inherent to Arab family values and traditions. Many factors contribute to these variations including religion, degree of cultural differences, age, gender, and family support.

Violence and Resilience

Arab families bring unique and diverse experiences with them as they immigrate to the United States. In many cases, depending on their country of origin, families have been impacted by ongoing political unrest, violence, and war in the Arab world. War and violence have devastated many Arab countries for centuries. Taking a closer look on the impact of war and violence on Arab Americans' well-being explains the development of resilience among this population and highlights the importance of family support to Arab Americans.

Most of the research on the effects of violence has focused on Israeli, Lebanese, and Palestinian families. In the study of relatives of the Hebron massacre, Elbedour, Baker, Shalhoub-Kevorkian, Irwin, and Belmaker (1999) found that family support was a significant factor in coping. Participants saw the struggle as a collective one rather than an individual experience, which helped with meaning making. Family and social support has also been correlated with health. Family members who reported satisfaction with their social support system have a more positive health outcome than those who did not, as well as fewer physical and mental health problems, and less marital conflict (Farhood, 1999).

War and violence often generate a different response in children compared to adults. Researchers have spent the most time examining children, trauma, and coping. Because family represents a protective barrier for children, witnessing humiliation and violence toward family members is especially harmful to children's well-being (Macksoud & Aber, 1996). Findings are not conclusive regarding resilience but there are some patterns. Strong maternal mental health is associated with positive psychological adjustment of the child (Qouta, Punamaki, & El Sarraj, 2005). Barber (1999) showed that a nurturing parenting style protected children's development and emotional well-being from the negative impact of military violence in Palestine and the Balkans. Children who perceived their parents as harsh and punitive were more likely to develop antisocial behavior, whereas parental acceptance provided a buffer between military violence and adolescents' depression (Barber, 1999). Garbarino and Kostelny (1996) provided evidence that Palestinian children with parents perceived as punitive were more vulnerable to the effects of chronic military violence when compared to children whose parents were nurturing. An additional study on Palestinians revealed that children who reported having accepting parents were more creative in problem solving than those who felt some rejection from their parents. The creativity could protect children's mental health during exposure to military violence (Punamaki, Qouta, & El Sarraj, 2001).

Family relationships are often impacted by war and trauma, yet play a significant role in the coping process. In one of the few studies focused on multiple family relationships, Joseph (2004) examined family relations in a small town in Lebanon after the 15-year civil war (1975–1990). She found that during a crisis of conflict, the families she witnessed were determined to try and maintain family relationships and functions. The trauma following the war also provided opportunities for change. Women challenged old structures and asserted new freedoms. Men and women expanded their notions of family in the name of protecting it even if that meant more equality for women.

Arab Americans have also faced traumatic events, including discrimination, while living in the United States. The attacks on the United States on September 11, 2001, greatly impacted many groups of people. As a result, Arab Americans experienced prejudice and discrimination. However, acts of discrimination against Arab Americans, predominantly Muslims, began before these attacks. Some historical events that provoked stereotypical thinking toward Arab Americans include the Arab trade restrictions implemented in the 1970s that resulted in increased gas prices in the United States and the 1983 bombing of the United States Marine barracks in Beirut, Lebanon (Cainkar, 1996; Orfalea, 1988).

Few studies have focused on the effects of discrimination on family values or overall health (El-Sayed & Galea, 2009). Of the few studies conducted, the experience of discrimination has increased psychological and emotional stress in this group (Padela & Heisler, 2010). Arab Americans have created many religious and cultural communities in the United States to increase their support network and happiness. Couples, who felt discrimination, became even more isolated after September 11, 2001, resulting in reinforcement of the nuclear family model they worked so hard to resist (Beitin & Allen, 2005).

Methodological Approaches

The empirical literature that studies Arab families in the Middle East, North Africa, North America, and Europe is predominantly quantitative survey based with large samples (Beitin et al., 2010). Studies on family values in Arab American families report the views of women and adolescents more often than those of other family members. Women and adolescents have been the dominant voices in samples, becoming the voice for all Arab families at the cost of silencing other members including men, elders, and other members. Men must be included in research so that struggles and strengths in the Arab American community are given a fuller context. If women become the voice, they are in effect problematized. Kulwicki and Miller (1999) assessed Arab American beliefs toward domestic violence and incorporated their findings into community education about domestic violence. The authors sampled 202 Arab Americans and 80 % were females. Read (2004) surveyed 416 Arab American women living across the United States about the relationships between family, religion, and women's labor force participation. By understanding men's views and their place in the application of theoretical constructs related to family values (i.e., patrilineality), practitioners can intervene at the level of family interactions rather than one person. For example, mothers are identified as significant factors in the adjustment of adolescents to the United States. Since research shows that some Arab men struggle to communicate with their children, this is neglected as a possible influence on adolescent adjustment and practitioners are less likely to address it. This is partly due to the patrilineal values of Arab families where mothers are viewed having a key role in balancing the family structure and responsible for the physical and emotional well-being of the family, especially upon immigration.

Research on Arab Americans has differed from the larger literature on the Arab world as a whole by grouping Arabs from different countries of origin into large samples. The larger Arab literature has tended to provide more homogenous samples by soliciting participants from the same country. This difference in sampling is likely a result of the diversity of the Arab population in United States as well as the dispersed populations of families originating from each Arab country. Britto and Amer (2007) examined adolescent identity in the context of family functioning and their sample consisted of Arabs identifying 11 different countries of origin. In their analysis, the researchers combined the participants as Arab Americans. There are advantages and limitations to this method. Grouping allows for a rich data set that includes the variations and nuances that exist from country to country in the Arab world. At the same time, within group differences that could have meaningful implications for the analysis and results are lost. For example, differences in patterns of identity development and immigration experiences may vary significantly based on religion, nationality, and gender. Further, there are many who trace their lineage to Arab countries but do not consider themselves Arabs (i.e., Armenians and Chaldeans). This has implications for studies which focus on Arab Americans from those countries. The samples are more likely to include those who represent one section of the population. Men and women who immigrated from those countries, speak Arabic, and practice many Arab traditions but do not identify as Arab do not have a voice in research on Arab Americans. The term "Arab" and its connotation can create divisions among people who nevertheless share so many cultural rituals and traditions.

Few studies examined family values by focusing on more than one family member in the sample. Sampling multiple members from a family can expand understanding of family constructs and dynamics since more perspectives provide greater depth in the data (Beitin, 2008). For example, Aroian et al. (2009) surveyed 530 mother–adolescent dyads to explore the relationship between parent–child relationships and adolescent behavior problems. Through the use of dyads, the authors found that even if mothers showed high levels of depression, it did not predict behavior problems in their adolescent children. Read and Oselin (2007) utilized ethnographic research with multiple family members to observe gender dynamics among Arab American men and women. As they observed interactions between parents and children, younger females were sometimes scolded for acting or dressing too American.

Critique

The literature on Arab American family values and traditions is scarce (Beitin et al., 2010). Studies in the larger literature on Arab family values are problem-focused emphasizing deficits rather than coping and strength. This is evident in the large percentage of articles reporting on domestic violence and mental illness. The Arab American empirical literature has shown early evidence of following a different path. Many researchers included a measure of support in coping even if their research is focused on problems (e.g., Ajrouch, 2007; Amer & Hovey, 2007; Ramaswamy et al., 2009).

The empirical literature focused on Arab American family values is most developed in the area of the impact of acculturation on Arab family values. Though immigration and acculturation have received the most attention, knowledge of the impact of these processes on family values is limited in scope and depth. Gender, as it relates to family values, is also a more developed area of study though it is limited by women composing a majority of samples.

Research on Arab American family values is centered on particular areas and needs more breadth. For example, there is little focus on the process of generational transmission of family values and traditions, which is a starting point in maintaining culture. Little is known about the impact of socioeconomic status on family values during adjustment in spite of the fact that socioeconomic status, often indicated by level of education, has shown to have some impact on Arab American families (Kulczycki & Lobo, 2002). Marital relationships are rarely studied yet their importance in coping is significant because of the loss of extended family (Aroian et al., 2010). The fallout from the attacks of September 11, 2001, continues yet there are limited studies which address the physiological and family effects of the fallout. Examination of family values has been conducted with one member of a family rather than dyadic or multiple family member surveys or interviews.

Implications

Family values and traditions are part of a foundation of Arab American communities. Professionals who work with Arab Americans need an understanding of family values in order to provide services that support the needs of their communities. From the literature, the theoretical constructs of collectivism, patrilineality, acculturation, violence, and resilience provide practitioners with a framework to inform their work. Further, these constructs have substantive effects on Arab American family values on several levels. They provide depth and understanding to family values in this group rather than initial responses which paint stereotypes of oppressive, violent men and submissive, exotic women. The theoretical constructs are interconnected with gender, religion, country of origin, SES, family relationships, parenting, and resilience.

On a practice level, Arab American families must be understood and approached with sensitivity to diversity of countries of origin, languages and dialects, religions, levels of acculturation, and incomes. Professionals should study the nuances of families that are seeking services. They should assess for acculturation, income, education, support, and religion in addition to standard needs questions. A family in a lower stage of acculturation needs more explanation and time earlier in the services, whereas a more acculturated family will be likely to have knowledge of social systems and need less guidance in the basic education of navigating society.

Multiple studies demonstrated that family and social supports reduce strain on families. Practitioners should seek ways to incorporate whole families into services by asking if a partner or other family members, including kin and religious leaders, can attend. Community practitioners can also create or reinforce social gatherings that support new immigrants. Professionals can increase their influence by making connections with religious and secular leaders in the community. These members may be particularly helpful in creating understanding if a family is struggling with rules or laws which contradict family values.

Marital relationships are under increased stress as couples must raise families with less support. Since marriage is strongly valued in Arab culture, reliance on a spouse is familiar and has been shown to increase successful coping and resilience in Arab American couples. Couples can access support from their partner with guidance from their communities, religious leaders, and practitioners. Religious leaders and practitioners can help couples identify their previously used strategies for coping as a couple, leverage cultural methods of coping from previous generations, or be given new tools focused on improving communication.

As youth enter adolescence, they require support to manage feeling supported and controlled by their families while negotiating their identity in US culture. Professionals should evaluate their own biases and cultural values and avoid imposing Western values of individualism and independence of children on Arab American families. A practitioner may react to shaming practices by parents toward adolescents in a way that negatively evaluates the situation and therefore seeks to stop it. Yet, this might only result in alienation since shaming is a method of protecting family honor. The possibility to introduce other methods of control may arise after joining with the family and evaluating behavior within a cultural context.

Religion is one aspect of identity to consider since some differences exist between the Arab American Muslim and Christian experiences. Since Christians seem to acculturate with less concern about religious practice, efforts should focus on helping them to navigate US society. Muslims also need similar support, though efforts should be made to minimize threats to religious preferences since they appear to fare better when able to remain connected to their religion. Muslim communities may be instrumental in this way, reaching out to fellow Muslims and developing programs with the purpose of keeping Muslims connected.

On a policy level, officials can provide funding and resources for programs which support Arab American family values. Because of Arab American family honor and social standing, they usually resist seeking professional family services to address struggles. There is a strong sense of shame and embarrassment associated with these services (Abu-Ras, 2003). Families are more likely to seek support from their religious community or physician. Arab Americans need funding for programs that support services provided in an integrated setting including doctors and religious leaders. Poor language skills have also correlated with the use of formal help by Arab American families; those with poor language skills are less likely to use services (Kulwicki, Miller, & Schim, 2000). Policies which provide ESL classes for immigrants as well as Arabic classes for children and adolescents would foster connections to culture, thereby supporting strong family bonds.

Overall, research on Arab American family values is scarce, but the available literature provides a more strength-based focus. Moreover, publications have increased in the field during the last 5 years. The understanding of family values and traditions would benefit from more qualitative research with more diverse samples in order to develop a deeper portrait of Arab American families as well as how to implement effective supports for health and stability. Collection of data on health and life satisfaction is needed on local and regional levels to provide relevant services to the unique needs of each geographical region. Finally, research studies that follow families and track family values and traditions over time would provide much needed insight into family change and continuity.

References

Abi-Hashem, N. (2008). Arab Americans: Understanding their challenges, needs and struggles. In A. J. Marsella, J. L. Johnson, P. Watson, & J. Gryczynski (Eds.), *Ethnocultural perspective on disaster and trauma: Foundations, issues, and applications* (pp. 115–173). New York: Springer.

Abraham, N., & Shryock, A. (2000). *Arab Detroit from margin to main-stream*. Detroit, MI: Wayne State University Press.

Abu-Baker, K. (2006). Arab/Muslim families in the United States. In M. Dwairy (Ed.), *Counseling and psychotherapy with Arabs and Muslims: A culturally sensitive approach*. New York: Teachers College Press.

Abu-Laban, S. M. (1991). Family and religion among Muslim immigrants and their descendants. In E. H. Waugh, S. M. Abu-Laban, & R. B. Qureshi (Eds.), *Muslim families in North America* (pp. 6–31). Edmonton, AB: The University of Alberta Press.

Abu-Ras, W. (2003). Barriers to services for Arab immigrant battered women in a Detroit suburb. *Journal of Social Work Research and Evaluation, 4*, 49–65.
Ajrouch, K. J. (2000). Place, age, and culture: community living and ethnic identity among Lebanese American adolescents. *Small Group Research, 31*, 447–469.
Ajrouch, K. J. (2004). Gender, race, and symbolic boundaries: Contested spaces of identity among Arab-American adolescents. *Sociological Perspectives, 47*, 371–391.
Ajrouch, K. J. (2007). Health disparities and Arab-American elders: Does intergenerational support buffer the inequality-health link. *Journal of Social Issues, 63*, 745–758.
Ajrouch, K. J., & Jamal, A. (2007). Assimilating to a white identity: The case of Arab Americans. *International Migration Review, 41*, 860–879.
Ajrouch, K. J., Yount, K., Sibai, A. M., & Roman, P. (2013). A gendered perspective on well-being in later life: Algeria, Lebanon, and Palestine. In S. McDaniel & Z. Zimmer (Eds.), *Global ageing in the 21st century*. Surrey: Ashgate Publishing.
Al-Haj, M. (1995). Kinship and modernization in developing societies: The emergence of instrumentalized kinship. *Journal of Comparative Family Studies, 26*, 311–328.
Al-Khawaja, M. (1999). Alshabab al A'rabi [Arab youth]. In K. Zakareya (Ed.), *Derasat fi almojtamaa' al A'rabialmoa'aser [Studies in the contemporary Arab society]* (pp. 255–304). Damascus: Al Ahali Publications.
Allen, K. R., Fine, M. A., & Demo, D. H. (2000). An overview of family diversity: Controversies, questions, and values. In D. H. Demo, K. R. Allen, & M. A. Fine (Eds.), *Handbook of family diversity* (pp. 1–14). New York: Oxford University Press.
Alwan, A., & Modell, B. (1997). *Community control of genetic and congenital disorders (Technical Publication Series 24)* (pp. 63–68). Alexandria: WHO/Eastern Mediterranean Region Office.
Amer, M. M., & Hovey, J. D. (2005). Examination of the impact of acculturation, stress, and religiosity on mental health variables for second-generation Arab Americans. *Ethnicity and Disease, 15*(1), 111–112.
Amer, M. M., & Hovey, J. D. (2007). Socio-demographic differences in acculturation and mental health for a sample of 2nd generation early immigrant Arab Americans. *Journal of Immigrant and Minority Health, 9*, 345–347.
Amin, S., & Al-Bassusi, N. (2004). Education, wage work, and marriage perspective of Egyptian working women. *Journal of Marriage and the Family, 66*, 1287–1299.
Arab American Institute Foundation. (2011). *Quick facts about Arab Americans*. Retrieved November 15, 2011, from http://www.aaiusa.org/page/-/AAIF/Educational/quickfacts.pdf
Aroian, K. J., Hough, E. S., Templin, T. N., Kulwicki, A., Ramaswamy, V., & Katz, A. (2009). A model of mother-child adjustment in Arab Muslim immigrants to the US. *Social Science & Medicine, 69*, 1377–1386.
Aroian, K. J., Templin, T. N., & Ramaswamy, V. (2010). Adaptation and psychometric evaluation of the multidimensional scale of perceived social support for Arab immigrant women. *Health Care for Women International, 31*, 153–169.
Aswad, B. C. (1991). Yemeni and Lebanese Muslim immigrant women in Dearborn Michigan. In E. Waugh & S. Abu-Laban (Eds.), *The Muslim family in America* (pp. 256–281). Alberta: University of Alberta.
Aswad, B. C. (1994). Attitudes of immigrant women and men in the Dearborn area toward women's employment and welfare. In Y. Y. Haddad & J. I. Smith (Eds.), *Muslim communities in North America* (pp. 501–519). Albany, NY: State University of New York Press.
Aswad, B. C. (1997). Arab American families. In M. K. DeGenova (Ed.), *Families in cultural context: Strengths and challenges in diversity* (pp. 213–237). Mountain View, CA: Mayfield.
Aswad, B. C., & Gray, N. A. (1996). Challenges to the Arab-American family and ACCESS. In B. C. Aswad & B. Bilge (Eds.), *Family and gender among American Muslims: Issues facing Middle Eastern immigrants and their descendants* (pp. 223–240). Philadelphia: Temple University Press.
Awad, G. H. (2010). The impact of acculturation and religious identification on perceived discrimination for Arab/Middle Eastern Americans. *Cultural Diversity and Ethnic Minority Psychology, 16*, 59–67.

Azaiza, F. (2005). Parent–child relationships as perceived by Arab adolescents living in Israel. *International Journal of Social Welfare, 14*, 297–304.
Barakat, H. (1993). *The Arab world: Society, culture, and state*. Berkeley: University of California Press.
Barber, B. K. (1999). Political violence, family relations, and Palestinian child functioning. *Journal of Adolescent Research, 14*, 206–230.
Beitin, B. K. (2008). Qualitative research in marriage and family therapy: Who is in the interview? *Contemporary Family Therapy, 30*, 48–58.
Beitin, B. K., & Allen, K. R. (2005). Resilience in Arab American couples after September 11th: A systems perspective. *Journal of Marital and Family Therapy, 31*, 251–268.
Beitin, B. K., Allen, K. R., & Bekheet, M. (2010). A critical analysis of western perspectives on families of Arab descent. *Journal of Family Issues, 31*, 211–233.
Ben-Ari, A., & Pines, M. A. (2002). The changing role of family in utilization of social support: Views from Israeli Jewish and Arab students. *Families in Society, 83*, 93–102.
Berry, J. W. (1997). Immigration, acculturation, and adaptation. *Applied Psychology, 46*, 5–34.
Britto, P. R., & Amer, M. (2007). An exploration of cultural identity patterns and the family context among Arab Muslim young adults in America. *Applied Development Science, 11*, 137–150.
Burgess, E. W., & Locke, H. J. (1945). *The family: From institution to companionship*. New York: American Book.
Cainkar, L. (1996). Immigrant Palestinian women evaluate their lives. In B. C. Aswad & B. Bilge (Eds.), *Family and gender among American Muslims* (pp. 41–58). Philadelphia, PA: Temple University Press.
Cohen, O., & Savaya, R. (2003). Lifestyle differences in traditionalism and modernity and reasons for divorce among Muslim Palestinian citizens of Israel. *Journal of Comparative Family Studies, 34*, 283–294.
Dhaher, E. A., Mikolajeczyk, R. T., Maxwell, A. E., & Krämer, A. (2010). Attitudes toward wife beating among Palestinian women of reproductive age from three cities in the West Bank. *Journal of Interpersonal Violence, 25*, 518–537.
Dwairy, M. (2003). Validation of multigenerational interconnectedness scale among Arab adolescents. *Psychological Reports, 93*, 697–704.
Dwairy, M. (2004). Parenting styles and psychological adjustment of Arab adolescents. *Transcultural Psychiatry, 41*, 233–252.
Dwairy, M. (2008). Parental inconsistency versus parental authoritarianism: Association with symptoms of psychological disorders. *Journal of Youth and Adolescence, 37*, 616–626.
Eisenlohr, C. J. (1996). Adolescent Arab girls in an American high school. In B. Bilge & B. C. Aswad (Eds.), *Family and gender among American Muslims: Issues facing Middle Eastern immigrants and their descendants* (pp. 250–270). Philadelphia: Temple University Press.
Elbedour, S., Baker, A., Shalhoub-Kevorkian, N., Irwin, M., & Belmaker, R. (1999). Psychological responses in family members after the Hebron massacre. *Depression and Anxiety, 9*, 27–31.
El-Sayed, A., & Galea, S. (2009). The health of Arab-Americans living in the United States: A systematic review of the literature. *BMC Public Health, 9*, 272–280.
Faragallah, M. H., Schumm, W. R., & Webb, F. J. (1997). Acculturation of Arab-American immigrants: An exploratory study. *Journal of Comparative Family Studies, 28*, 182–203.
Farhood, L. (1999). Testing a model of family stress and coping based on war and non-war stressors, family resources, coping and family adaptation among Lebanese families. *Archives of Psychiatric Nursing, 13*, 192–203.
Fronk, C., Huntington, R. L., & Chadwick, B. A. (1999). Educational attitudes and trends in Palestine. *Educational Studies, 25*, 217–243.
Garbarino, J., & Kostelny, K. (1996). The effects of political violence on Palestinian children's behavior problems: A risk accumulation model. *Child Development, 67*, 33–45.
Haj-Yahia, M. M. (2000). Wife abuse and battering in the sociocultural context of Arab society. *Family Process, 39*, 237–255.

Haj-Yahia, M. M. (2011). Contextualizing interventions with battered women in collectivist societies: Issues and controversies. *Aggression and Violent Behavior, 16*, 331–339.

Hakim-Larson, J., Kamoo, R., Nassar-McMillan, S. C., & Porcerelli, J. H. (2007). Counseling Arab and Chaldean American families. *Journal of Mental Health Counseling, 29*, 301–332.

Hatab, Z., & Makki, A. (1978). *Al-solta el-abawiawal-shabab.* Beirut: Ma'had El-Inmaa' El-Arabi. Beirut: Arab Development Institution (in Arabic).

Hattar-Pollara, M., & Meleis, A. I. (1995). Parenting their adolescents: The experiences of Jordanian immigrant women in California. *Health Care for Women International, 16*, 195–211.

Joseph, S. (1993). Gender and relationality among Arab families in Lebanon. *Feminist Studies, 19*, 465–486.

Joseph, S. (1999). *Intimate selving in Arab families: Gender, self and identity*. Syracuse, NY: University of Syracuse Press.

Joseph, S. (2004). Conceiving family relationships in post-war Lebanon. *Journal of Comparative Family Studies, 35*, 271–293.

Kandiyoti, D. (1988). Bargaining with patriarchy. *Gender and Society, 2*, 274–290.

Khalaila, R. (2010). Development and evaluation of the Arabic Filial Piety Scale. *Research on Social Work Practice, 20*, 356–367.

Khalifa, M. A. (1988). Attitudes of urban Sudanese men toward family planning. *Studies in Family Planning, 19*, 236–243.

Kulczycki, A., & Lobo, A. P. (2002). Patterns, determinants and implications of intermarriage among Arab Americans. *Journal of Marriage and the Family, 64*, 202–210.

Kulwicki, A. D., & Miller, J. (1999). Domestic violence in the Arab American population: Transforming environmental conditions through community education. *Issues in Mental Health Nursing, 20*, 199–215.

Kulwicki, A. D., Miller, J., & Schim, S. M. (2000). Collaborative partnership for culture care: Enhancing health services for the Arab community. *Journal of Transcultural Nursing, 11*, 31–39.

Laffrey, S. C., Meleis, A. I., Lipson, J. G., Solomon, M., & Omidian, P. A. (1989). Assessing Arab American health care needs. *Social Science & Medicine, 29*, 877–883.

Lev-Wiesel, R., & Al-Krenawi, A. (1999). Attitudes toward marriage and marital quality: A comparison among Israeli Arabs differentiated by religion. *Family Relations, 48*, 51–56.

Lijtmaer, R. M. (2001). Splitting and nostalgia in recent immigrants: Psychodynamic considerations. *Journal of the American Academy of Psychoanalysis, 29*, 427–438.

Macksoud, M., & Aber, J. (1996). The war experiences and psychosocial development of children in Lebanon. *Child Development, 67*, 70–88.

May, K. M. (1992). Middle-Eastern immigrant parents' social networks and help-seeking for child health care. *Journal of Advanced Nursing, 17*(8), 905–912.

Meleis, A. I. (1991). Between two cultures: Identity, roles, and health. *Health Care for Women International, 12*, 365–377.

Moghadam, V. M. (2004). Patriarchy in transition: Women and the changing family in the Middle East. *Journal of Comparative Family Studies, 35*, 137–163.

Obeid, N., Chang, D. F., & Ginges, J. (2010). Beliefs of wife beating: A Lebanese case. *Violence Against Women, 16*(6), 691–712.

Olmsted, J. (2005). Gender, aging, and the evolving Arab patriarchal contract. *Feminist Economics, 11*(2), 53–78.

Orfalea, G. (1988). *Before the flames: A quest for the history of Arab Americans*. Austin, TX: University of Texas Press.

Padela, A., & Heisler, M. (2010). The association of perceived abuse and discrimination after September 11, 2001, with psychological distress, level of happiness, and health status among Arab Americans. *American Journal of Public Health, 100*, 284–291.

Phinney, J. S., Horenczyk, G., Liebkind, K., & Vedder, P. (2001). Ethnic identity, immigration, and well-being: An interactional perspective. *Journal of Social Issues, 57*, 493–510.

Punamaki, R. L., Qouta, S., & El Sarraj, E. (2001). Resiliency factors predicting psychological adjustment after political violence among Palestinian children. *International Journal of Developmental Behaviour, 25*, 256–267.

Qouta, S., Punamaki, R. L., & El Sarraj, E. (2005). Mother-child expression of symptoms in life-endangering situation. *Journal of Clinical Child Psychology, 10*, 151–165.

Ramaswamy, V., Aroian, K. J., & Templin, T. N. (2009). Adaptation and psychometric evaluation of the multidimensional scale of perceived social support for Arab American adolescents. *American Journal of Community Psychology, 43*, 49–56.

Raz, A. E., & Atar, M. (2004). Cousin marriage and premarital carrier matching in a Bedouin community in Israel: Attitudes, service development, and educational intervention. *The Journal of Family Planning and Reproductive Health Care, 30*, 49–51.

Read, J. G. (2003). The sources of gender role attitudes among Christian and Muslim Arab American women. *Sociology of Religion, 64*, 207–222.

Read, J. G. (2004). Family, religion, and work among Arab-American Women. *Journal of Marriage and the Family, 67*, 1042–1050.

Read, J. G., & Oselin, M. (2007). Gender and the education-employment paradox in ethnic and religious contexts: The case of Arab Americans. *American Sociological Review, 73*, 296–313.

Rudy, D., & Grusec, J. E. (2006). Authoritarian parenting in individualist and collectivist groups: Associations with maternal emotion and cognition and children's self-esteem. *Journal of Family Psychology, 20*(1), 68–78.

Shabib, M. (2001). Baa'danmat al tafaa'ul al walidikamayudrikha al abnaa (Some parental interaction styles as perceived by the children). *Majallat Al Tarbeyah: Education Faculty in Al Azhar University, 102*, 232–265.

Shah, N. M. (2004). Women's socioeconomic characteristics and marital patterns in a rapidly developing Muslim society, Kuwait. *Journal of Comparative Family Studies, 35*, 163–183.

Shalhoub-Kevorkian, N. (1997). Tolerating battering: Invisible way of social control. *International Review of Victimology, 5*, 1–21.

Sibai, A. M., Beydoun, M. A., & Tohme, R. A. (2009). Living arrangements of ever-married older Lebanese women: Factors behind co-residence with an adult child. *Journal of Cross-Cultural Gerontology, 24*, 5–17.

Smith, M. D. (1990). Patriarchal ideology and wife beating: A test of a feminist hypothesis. *Violence and Victims, 5*, 257–274.

Sugarman, D., & Frankel, S. (1996). Patriarchal ideology and wife-assault: A meta-analytic review. *Journal of Family Violence, 11*, 13–39.

Thornton, A. (2005). *Reading history sideways: The fallacy and enduring impact of the developmental paradigm on family life*. Chicago: University of Chicago Press.

Tillion, G. (1983). *The republic of cousins: Women's oppression in Mediterranean society*. London: AI Saqi Books.

Tohme, R., Yount, K. M., Yassine, S., & Sibai, A. (2011). Socioeconomic resources and living arrangements of older adults in Lebanon: Who chooses to live alone? *Ageing & Society, 31*, 1–17.

United Nations. (2007). *World marriage data 2006*. POP/DB/Mar/Rev.2007.

Waugh, E. H., Abu-Laban, S. M., & Qureshi, R. B. (Eds.). (1991). *Muslim families in North America*. Edmonton, AB: The University of Alberta Press.

Chapter 5
Arab Americans and Gender

Louise Cainkar and Jen'nan Ghazal Read

Gender is a major organizing feature in all societies across time and space. In the contemporary US context, research increasingly acknowledges the importance of gender relations in the settlement experiences of immigrant populations. Most of this research has focused on Hispanic groups, and to a lesser extent, Asian populations. In this chapter, we extend this research to discuss the role of gender relations in the assimilation and adaptation experiences of Arab Americans, particularly in the latter half of the twentieth century. We discuss research findings on Arab Americans that identify gender as a key explanatory variable for differential experiences and outcomes in the United States using three theoretical constructs: segmented assimilation, agency, and social capital. Segmented assimilation, advanced by Portes, Zhou, and others (Portes, 1996; Portes & Rumbaut, 2006; Portes & Zhou, 1993; Zhou & Bankston, 1998), suggests that different types of assimilation processes take place, depending on the characteristics immigrants bring with them as well as the conditions of the host society in which they settle. This theory specifically recognizes that immigrants will assimilate into different segments of society depending on such factors, instead of following a single normative pattern (Ajrouch & Kusow, 2007; Zhou, 1997). Many Arab Americans today embrace a selective acculturation strategy, where they choose which components of American culture and which of their "homeland" cultures they desire to adopt or maintain (Cainkar, 2011), producing some measurable successes in their American experience while maintaining their cultural differences from mainstream society. Agency,

L. Cainkar (✉)
Department of Social and Cultural Sciences, Marquette University,
LaLumiere Hall, 359, P.O. Box 1881, Milwaukee, WI 53201-1881, USA
e-mail: Louise.Cainkar@mu.edu

J.G. Read
Department of Sociology, Duke University, 275 Soc/Psych Building,
Durham, NC 27708, USA
e-mail: jennan.read@duke.edu

S.C. Nassar-McMillan et al. (eds.), *Biopsychosocial Perspectives on Arab Americans: Culture, Development, and Health*, DOI 10.1007/978-1-4614-8238-3_5,

a concept brought to the forefront in sociology by Giddens (1984), acknowledges that individuals possess autonomy to act, but within the constraints of larger social and historical forces. Finally, social capital "is created when the relations among persons change in ways that facilitate action" (Coleman, 1990, p. 304). In other words, resources emanate from the relationships between individuals. Each concept lends insight about the ways that gender relations play out and shape the Arab American experience.

To illustrate the dynamics of gender relations, we begin by highlighting the importance of family in Arab culture, and then using the theoretical constructs of segmented assimilation, agency, and social capital, discuss the extent to which these values have transferred (successfully or not) to the American context, including their impact on women's education and employment. We further apply the notion of agency to focus on the post-9/11 context and conclude with implications from our review for Arab American health.

The Role of Family in Cultural Reproduction

In Arab culture, as with other western Asian cultures, family is the single most important social institution. As noted by Aswad (2005) "Other institutions, political, religious and social, may compete for importance, but seldom succeed. Women play an extremely important role in the family … and the ideology of family rules" (p. 147), which includes norms concerning the different roles, practices, and expectations that should be placed on women and men. As a result, an individual raised in an Arab American family that observes the gendered norms, modes of deference, and expectations that are foundational to Arab culture and social organization will find his/her experience of gendered differences heightened when compared to white, American middle class culture.

Precisely because family is the cornerstone of Arab culture, marriage is revered and divorce is highly frowned upon. In general, marriages are approached as matters that begin with compatibility rather than love, which is assumed to emerge over time, a perspective that supports those who believe that marriage by arrangement can be as successful as marriage for love, with both patterns found among Arab Americans. Allowing for significant variation in content and emphasis, gendered expectations are foundational to compatibility. Divorce is another area of asymmetry, where the stigma is greater for women than men, although as pointed out by Aswad (1999), there are regional differences. "Divorce does not carry the stigma for Yemeni that it does for Levantine women" (p. 182). Natal and extended family members will pressure married couples to stay together even if one or both partners are not happy, and especially if there are children. Nonetheless, as suggested by Aswad, the pressure on women to remain in a marriage is stronger than for men. This condition applies even in cases of domestic violence, where the family may intervene to halt the violence but will also encourage the couple to make the marriage work. A study conducted in Chicago of barriers and resources for domestic violence interventions among Arab Americans found that the number one reason women did not leave a situation of domestic violence, as reported by survivors, their relatives, and social workers, was "pressure to remain in the marriage," followed by viewing "marriage as a family matter" and, thirdly, "the presence of children" (Cainkar & Del Toro, 2010). One survivor told the researchers:

> To walk out of your house on your husband is bad. This is how we're brought up and how we think ... It's not just walking out on your husband. It's walking out culturally. Maintaining a home is the cornerstone of our culture ... You're the guardian of all those responsibilities. (p. 24)

In addition to stigma and family pressures, woman's reticence to leave a marriage is exacerbated if she lacks job skills or other economic resources, has difficulty locating and maintaining alternative domestic arrangements, and fears losing her children to her husband's family (Cainkar & Del Toro, 2010; Hajjar, 2004). These problems are intensified for immigrant women, who may not speak English, may be living at great distances from their natal family, and may be disinclined to take their problems outside of the family. They may not seek the support of social workers or domestic violence shelters because of "fear, cultural differences, language barriers, and lack of understanding and capacity to negotiate the 'system'" (Cainkar & Del Toro, 2010, p. 6). These fears are only compounded when women who have initiated steps report being greeted by professionals acting on stereotypes, who assume that violence is endemic to their culture and offer an inadequate degree of compassion (Cainkar & Del Toro, 2010). In addition, some immigrant women may believe that their husbands will be deported if they call the police (Cainkar, 2000; Kulwicki & Miller, 1999) or that they will lose their own US permanent residency upon divorce (Cainkar & Del Toro, 2010). All of these factors highlight the importance of women's access to bilingual, culturally informed, and immigration law and VAWA (Violence Against Women Act) knowledgeable case-workers.

Just as families can pose barriers to women seeking to leave a violent marriage, the support of family was found to be the single most important factor leading to the successful conclusion of a domestic violence case, according to interviews with survivors, relatives, and social workers. As one survivor stated: "Family support is very important. Women who get support from their families can leave their husband" (Cainkar & Del Toro, 2010, p. 32). Social workers from within the Arab American community agreed that their most successful strategy has been helping women find one person in their or their husband's family who will advocate within the family on their behalf. Where this fails, culturally competent shelters and support services are the next most promising resources, but they are in limited supply in the United States.

The ways in which men and women experience family life shape gender relations in Arab culture. Differences between what boys and men and girls and women can or should do produce gendered variations in identity management, expressions of agency, and access to support in troubled times. There are further variations by family social class background, immigrant generation, and the degree to which the family and local ethnic community subscribe to traditional gender norms.

Expectations associated with roles within the family permeate the daily experiences of Arab Americans in ways that spill over into various life arenas including social relationships, education, and occupational pursuits. We turn next to relevant issues for gendered roles and relationships in the US context.

Arab Gendered Roles and Relationships in the US Context

The transference of traditional gender relations from other parts of the world to the United States has had mixed outcomes for many immigrant groups. Immigrants, in general, often maintain more traditional family lives than the American mainstream because there is a strong desire to maintain ethnic culture—something that happens primarily within the home (i.e., through the cooking of ethnic meals, socialization of the children, etc.). Immigrant groups also view the preservation of female chastity and traditional gender roles as mechanisms for asserting moral superiority over mainstream American culture, and co-ethnic communities often exert pressure on families to keep women out of the labor market altogether or only work intermittently in order to maintain these boundaries (Espiritu, 2001; Gibson, 1988). At the same time, women often make modest gains in independence and decision-making ability that reflect an improvement in status vis-à-vis gender relations in their countries of origin. Conversely, men often lose status and power with migration, putting even greater pressure on women to conform to traditional roles in order to maintain family stability.

The degree to which Arab cultural values influence attitudes and behaviors among Arab American women is less clear, however. This group is not monolithic, and variations in Arab American attitudes on social issues suggest mixed outcomes for women's achievement. For example, some Arab Americans feel that adhering to cultural traditions is essential for maintaining an ethnic identity and believe that women should remain in the home, with primary responsibility for the family (e.g., Aswad & Bilge, 1996; Ghanea Bassiri, 1997; Haddad & Lummis, 1987). Other Arab Americans evince attitudes more in keeping with American ideals of gender egalitarianism, supporting women's education and employment (e.g., Haddad & Smith, 1994; Keck, 1989).

Immigrant parents' ability to transmit culture and national and/or religious identity to their children often hinges on these gender roles (Ajrouch, 1999; Cainkar, 1988, 2004; Read & Oselin, 2008). Arab families supported by the social capital found in co-ethnic community members transmit familiar and personally experienced gendered norms and behavioral codes to their children and identify them as ways of being Arab, or Palestinian, or Lebanese, or Egyptian (in other words, a national identity), and/or of being Muslim. In doing so, they are instilling in their children both ways of being (acting) and ways of belonging to the group(s) (membership) their parents have chosen to prioritize (Levitt & Glick Schiller, 2004), while setting them apart from the dominant American culture in which they live (selective acculturation). A greater number of behavioral prescriptions are imposed on females than males, especially in the American context where distancing is expected, requiring that young women engage in more complex "negotiation between sets of values and cultural ideals that often seem incompatible" than young men (Shakir, 1997, p. 10).

Additionally, the behaviors of women are embedded with substantially more meaning for the honor of the family then those of men, placing a far greater burden of optimum performance on females. Research by Ajrouch (2004) among Lebanese American Muslims in the Detroit area found that second generation children of Arab immigrants used gendered behavior codes as boundary markers to differentiate between themselves and other Americans and to articulate their Arab Americanness. According to Ajrouch (2004, p. 380), "The boundaries that signify ethnic identity for the adolescents draw heavily on articulations about appropriate feminine behavior" a pattern of ethnic identity formation not unique to Arab Americans. Put succinctly, Arab American girls and women are understood by Arab American community members as different from and better than "American" girls and women because Arab females control their sexuality. They show they are doing so (perform by the rules) by limiting their (observable) contacts with males outside of the family, by their demeanor in public, and by dressing modestly, which can range from shunning provocative clothing to wearing concealing clothing, such as a *jilbaab*, *baltu*, and/or *hijab* (long coat, long wrap, head covering, respectively).

Sarroub's (2005) research on Yemeni American girls in Dearborn, MI, found that these girls spoke, walked, sat, and studied in ways that bridged the two worlds in which they lived—Yemeni and American—and that they remained vigilant to Yemeni expectations of honor and modesty and limited their relationships with non-Yemenis and Yemeni males. Sarroub narrates the "in-betweenness" that characterizes these girls' daily lives as they negotiate between varying and sometimes conflicting expectations emerging from the family, the Yemeni community, their own aspirations, and the norms and values of mainstream American society. Yemeni American girls "maintained dual identities according to the gendered, economic, and cultural spaces they inhabited" (p. 44), illuminating their own agency. At junctures that required reflection on how their choice of action might affect other Yemenis' perceptions of them, the girls "were forced to imagine Yemen as their homeland," a device that allowed them to make appropriate decisions. Although the Yemeni American community is not normative for Arab Americans because it is more conservative, has lower-income, and a lower rate of family migration than other Arab American groups, these insights are instructive: the school-based experiences identified by Sarroub convey a flavor of the social pressures that bear on many Arab American girls, influencing their formation of social relationships.

The other side of this cultural dance lies in the requirement that males behave in ways that do not thwart the efforts of girls and women to perform honorably. A normative mode of young Arab American male behavior is to have two sets of codes, one for Arab women and girls and one for everyone else. Although both young men and women are subject to family and community views regarding dating and marriage, boys are much freer to do as they wish outside the Arab American community and prior to marriage. Yet the state of "in-betweenness" that is created when one moves daily within two cultures, a condition that nonetheless applies to both male and female Arab Americans, can provoke a sense that one is an outsider in both cultures. In her Epilogue to *Bint Arab*, the anthology of Arab and Arab American women's writing, Evelyn Shakir (p. 196) writes a letter to her deceased mother that expresses well the challenges for second generation Arab Americans, and especially women, who negotiate two cultural places:

> This house, this text, is full of voices tumbling over one another. ... Issues worried in every room, on every story (in every story) from generation to generation: how to be a good daughter, sister, wife, mother, how to be a good Arab, how (pay good heed) to survive. ... Hearts divided between two urges. The need to make a getaway (crash out the back door, run for your life), the need to belong (pull up to the table with women who you call "sister" and know your people for three generations back). ... And finally, after half a lifetime staring out the window, planting in the garden, smiling at the neighbors, passage into a new identity, neither *arab* nor *ameerkan* (italics in original).

Two major methodological limitations must be addressed in considering the research on gender and Arab Americans. First, is the fact that the majority of studies on dynamics of gender relations have been addressed primarily in community-based studies that focus on one national origin or religious group (Ajrouch, 2004; Cainkar, 1999; Sarroub, 2005). As a result, generalizations about Arab American experiences tend to be skewed toward those of individuals living in higher concentration areas with those of the same national origin or religious background. An exception is the work carried out by (Read, 2004; Read & Oselin, 2008), who uses both the US Census data as well as other survey data to document the situation of women. These more nationally representative portraits suggest that women living in ethnic enclaves experience greater pressure to conform to traditional gender norms than do those living in more ethnically diverse areas. Second, much of the work on gender and Arab Americans emphasizes the experiences of women. We know little about how masculinity ideals inform the lives of Arab American boys and men and even less about negotiations of gender identity and sexuality. This is problematic because it contributes inadvertently to the perpetuation of stereotypes of Arab women by disproportionately emphasizing their individual experiences relative to those of men and to those of other family members. Nevertheless, an increasing number of studies are debunking common myths of Arab women by highlighting their achievements in the public sphere, as detailed in the next section.

Achievements in Education and Employment

Despite a persistent respect for certain norms and values, neither Arab culture nor Arab American culture is monolithic or static. Additionally, every generation evidences changes, so that, for example, women generally see their lives as better than those of their mothers (Cainkar, 1996).

Moreover, statistics show that Arab Americans (men and women) surpass the overall American population on a range of measures of success. It is likely that it is here where the positive impacts of strong family, collective responsibility, and selective acculturation are most strongly observed and quantified. Arab Americans post higher rates of educational attainment than the US population as a whole, and this exceptional pattern applies to both women and men and to every Arab nationality group. Census 2000 found that 41 % of Arab Americans age 25 and older, and 36 % of Arab American women, held a bachelor's degree or higher, compared to 24 % of the American population as a whole (Census, 2000; Read & Oselin, 2008).

Estimates derived from the 2009 American Community Survey (ACS) indicated even larger discrepancies between Arab Americans and the US population as a whole: 41.5 % of Arab American women and 48 % of Arab American men had a bachelor's degree or higher, compared to 28 % and 27 %, respectively, of the US population as a whole (Census, 2010). These rates of educational attainment reflect a mix of values, ambitions, and strategies acted upon in a place where educational opportunity is widely available, and to some degree the selective migration of highly educated Arabs. Even within Arab American communities that are particularly conservative and where there is pressure on girls to marry young, continuing education after high school is considered a legitimate female strategy to delay marriage, whereas working for pay or staying at home would likely propel one quickly into the marriage market (see, e.g., Malek, 2005). One outcome of this female strategy is gendered imbalances in educational attainment in some Arab American communities, where girls may study more diligently and become more educated than their male counterparts, who face pressures to work to support the family during and after high school. Sarroub's (2005) study of Yemeni American high school girls in Dearborn, MI, found that their mean GPAs were higher than those of non-Arab girls and much higher than those of Yemeni boys, for whom grades were not as important as working. Sarroub also found that Yemeni families valued high grades and diligent study habits for girls, which were interpreted as reflecting self-discipline. Arab American families closer to the norm are middle class and less likely to pressure young men to work before completing college, while exhibiting family level variation on whether girls are encouraged to complete college before marriage or vice versa. High socioeconomic status generally correlates with high premarital educational attainment for males and females alike.

The expected relationships between educational attainment and labor force participation, however, do not play out for Arab Americans. Two unique and gendered patterns are particularly salient. First, research has shown that for many Arab Americans education is not necessarily viewed primarily as an instrumental means to a specific career, although it can be. University education may instead be viewed as a family resource that serves different purposes for women and men. Read and Oselin (2008, p. 301) studied this phenomenon as it applies to Arab American women, piqued by the large discrepancy in Census 2000 data between their educational attainment and labor force participation rates, where the former are quite high but the latter, at 66.5 %, were "below that of most other US ethnic groups of women." Normative American patterns and gender theory posit a direct and positive relationship between women's educational attainment and their labor force participation rates, yet this relationship does not hold for Arab American women. Among Arab

American women, whether Christian or Muslim, education is interpreted as having mainly instrumental parenting and family value. "Lower employment rates are almost entirely due to cultural preferences for traditional gender roles, which are maintained through relationships and ethnic networks," according to Read and Oselin (2008, p. 302). Arab women who are immigrants and native-born Arab American women who live in ethnic enclaves are the most likely to subscribe to these cultural preferences that view women's education as a family resource that "ensures the transmission of Arab cultural values and religious beliefs (Muslim or Christian) to the children, provides status and honor to the family, and works to maintain ethnic and religious boundaries with the American mainstream" (p. 307).

In light of the fact that educated Arab American women, whether immigrant or US-born, may choose not to enter the paid labor force even with a college education, it is quite incorrect to interpret that a stay at home Arab American mother is an uneducated woman, or a woman lacking in aspirations. Yet Arab American women have repeatedly described being treated this way in a range of settings during interviews that span Cainkar's research career. Similarly, Arab American women who aspire to domesticity, whether highly educated or not, should not be instantly understood as oppressed by their male kin; they may be acting with agency on a value system they believe in, one that prioritizes family. Read and Oselin (2008, p. 309) found that the many of the women they interviewed were "satisfied with their roles" and should therefore be expected to transmit these values to their daughters. At the same time, Read and Oselin surmised that the higher overall labor force participation rate of US-born second generation Arab American women (78 %, compared to 59 % for immigrant Arab American women), which was nearly parallel to the overall US rate for women, indicated that interactions with mainstream American society are causing some traditional gender "cultural schemas" to lose their force. Read (2004) concluded that traditional gender ideologies are most likely to be found among women who remain within Arab ethnic social circles, subscribe mainly to ethnic organizations, and have an Arab spouse. It appears that women exhibiting social capital with high ethnic traits are most likely to adhere to traditional gender ideologies, in part because these gender ideologies promote the attainment of social capital for women in order to provide greater stability to the family (Read & Oselin, 2008). She further concluded that cultural assimilation is occurring: comparing Arab women who migrated more recently to women who were born in the United States and women who migrated more than 20 years ago, support for traditional gender roles is lowest among American-born women and somewhat lower among women who have been in the United States for decades. Indeed, length of time in the United States appears to have more influence on women's gender ideologies than other factors, intimating more of an overall cultural assimilation as opposed to segmented assimilation.

When Arab American women enter the labor force, both in the United States and the Arab world, the type of work they prefer is significantly influenced by cultural notions about appropriate work for women, which generally preclude hard manual labor and work seen as dangerous; although less limiting, Arab men are not immune from cultural prejudices about dignified work. While women have always engaged in hard manual agricultural work, such work is seen as family work and therefore private. In the United States and the Arab world, women engaged in formal, paid work are most likely to be in the fields of teaching (much less so in the United States), in the sales and service sectors catering to women, and in arenas such as banking, restaurant management, government employment, and for those with the appropriate degrees, medical, dental, pharmaceutical, and legal professions. Notions about appropriate work and work contexts for women pose the largest challenges for Arab American women seeking work who have a high school or less education and for Arab refugees (e.g., Iraqis, Sudanese, and Somalis), who are required to work for pay shortly after arrival in the United States in order to qualify their families for social welfare benefits. Refugee resettlement agencies generally place new refugees in companies where they have built ongoing relationships, and these are highly likely to be in the manufacturing, meat slaughtering, and cleaning industries. Between little experience of such work in the Arab world and a general cultural disdain for the type of work, both male and female refugees experience loss of dignity in these jobs (Cainkar, 1999).

While Arab American men do not exhibit the same divergences from US labor force norms as Arab American women, they exhibit their own anomalies. Many college-educated and a substantial proportion of noncollege-educated Arab American men ultimately become entrepreneurs, working in commercial and professional sectors of the economy (Cainkar, 1999). Census 2000 data indicated that some 42 % of employed Arab Americans aged 16 and older worked in management, professional, and related occupations, compared with 34 % of the overall US population, and another 30 % worked in sales and office occupations, compared with 27 % of the overall US population, accounting for more than 70 % of Arab American workers (Brittingham & de la Cruz, 2005). More recent 2009 ACS data showed that 42 % of Arab American men worked in management, professional, and related occupations, as compared to 33 % of the male US population overall, and 27 % of Arab American men were in sales and office occupations, as compared to 18 % of the US male population overall, these two occupational sectors accounting for nearly 70 % of Arab American male workers. Arab American women show similarly high rates of management, professional, and related occupations, 48 % as compared to 39 % for the US female population overall, but fall below the US norm in sales and office occupations (30.5 % as compared to 33 %), a statistic that is not surprising in light of the fact that a large proportion of non-Arab American females in these sectors are sales clerks and secretaries rather than entrepreneurs (2009 ACS data). The propensity for entrepreneurial work is characteristically Arab American (as well as in the global Arab diaspora) and has been documented throughout 100 years of Arab American history (e.g., Cainkar, 2009; Elkholy, 1966; Hooglund, 1985, 1987; Naff, 1985; Orfalea, 2006). The social capital embedded in ethnic social networks that transmit skills, provide loans, and identify entrepreneurial opportunities drives the continuing Arab American presence in these economic niches, along with, some believe, a cultural tendency for self-employment and trade, as well as perceptions of discrimination in mainstream employment sectors.

Prior research in the Chicago metropolitan area identified important variations among Arab Americans working in the retail sector that were correlated with immigrant generation, social class, and education, as well as gendered patterns of work related to work hours and business locations (Cainkar, 1999). Arab American men who work as clerks in the retail sector tend to be immigrants who are employed by Arab American small business owners (who may also be immigrants). While Arab American business owners may expect moderate to high incomes from these enterprises, clerk employees work very long hours, and are away from home a substantial amount of time, at wages that place their families below the poverty level. Some scholars believe that the absence of the male head of family from the home for long hours results in stricter households with inflexible rules, especially for teenage girls, although no systematic study has been conducted on this matter. College-educated men with family financial resources may engage in a period of clerkship as training for their own family business and later experience upward economic mobility, but men with a high school education or less and few family financial resources often remain stuck in this low-income occupation, unable to pull their family out of poverty. In this scenario and with welfare reform, immigrant Arab American women who seek to raise their families out of poverty have begun working in various low-skill sales and service occupations, although many do so quite hesitantly because of the aforementioned belief that women should be at home to guide their children's upbringing. These women are not as likely as Arab American men to be working at Arab American retail businesses largely due to the long work hours required and because a preponderance of Arab American retail businesses are located in low-income urban neighborhoods perceived as dangerous. In light of an increase in Arab American immigrant women seeking work for economic reasons yet unable to tap into Arab ethnic networks for jobs, the job discrimination they report (particularly women in *hijab*) is particularly economically damaging.

The 2009 ACS reported a poverty rate of 14.5 % for Arab American families, compared to 10.5 % for the overall US population. Similarly, Census 2000 reported that some 17 % of Arab Americans lived in poverty, compared with 12 % of the overall US population. Arab Americans at the lower end of the income curve tend to be members of refugee families and recent immigrants without college education; the highest rates of poverty in Census 2000 were shown for Iraqis and especially Iraqi children (41%). Overall, however, Arab Americans report higher median household and family incomes than the US population as a whole. According to 2009 ACS data, the Arab American median household income was $54,749 and the median family income was $65,843, as compared to $50,221 and $61,082, respectively, for the US population as a whole. Census 2000 data showed similar economic advantages for Arab Americans and found that Arab men and women earned more than men and women in the general population. In 1999, median earnings for Arab American men working year-round, full-time were $41,700 as compared to $37,100 for men in the general population. Arab American women posted median earnings of $31,800 as compared to $27,200 for women in the general population. There were substantial variations among Arab Americans: men of Lebanese and Syrian ancestry earned significantly more than Iraqi, Jordanian, and "other

Arab" men; women of Egyptian ancestry had the highest earnings and women of Moroccan ancestry the lowest; and as indicated in the above data, there is a significant gender gap between male and female earnings.

While Census data have been invaluable in identifying trends and profiles of educational levels and occupational status for men and women, they have their limitations. First, it is unclear the extent to which the events of September 11, 2001, affected the responsiveness of Arab Americans to data collection efforts by government agencies (e.g., the ACS). Those of lower socioeconomic backgrounds and/or newer immigrants are likely to be the most cautious in participating, thus the data may be skewed toward those in higher socioeconomic categories. Second, as is the case with quantitative data more generally, Census data do not provide a means for understanding the processes and motivations behind educational and occupational trajectories. As Read and Oselin (2008) found in their qualitative study of women, the meaning of education in Arab communities can diverge drastically from traditional western conceptions that view it as an individual commodity to be used in the market for profit. Rather, women's education provides social capital for the family, which results in benefits for the collective rather than the individual (via boundary maintenance, socialization of children, etc.).

Arab American Women and Men: Challenges After 9/11

A chapter on Arab Americans and gender would be incomplete without addressing the contemporary historical context in our post-9/11 era. Commonly held understandings in American culture about Arab and Muslim women and men have evolved into negative stereotypes that have at certain historic moments been used by parties with specific interests to provoke hatred, as blunt instruments of repression, and to build support for war. As anthropologist Nadine Naber (2000, p. 44) has stated: "imaginary portrayals of gender relations among both the dominated and the dominant group are used to further justify lived colonialist, imperialist, racist and patriarchal practices." The alleged relationship between *hijab* and oppression and the notion of saving Muslim women from Muslim men was a core theme invoked to garner public support the US invasion of Afghanistan after the 9/11 attacks (Abu-Lughod, 2002). Indeed, photos of women in *hijab* have been central to constructing Arab and Muslim societies as places where the American ideals of freedom and individual liberty are absent (a premise whose falsity was revealed by the revolutions for freedom occurring across the Arab World in 2011).

In addition, the more recent revival of religiosity and heightened adherence to religious prescriptions among Muslims globally has brought about gendered cultural changes that many in the West view as "backward," such as increasing use of *hijab* (modesty, covering) among Muslim women. Often viewed simplistically from the outside as a condition forced on women by men, the assumption of compulsion hides the complexities of social belonging and women's agency that exist around veiling (Bartkowski & Read, 2003; El Guindi, 1999; Read & Bartowski, 2000) as well as the ways in which "veiled women" express their individuality and style (Tarlo, 2010). El Guindi (1999, p. 184) described women's decisions to wear *hijab* in Egypt as statements of "liberation from imposed, imported identities, consumerist behaviors, and an increasingly materialist culture." Embedded within wearing *hijab*, continues El Guindi, "is imagery that combines notions of respectability, morality, identity, and resistance." Scholars long ago observed that asserting the dignity of components of self, including one's cultural choices and expressions of religious faith, has largely positive psychological and social consequences, whereas rejecting integral parts of the self because of social prejudices may be psychologically damaging and socially disruptive (Du Bois, 1903; Fanon, 1952/1967).

Arab American males and females may verbalize support for and comply with gendered cultural norms in part because they agree with them, but also because *not* doing so implies capitulation to the prejudices of others, and in such capitulation lays a loss of personal self-dignity. Such tensions illustrate the agency of Arab Americans. This principle may apply to a whole range of behaviors such as taking personal responsibility for the care of other family members, respecting parental authority, acknowledging that one's public behavior reflects upon family, agreeing that one's primary role in the family is dictated by gender, and accepting an arranged marriage and/or that one should marry within the extended family. Thus, a Muslim woman wearing a headscarf might be understood similarly through both meanings, religious and social, the former expressing the dignity of the individual in the presence of God, the latter expressing the dignity of Muslims in the context of social derision. The social meaning is perhaps better understood in its negation: removing a headscarf largely because doing so reduces prejudice and discrimination contains within it an element of accepting its "wrongness." A fundamental question around these issues of choice, or agency, is whether everyone has access to American freedom or whether it has culturally bound limits that can exclude certain practices.

Nevertheless, many in the United States view wearing *hijab* as symbolic of women's submission to patriarchal men and assume that once Muslim women migrate to the United States they will exercise their new freedom and remove their "veils." When women don't do this, it is taken as further proof of male domination, now carried across the ocean and poised to threaten the American way of life. On the other hand, when women say they wear *hijab* by choice it is interpreted as rejection of American freedom. *Hijab* is counterposed to being American and it is such ideas that led to widespread attacks on women in *hijab* after 9/11 (Cainkar, 2009; Read, 2007). One in-depth sociological study found that women reported experiencing hate acts at a rate more than double that of men, 64 % vs. 30 %, and that a woman wearing *hijab* (in these cases a head scarf) was present in more than 90 % of the hate incidents reported by Arab Muslim women and more than half of those reported by men (Cainkar, 2009). Women were subjected to assault, road rage, spitting, hostile graffiti on their homes, and a host of hostile hand signals and comments. As one woman stated, "Literally, I could not leave my apartment because I was scared to leave and lived in fear. For the first time in my life, I was fearful for my life." Arab and Muslim men did not escape this period without harm, as gendered notions cast them as security threats, placing them under the watchful eye of government and resulting in tens of thousands (if not more) being subjected to arrest without charge, interrogation, special registration, deportation, frozen bank accounts, and other security measures. Thus, even post-9/11 backlash was gendered, with Arab/Muslim men pinned with being inherently violent and anti-American, and Arab/Muslim women, especially women wearing *hijab*, perceived as threats to American culture and its way of life.

Again, there are methodological issues related to data collection efforts in a post-9/11 world. First, we have seen the emergence of new sources of funding from governmental entities such as the Department of Homeland Security and the Department of Defense, but these are difficult for researchers to use because of the fear and mistrust it would likely invoke among Arab Americans. In addition, and as mentioned previously, research about gender is disproportionately focused on the experiences of women, with much less attention on Arab men, who continue to be stereotyped as violent and oppressive. Without empirical data, we may assume that these stereotypes will continue to hinder the assimilation of Arab American men and women, alike.

Conclusions for Health

The literature reviewed above has multiple implications for Arab American health. Perhaps the single most important implication is that Arab Americans are not monolithic on numerous factors known to be associated with health: immigrant status, educational attainment, occupation, and so on. In terms of the focus of this chapter, we know that gendered roles are important for health outcomes among all Americans, regardless of nativity or ethnicity (Read & Gorman, 2010). Men and women in the United States occupy different social roles that shape their experiences of health and their interactions with the health care system. For men in general, research consistently finds that pressures to conform to hegemonic ideals of masculinity make them reluctant to seek health care. We need more research to verify that similar factors influence health-seeking behavior among Arab American men.

For women, evidence suggests that women's multiple role combinations have implications for their health, often in more concrete ways than suggested by psychosocial explanations alone. Women's domestic and familial roles place them in contact with the health care system more frequently than men to seek care for themselves as well as their children and elderly family members, which in turn might make women more aware of their health problems than men (Lillard & Waite, 1995). Given women's key role in upholding culture among Arab Americans, especially in family relations, we would expect Arab American women to mirror the situation of other women in US society. Thus apparent disparities in men's and women's health may partly reflect differences in their utilization of care, which in turn affects knowledge of their health conditions. Again, agency is a key factor in these experiences. As Bird and Rieker (2008) argue, health outcomes are shaped by the constraints that are placed on men's and women's health-related choices. Women's (and men's) decisions are made within a context of constraints that often inhibit their expression of agency.

This can be particularly true for immigrants entering into new contexts with new, less familiar constraints. Immigrant men are often charged with the economic security of the family, leaving immigrant women responsible for other domains of social life, including the well-being of household members. In this context, obstacles such as lack of health insurance and poor language skills become less of a barrier to seeking health care for immigrant women because their status within the home and community depends, in large part, on fulfilling these duties, thus women are more likely than men to seek care for themselves or other family members, regardless of the obstacles (Hattar-Pollara & Meleis, 1995). At the same time, strict interpretations of gender relations that include preventing any physical contact between women and men (other than immediate family members) might serve as obstacles to women seeking care in a health care environment heavily dominated by males.

Further, gender plays an important role in the decision to migrate. Women's motivations for migrating are more likely to be based on family and less likely to be based on employment than are men's, implying that the likelihood of selectively migrating based on good health is weaker among Arab American women than men. Arab women's education and employment rates are extremely low across countries in the Middle East, and many remain low after arriving in the United States, leaving women with fewer resources needed to prevent and cure disease.

Another important implication for health is the role of family in Arab culture. The social capital found in Arab families can serve as barriers or resources, depending on the circumstances. Families with high social capital in tight-knit ethnic communities may feel greater pressure to restrict women's interactions in a largely male US health care system, whereas those in more ethnically diverse communities may be free of those expectations. The role of Arab families also varies extensively by social class, nativity, and national origin, thus it is critical to acknowledge this diversity. Wealthy Arab families can look completely different than Arab families in poverty, even if they share the same national origin and generational status. Moreover, the extent to which Arab families enforce a strict division of gender roles is contextual and circumstance-specific, such that behaviors in one setting may differ from those enacted in another. Furthermore, the agency identified among women in particular illustrates circumstances in which they navigate two worlds, that of the immigrant and that of mainstream America. Such tensions may inform experiences of psychological distress. Indeed, segmented assimilation may be somewhat gendered in that men are pressured to succeed and achieve the American dream while women are encouraged to become cultural carriers for the Arab American community. Such divergent expectations may yield health behaviors that vary with men adopting lifestyle and habits more in line with mainstream American culture while women retain more of the practices found in the homeland (e.g., diet). The main conclusion from this is that health care providers need to be aware of these nuances. As Aswad (2005) stressed, counselors unfamiliar with the Arab American community need to be cognizant of the important role family plays in the lives of Arab American women and men and avoid imposing American cultural norms that assume independence on their Arab American clients. Moreover, the various roles that men and women hold in families may be illuminated through the concepts of social capital, segmented assimilation, and agency, each revealing key insights into various health issues.

Finally, the horrific events of September 11, 2001, and the continued acts of violent extremism globally that are often incorrectly associated with Arabs have had serious physical and mental health ramifications for Arab Americans. Health researchers increasingly find that mental and physical health are intricately connected and can influence each other over time. Studies show that physical health problems increase the likelihood of depression over time, and depression increases the likelihood of developing a physical health condition. Many Arab Americans continue to struggle with issues of identity and feelings of marginalization and disempowerment in the post-9/11 era. The nature and quality of social capital available may serve as important coping mechanisms, or conversely exacerbate health as it becomes overly strained in attempts to attenuate such stress. The extent to which a sense of agency may be exercised to navigate such tensions may vary by gender where women and men face unique challenges (e.g., men profiled as terrorist; women viewed as subservient). For health researchers and practitioners, this requires additional attention to the complex link between mental and physical well-being.

References

Abu-Lughod, L. (2002). Do Muslim women really need saving? Anthropological reflections on cultural relativism and its others. *American Anthropologist, 104*(3), 783–790.

Ajrouch, K. J. (1999). Family and ethnic identity in an Arab American community. In M. Suleiman (Ed.), *Arabs in America: Building a new future* (pp. 129–139). Philadelphia: Temple University Press.

Ajrouch, K. J. (2004). Gender, race, and symbolic boundaries: Contested spaces of identity among Arab American adolescents. *Sociological Perspectives, 47*(4), 371–391.

Ajrouch, K. J., & Kusow, A. (2007). Racial and religious contexts: Situational identities among Lebanese and Somali Muslim immigrants. *Ethnic and Racial Studies, 30*(1), 72–94.

Aswad, B. (1999). Attitudes of Arab immigrants toward welfare. In M. Suleiman (Ed.), *Arabs in America: Building a new future* (pp. 177–191). Philadelphia, PA: Temple University Press.

Aswad, B. (2005). Family relations: The United States. In S. Joseph (Ed.), *Encyclopedia of women and Islamic cultures* (pp. 147–151). Leiden, NL: Brill.

Aswad, B., & Bilge, B. (Eds.). (1996). *Family and gender among American Muslims: Issues facing Middle Eastern immigrants and their descendants*. Philadelphia, PA: Temple University Press.

Bartkowski, J. P., & Read, J. G. (2003). Veiled submission: Gender, power, and identity among evangelical and Muslim women in the United States. *Qualitative Sociology, 26*(1), 71–92.

Bird, C. E., & Rieker, P. (2008). *Gender and health: The effects of constrained choices and social policies*. New York: Cambridge University Press.

Brittingham, A., & de la Cruz, G. P. (2005). *We the people of Arab ancestry in the United States*. Washington, DC: U.S. Census Bureau.

Cainkar, L. (1988). *Palestinian Muslim women in the United States: Coping with tradition, change, and alienation.* Unpublished doctoral dissertation, Northwestern University, Evanston, IL.

Cainkar, L. (1996). Palestinian women: A generational perspective. In B. Aswad & B. Bilge (Eds.), *Family and gender among American Muslims* (pp. 41–58). Philadelphia, PA: Temple University Press.

Cainkar, L. (1999). The deteriorating ethnic safety net among Arabs in Chicago. In M. Suleiman (Ed.), *Arabs in America: Building a new future* (pp. 192–206). Philadelphia, PA: Temple University Press.
Cainkar, L. (2000). *The Iraqi community in Chicago*. Washington, DC: The Iraq Foundation Community Assessment Project.
Cainkar, L. (2004). Islamic revival among second-generation Arab Americans: The American experience and globalization intersect. *Bulletin of the Royal Institute for Inter-Faith Studies, 6*(2), 99–120.
Cainkar, L. (2009). *Homeland insecurity: The Arab American and Muslim American experience after 9/11*. New York, NY: Russell Sage Foundation Press.
Cainkar, L. (2011, August). *The role of transnational selective acculturation in American being, belonging, and success*. Paper presented at the Annual American Sociological Association Meetings, Las Vegas, NV.
Cainkar, L., & Del Toro, S. (2010). *Barriers, resources, and best practice strategies for working with domestic violence cases in Arab and Muslim American communities*. Chicago: Arab American Action Network.
Coleman, J. S. (1990). *Foundations of social theory*. Cambridge, MA: Harvard University Press.
Du Bois, W. E. B. (1903). *The souls of black folk*. New York, NY: Bantam Classic.
El Guindi, F. (1999). *Veil: Modesty, privacy and resistance*. Oxford: Berg.
Elkholy, A. (1966). *The Arab Moslems in the United States*. New Haven, CT: College.
Espiritu, Y. L. (2001). 'We don't sleep around like white girls do': Family, culture, and gender in Filipina American lives. *Signs, 26*, 414–440.
Fanon, F. (1967). *Black skin, white masks* (C. L. Markmann, Trans.). New York: Grove Press. (Original work published 1952)
Ghanea Bassiri, K. (1997). *Competing visions of Islam in the United States: A study of Los Angeles*. Westport, CT: Greenwood.
Gibson, M. A. (1988). *Accommodation without assimilation: Sikh immigrants in an American high school*. Ithaca, NY: Cornell University Press.
Giddens, A. (1984). *The constitution of society: Outline of a theory of structuration*. Berkeley, CA: University of California Press.
Haddad, Y., & Lummis, A. (1987). *Islamic values in the United States: A comparative study*. New York: Oxford University Press.
Haddad, Y., & Smith, J. I. (Eds.). (1994). *Muslim communities in North America*. Albany, NY: SUNY Press.
Hajjar, L. (2004). Religion, state power, and domestic violence in Muslim societies: A framework for comparative analysis. *Law & Social Inquiry, 29*(1), 1–38.
Hattar-Pollara, M., & Meleis, A. (1995). The stress of immigration and the daily lived experiences of Jordanian immigrant women in the United-States. *Western Journal of Nursing Research, 17*, 521–539.
Hoogland, E. (1985). *Taking root: Arab-American community studies* (Vol. II). Washington, DC: ADC Research Institute, The American-Arab Anti-Discrimination Committee.
Hooglund, E. (Ed.). (1987). *Crossing the waters, Arabic-speaking immigrants to the United States before 1940*. Washington, DC: Smithsonian Institution Press.
Keck, L. (1989). Egyptian Americans in the Washington, DC area. In B. Abu-Laban & M. Suleiman (Eds.), *Arab Americans: Continuity and change* (pp. 103–126). Belmont, MA: Association of Arab-American University Graduates.
Kulwicki, A., & Miller, J. (1999). Domestic violence in the Arab American population: Transforming environmental conditions through community Education. *Mental Health Nursing, 20*(3), 199–216.
Levitt, P., & Glick Schiller, N. (2004). Conceptualizing simultaneity: A transnational social field perspective on society. *International Migration Review, 38*(3), 1002–1039.
Lillard, L. A., & Waite, L. J. (1995). 'Til death do us part': Marital disruption and mortality. *The American Journal of Sociology, 100*, 1131–1156.

Malek, A. (2005). Why are we always fighting and what are we fighting for? Alternating defensive postures and the relevance of rights to Arab and Arab-American women. *The MIT Electronic Journal of Middle East Studies, 5*, 169–181.

Naber, N. (2000). Ambiguous insiders: An investigation of Arab American invisibility. *Ethnic and Racial Studies, 23*(1), 37–61.

Naff, A. (1985). *Becoming American: The early Arab immigrant experience*. Carbondale, IL: Southern Illinois University Press.

Orfalea, G. (2006). *The Arab Americans: A history*. Northampton, MA: Interlink.

Portes, A. (1996). *The new second generation*. New York: Russell Sage.

Portes, A., & Rumbaut, R. G. (2006). *Immigrant America: A portrait*. Berkeley, CA: University of California Press.

Portes, A., & Zhou, M. (1993). The new second generation: Segmented assimilation and its variants. *The Annals of the American Academy of Political and Social Science, 530*(1), 74–96.

Read, J. G. (2004). *Culture, class, and work among Arab American women*. New York, NY: LFB Scholarly.

Read, J. G. (2007). The politics of veiling in comparative perspective. *Sociology of Religion, 68*, 231–236.

Read, J. G., & Bartowski, J. P. (2000). To veil or not to veil? A case study of identity negotiation among Muslim women in Austin, Texas. *Gender and Society, 14*, 395–417.

Read, J. G., & Gorman, B. (2010). Gender and U.S. health inequality. *Annual Review of Sociology, 36*, 371–386.

Read, J. G., & Oselin, S. (2008). Gender and the education-employment paradox in ethnic and religious contexts: The case of Arab Americans. *American Sociological Review, 73*, 296–313.

Sarroub, L. (2005). *All American Yemeni girls, being Muslim in a public school*. Philadelphia, PA: University of Pennsylvania Press.

Shakir, E. (1997). *Bint Arab. Arab and Arab American women in the United States*. Westport, CT: Praeger.

Tarlo, E. (2010). *Visibly Muslim: Fashion, politics, faith*. Oxford: Berg.

U.S. Bureau of the Census. (2000). *Census of population and housing. Public-use microdata samples*. Washington, DC: U.S. Government Printing Office.

U.S. Bureau of the Census. (2010). Selected population profile in the United States: Arabs (400–415, 417–418, 421–430, 435–481, 490–499) Table: S0201, 2010 American Community Survey 1-year estimates. American Community Survey.

Zhou, M. (1997). Segmented assimilation: Issues, controversies, and recent research on the new second generation. *International Migration Review, 31*(4), 825–858.

Zhou, M., & Bankston, C. (1998). *Growing up American: How Vietnamese children adapt to life in the United States*. New York, NY: Russell Sage.

Chapter 6
Arab Americans and the Aging Process

Sawsan Abdulrahim and Kristine J. Ajrouch

Background

Aging may be viewed as a developmental process marking human experience from the moment we arrive into the world until we die. The study of aging, however, generally draws our attention to the latter part of the life course. We use chronological age (i.e., birth date) to identify adults as relatively older. Though legally in the USA adults aged 65 and above are traditionally considered to have entered old age, we use 60 years as the beginning point in our discussion of research on the Arab American aging experience. This demarcation recognizes that ethnic minorities often use other indicators such as social roles (e.g., becoming a grandparent) to mark entrance into later life.

Perceptions of aging are culturally constructed. The status of older adults and their well-being in any society is an outcome of an intricate relationship between cultural norms and social constraints. In traditional Arab culture, where family and religion play a central role in social organization, aging is viewed positively and older family members are held in high esteem and revered (El-Kholy, 1988). The traditional view of Arab families is that they are extended, patriarchal, and intact (Barakat, 1985), allowing parents to age in a multigenerational family environment and to receive needed support from adult children. One theoretical framework advances that Arab families operate through patriarchal connective arrangements whereby the personal self fits into fluid gendered and aged structures (Joseph, 2000).

S. Abdulrahim (✉)
Faculty of Health Sciences, American University of Beirut,
PO Box 11-0236, Riad El Solh, 1107 2020 Beirut, Lebanon
e-mail: sawsan.abdulrahim@gmail.com

K.J. Ajrouch
Sociology, Anthropology, Criminology, Eastern Michigan University,
712 Pray-Harrold, Ypsilanti, MI 48197, USA
e-mail: kajrouch@emich.edu

S.C. Nassar-McMillan et al. (eds.), *Biopsychosocial Perspectives on Arab Americans: Culture, Development, and Health*, DOI 10.1007/978-1-4614-8238-3_6,

Patriarchal connectivity provides a kin "contract" that protects (and privileges) men and older women who, with age, come to exert social control over younger men and women in the family. As the contract ascribes age–gender-based rules of exchange, an older adult invests her/his well-being in the actions of younger people to whom he/she is connected. Ultimately, older men are thought to wield a large amount of control in family relations because of cultural sanctions that allow men to direct the lives of women and youth. Hence, their sense of well-being rests heavily on relations with women and younger adults. Other work suggests that there may indeed be a gender crossover effect in old age. The strong role of older women in families suggests that there are certain perceived (but not guaranteed) "benefits" which motivate women to conform to the system in order to maximize their security in old age. In this way, women invest heavily in their children (particularly sons) in the hopes of receiving dividends in old age, especially those married and with male children (Kandiyoti, 1998; Olmsted, 2005; Yount, 2005). Indeed, women in Arab societies are thought to be generally advantaged over men in the informal economic exchanges that they receive in old age (Yount, 2005; Yount & Sibai, 2009). Migration, however, influences the structure of Arab families, interactions between members, and the well-being of older adults in them.

Arab American aging should be understood within the context of immigration so as to draw attention to cultural and social factors. Most of those who have researched and written on Arab immigration describe at least two separate waves (Abu-Laban, 1991; Naff, 1985; Orfalea, 1988). The first wave of Arab immigration to the USA began in the early 1900s (Naff, 1985; Orfalea, 1988). The majority were of the Christian faith, originating from modern-day Syria and Lebanon. Older adults descending from this wave were born in the USA, and though they often relate to their Arab ancestry, acculturated during a time where expectations mandated one to follow a European model of cultural assimilation as white ethnics. The second wave of Arab immigration began with changes in immigration law during the 1950s and mid to late 1960s, representing a markedly different group. They were more educated, more financially adept, more likely to be Muslim, and left their home countries under duress, due to political disputes and all-out warfare (Abu-Laban, 1991; Orfalea, 1988; Zogby, 1990). Whereas the first wave embraced American mores, the second wave waited much longer before settling in. Continuing political instabilities, wars, and occupations in the Arab region have been a factor in the near-constant stream of Arabic-speaking immigrants that have arrived since 1967, beginning with Palestinian and Lebanese immigrants (Abu-Laban, 1991; Orfalea, 1988). The latest group of migrants was Iraqi refugees whose numbers increased markedly since 1990 due to the succession of wars (Sirkeci, 2005). Older Arab Americans from this wave are immigrants, with some having grown old here while others arrived after the age of 60. With more attention to ethnicity in a post-civil rights era, descendants from this wave escaped pressure to shed all their cultural ways and hence are likely to retain more aspects of homeland culture including language, food preferences, and family relations.

Demographically, like other immigrants in the USA, those from Arabic-speaking countries tend to be younger compared to the general population (Brittingham &

de la Cruz, 2005). The 5 % Public Use Microdata Sample (PUMS) from 2000, which allows for gathering sociodemographic data on persons of Arab ancestry, revealed that out of 53,874 Arab Americans counted, 4,225 reported being aged 65 or older (Dallo, Al-Snih, & Ajrouch, 2009). Therefore, approximately 8 % of Arab Americans were legally defined as old in 2000 compared to 12 % in the overall population. According to the most recent Census data available via the American Community Survey (2007–2009), Arab Americans aged 65 or older comprise approximately 7.3 % of the national Arab American population (Arab American Institute Foundation, 2008).[1] Recent evidence, however, has highlighted a trend towards aging among Arab Americans (Kusow & Ajrouch, 2011). For example, the US Census data show immigrants from Lebanon reported a median age of 30 years old in 1980 and 39 years old in 2000. Similar patterns were observed among immigrants from Jordan (26 years old in 1980 and 36 years old in 2000), Egypt (35 years old in 1980; 42 years old in 2000), and Morocco (27 years old in 1980; 37 years old in 2000). This pattern parallels the general US population, which in 2000 reported a median age of 35 years old (Meyer, 2001).

Aging among Arab Americans in the USA represents a new and evolving area of study in need of deeper understanding. To situate the experience of aging Arab Americans and well-being, this chapter first presents a review of the literature on immigration, aging, and well-being followed by a discussion of four theoretical frameworks employed in the scholarship on social aspects of aging—(a) the life course perspective, (b) the convoy model of social relations, (c) intergenerational solidarity and ambivalence, and (d) successful aging. By juxtaposing these literatures, we identify gaps and limitations in the existing body of knowledge on aging and the well-being of Arab Americans. The chapter concludes with a section on the specific needs for future research and practice.

Immigration, Aging, and Well-Being

Links between immigrant status and well-being have been well-researched. Findings point to clear health differentials between immigrants and their US-born counterparts, though who is advantaged often depends on the well-being outcome measured. The majority of this research has focused on immigrants from Asia and Latin America. We summarize these findings to illustrate theoretical developments as they relate to aging and then present relevant scholarly work conducted on Arab Americans.

[1] It should be noted, however, that Census numbers do not always coincide with community population statistics. For instance, 1990 Census data using the ancestry question suggested there were 151,493 Arab Americans in Michigan; however, community-based estimates suggested the number to be closer to 490,000 (The Zogby Study, 1997). Moreover, while the 2000 Census data suggested that 11 % of the Arab American population in Michigan was 55 years old or more, a representative sample of the metropolitan Detroit area of those aged 20 and over reported that 27 % of the Arab American population was 55 years old or more (Ajrouch & Jamal, 2007).

A large body of evidence suggests that immigrants in the USA have better health than the native-born population (Abraído-Lanza, Dohrenwend, Ng-Mak, & Turner, 1999; Frisbie, Cho, & Hummer, 2001; Lucas, Barr-Anderson, & Kington, 2003; Read, Emerson, & Tarlov, 2005). This trend appears strongest for Latino immigrants and when examining mortality as the outcome. Immigrants overall have longer life expectancies than the US born, and therefore are more likely to live into the latter part of the life course. A number of hypotheses have been advanced to explain the immigrant health advantage. First, "the healthy migrant effect" hypothesis suggests that immigrants are naturally a self-selected group who are younger and healthier compared to both those who remain behind and the general population in the host country (Abraído-Lanza et al., 1999). As such, the mortality advantage is more pronounced among those who immigrate at a young age and lower among those who immigrate in old age to join their children (Hummer, Benjamins, & Rogers, 2004). The second hypothesis suggests cultural change as an explanatory pathway, though this hypothesis has recently come under critique. Whereas immigrants arrive to the USA with healthy lifestyle habits and strong social networks, these health-promoting factors are eroded in future generations as members of the group integrate into mainstream society (Lara, Gamboa, Kahramanian, Morales, & Bautista, 2005). This pattern has been most strikingly observed among Latino Americans and may be an outcome of the structural and socioeconomic conditions descendants of immigrants face in the process of becoming American. A third explanation advances that some immigrant group members who spend their adult life in the USA ultimately return to their country of origin in old age. This return migration is speculated to bias the health profile of immigrant groups because a proportion of mortality in old age takes place for immigrants in their country of origin and is therefore not accounted for in the USA (Abraído-Lanza et al., 1999).

Although the data on mortality are provocative, whether the immigrant health advantage persists in old age is an open question. A review by Markides, Salinas, and Sheffield (2009) showed that the mortality advantage does not necessarily translate to health status advantage in old age. Their review illustrated that compared to the US-born whites, Asian immigrants experience high rates of disability in old age, and Asian and Latino immigrant elders exhibit poorer mental health (Markides et al., 2009). Furthermore, immigrant women, who are presumed to be less self-selective than their male counterparts, do not fare well when the health outcome is disability (Markides & Wallace, 2007 as referenced in Markides et al., 2009). In the area of cognitive function, recent research showed that cognitive decline in old age is slower among Latino immigrants compared to the US-born Latino Americans (Hill, Angel, Balistreri, & Angel, 2010). Gender and age at migration are also important to take into account when examining the health of immigrants in old age. The healthy migrant effect holds for those who migrate to the USA young and not for those who immigrate after the age of 50 (Hill et al., 2010). Moreover, immigrants in general and older immigrants specifically are more likely to be uninsured and to underutilize health care services (Jenkins, Le, McPhee, Stewart, & Ha, 1996). Naturally, undocumented immigrants are at an even heightened disadvantage with respect to health care access (Berk, Schur, Chavez, &

Frankel, 2000). In sum, a health advantage among immigrants is not straightforward, complicated by multiple social factors.

Given data limitations, it is not possible to confirm whether an immigrant health advantage exists among Arab American elders. In fact, some evidence on Arab Americans in general runs in contrast to the immigrant health advantage. A study conducted in the metropolitan Detroit area suggests that the health status of the US-born Arab Americans is better than Arab immigrants (Abdulrahim & Baker, 2009). This pattern extended to a national sample of older adults identified from the 2000 US Census. Analysis revealed that immigrant Arab American elders had a higher sex- and age-adjusted prevalence of having a physical (limited in one or more basic physical activities such as walking, climbing stairs, reaching, lifting, carrying) or self-care (dressing, bathing, or getting around inside the home) disability compared to the US-born Arab Americans (Dallo et al., 2009). Advantages in health appear accounted for by the US-born generation's possession of more human capital, specifically higher education levels and better English language skills. National origin diversity also arose as an important factor for health status among Arab American elders. Dallo and colleagues showed that older adults from Iraq and Syria reported the highest estimates of having a physical disability compared to individuals from other Arab countries. Individuals from Iraq and Lebanon reported the highest estimates of having a self-care disability compared to other countries.

Other studies parallel findings in the immigrant aging literature to suggest advantages among the US-born Arab Americans in psychological health. The US-born Arab American elders reported less depression and higher life satisfaction compared to Arab immigrant elders (Ajrouch, 2007a). Furthermore, higher education and English language skills (factors which are associated with experiencing lower acculturative stress) are also associated with lower depression among Arab American elders (Wrobel, Farrag, & Hymes, 2009).

The limited literature further reveals that immigrant status is not the only determinant of Arab American well-being in old age. Social support exhibits important health-promoting effects. For example, receiving emotional support from the child upon whom older adults relied most buffered the association between low education levels and self-reported chronic conditions and functional disability (Ajrouch, 2007b). In other words, those who reported the ability to confide in their child reported health outcomes that were on par with their higher educated counterparts, regardless of immigrant status. In sum, preliminary evidence suggests that though immigrant status is associated with various well-being outcomes, additional factors such as human (e.g., language, education level) and social (relationship type and quality) capital play an important role in the well-being of older Arab Americans.

Overall, findings concerning links between immigrant status and well-being among Arab Americans suggest they may be a special case. Immigrant Arab Americans appear vulnerable compared to their US-born counterparts both physically and mentally, even in old age. Vulnerabilities reported by immigrant Arab Americans may be explained by the fact that immigration to the USA from Arabic-speaking countries often occurs due to war or political instability. As such, immigrants may come with both physical and mental health challenges, making them quite distinct from other immigrant groups in the USA. Moreover, both human and social capital obviously hold due importance for older Arab Americans, much as they do for other immigrant and ethnic groups in the USA. Human capital refers to characteristics that an individual holds (e.g., education) and social capital refers to the relationships one forges with others. Each represents qualitatively distinct resources, and their associations with well-being highlight the pathways through which immigrant status may influence well-being among Arab American elders. Finally, given the difficulty of identifying Arab Americans in large data sets, such limitations should be acknowledged as a potential barrier to discerning a complete understanding of the Arab American experience with regard to immigration, aging, and well-being. Next, we turn to key theoretical constructs in the study of aging.

Theoretical Constructs on Aging

Theoretical developments in the field of aging have evolved over the years. Early thinking introduced the notion of disengagement theory (Cumming, Dean, Newell, & McCallfrey, 1960; Cumming & Henry, 1961). Taking a functional perspective, disengagement theory advanced the idea that as people age, a mutual process of disengagement occurs whereby both the individual and society slowly begin to withdraw from one another. This theory was later challenged with the advancement of activity theory (Havighurst, Neugarten, & Tobin, 1968). Contrary to the proposition that older adults preferred disengagement, activity theory proposed that life satisfaction and well-being were enhanced when older adults were in fact engaged, active members of society. These theories may seem somewhat basic today, but they represent the starting point from which many current perspectives have emerged. In the paragraphs below, we discuss contemporary theoretical perspectives concerning social aspects of aging in the USA including the life course perspective, the convoy model of social relations, intergenerational solidarity/ambivalence, and successful aging.

The Life Course Perspective

A life course perspective is perhaps best known by the early work of Glen Elder (1999/1974). It refers to a dynamic and process-based approach to understanding aging by examining how human lives are socially organized and evolve over time. The life course perspective emerged during the 1960s in response to limitations identified in existing theories about human development, particularly the conceptual and methodological issues associated with aging. The noteworthy aspect of a life course perspective involves highlighting the significance of context to human aging. The personal and biographical level of human experience is examined with simultaneous consideration of timing, social institutions/policies, and structural position (i.e., race, class, gender) within a historical time period. The roots of a life course perspective may be found in the tenets of multiple disciplines. Assumptions within the fields of psychology (Baltes & Baltes, 1990), sociology (Riley, Kahn, & Foner, 1994), and history (Hareven, 2001) each contribute to link individual experiences within the context of changing historical and social conditions. A life course perspective combines multiple sets of assumptions from each discipline to provide an all-encompassing interdisciplinary framework for understanding human aging. Social institutions and policies shape life experiences over time, influencing social roles, positions, and statuses as well as providing meaning to such experiences. Moreover, attention to general patterns between and within birth cohorts is key to applying a life course perspective. A life course perspective underscores the importance of studying life events (e.g., marriage) and life phases (e.g., old age) in tandem, at multiple levels of analysis, and within the context of previous life experiences (Phillips, Ajrouch, & Hillcoat-Nalletamby, 2010).

The life course perspective is broad in range and is suitable to exploring immigration and the diverse aging experiences of Arab Americans. Some of the most important life course factors to consider are nativity status and, for immigrants, age at migration and length of residence in the USA. The limited evidence on Arab Americans highlights that the mental health of older adults born in the USA is better than the mental health of immigrants (Ajrouch, 2007a). This finding is complicated by the fact that Arab immigrant older adults are a heterogeneous group, some who immigrated young and experienced transitioning from adulthood to old age in the USA and others who immigrated in old age to join family members. Moreover, Arab immigrants who arrive to the USA after having lived through wars and civil strife would be more likely to experience a negative aging trajectory compared to those who arrive from relatively politically stable countries. Even if one focuses on immigrants from one country such as Iraq, for example, it is safe to assume that Iraqis who immigrated to the USA in the 1980s will experience better health in old age compared to those who arrived more recently after experiencing the trauma of war and living in a refugee camp.

The experience of war, of course, draws attention to sociohistorical context. Recent sociohistorical events may impact identity formation differently among Arab Americans depending on age, which have enormous implications for well-being over the life course. Ajrouch and Jamal (2007) found that older Arab Americans are more likely than younger Arab Americans to identify as white. There has never been a time in the US history when race was not a salient marker of difference, and though Arab Americans fought for the right to identify as white in the early 1900s (Gualtieri, 2001), recent research suggests that not all Arab Americans identify with being white; instead, there is diversity in how members of this group subjectively interact with racial categories (Abdulrahim, 2008; Ajrouch, 2004).

A sociohistorical event, such as 9/11 and the War on Terror that followed may influence racial identification patterns among younger and older Arab Americans. Ajrouch and Jamal (2007) provide a potential example: being a 15-year-old son versus a successful 50-year-old father when 9/11 occurred is likely to produce divergent effects among Arab Americans. The 50-year-old has had a lifetime as a member of an invisible ethnic group, while the 15-year-old is forging into adulthood as a member of a very visible negatively targeted ethnic group. Such experiences among younger cohorts may influence the likelihood of feeling marginalized, and hence distance themselves from dominant society. The consequential effect may be to reject a white identity and instead take on a racial identity that incurs minority status elements. Implications for the aging experience may include new mistrust of mainstream institutions meant to aid and provide support to aging individuals and families.

Detected age differences in whether or not one identifies as white may represent developmental changes, cohort differences, or period effects. True age differences reflect developmental changes, yet attention to cohort effects allows researchers to determine whether characteristics and outcomes result from having been born during a specific span of years (e.g., Baby boomers) while period effects draw attention to historical events (e.g., 9/11) at time of measurement as influencing characteristics and outcomes. Disentangling age, cohort, and period effects will allow for a deeper and more accurate understanding of aging but will be achieved only with the availability of cross-sequential longitudinal panel data, that is, following multiple samples of the same people over time (Schaie & Strother, 1968). Nevertheless, findings from research on older Arab Americans provide important preliminary understandings of potential age differences, pointing to the need for future studies that incorporate a longitudinal design. In sum, a life course perspective provides an important framework for understanding links between individuals, their social relations over time, and larger sociohistorical events. We turn next to a discussion of social relations.

The Convoy Model of Social Relations

The convoy model of social relations is informed to a large extent by the life course perspective. This model focuses on links between social relations and health, recognizing that social relations are both individual and cumulative, and that they reflect a lifetime of experiences and exchanges (Antonucci, 1985; Kahn & Antonucci, 1980). Social relations are conceptualized as multidimensional and longitudinal in nature, shaped by personal (e.g., age, gender, personality) and situational (e.g., role expectations, resources, demands) characteristics, which influence both the structure of the support network and the exchange of social support. Historical change influences social relations through changes in personal (e.g., higher education levels) and situational (e.g., occupying the roles of both mother and daughter) characteristics, which in turn influence the structure, function, and evaluation of social relations. The nature and function of social relations are thought to change over time and with age. Moreover, not all people receive support from those who surround them and not all support is positive (Rook, 1992). Some support networks may produce a negative effect by making demands or getting on nerves to ultimately irritate a person. Convoys of social relations may include family, friends, neighbors, and additional important and close others. Research in the tradition of the convoy model of social relations shows that though family usually occupies a prominent place in one's network, the proportion of one's network who is family is greater in later life (Ajrouch, Antonucci, & Janevic, 2001).

The family unit is central to Arab American daily life. In particular, social identity and responsibility are determined by family affiliation (Aswad, 1997), yet little is known about the influence of family relations on well-being. Arab Americans often refer to family as an ideal situation where elders are respected and secured a space at the center of family life (Ajrouch, 1997; El-Kholy, 1988). Such ideal notions, however, may not represent lived experience. Over time, family relations may change as social and economic demands affect expectations, relationships, and lifestyles. For instance, Ajrouch (2007b) found that key aspects of the spousal relationship varied among older Arab Americans living in the Metro Detroit area. The US-born elders reported more often that their spouse gets on their nerves and makes too many demands than did their immigrant counterparts, while immigrants reported a higher likelihood of feeling that they may confide in their spouse. Relations with adult children also varied. The US-born elders reported on average better relationships with the child they relied upon most than did their immigrant counterparts. This finding regarding relations with an adult child reflects a pattern found within other immigrant groups in that relationships with adult children may be more strained among elder immigrants due to conflicting expectations (Yee, 1994). Finally, whereas immigration signals that a higher proportion of younger people leave parents behind, increasingly, older adults are immigrating to join their children (Jackson, 2002). This trend raises questions related to the parent–adult child relationship.

Intergenerational Solidarity and Ambivalence

The concepts of intergenerational solidarity and ambivalence speak to theoretical developments that address the type and quality of relationships that exist between older adults and their children. Intergenerational solidarity advocates first proposed that positive aspects including affection and filial obligation are normative and dominate the nature of relations between parent and child generations (Bengtson & Schrader, 1982). An update to this notion is the intergenerational stake hypothesis that suggested older adults invest heavily in their children, and hence view relations more positively and more congruent than do their children (Bengtson & Kuypers, 1971; Giarrusso, Feng, & Bengtson, 2004). Later iterations included conflict as a dimension of intergenerational relations, though in the context of solidarity (Parrott & Bengtson, 1999; Silverstein, Gans, Lowenstein, Giarusso, & Bengtson, 2010).

Intergenerational solidarity may function differently among well-established Arab Americans than among recent cohorts of Arab immigrants for whom the context of immigration may have led to the severing of family networks and the disruption of intergenerational ties. In Arab families, which are extended and multigenerational, members from the young adult generation initially migrate for economic reasons, leaving parents behind. The increasing age profile of persons of Arab ancestry in the USA (Kusow & Ajrouch, 2011) may be partly an outcome of parents joining their immigrant children through family reunification. This reunification can enhance intergenerational solidarity and provide benefits to both parents and adult children. However, it may also come at the expense of severing connections with same-age peers and relatives in the country of origin, leading to less than optimal well-being in old age.

Ambivalence emerged as a challenge to solidarity to suggest that positive sentiments coupled with simultaneous irritations better reflect the nature of relationships between generations (Luscher & Pillemer, 1998). In other words, parent–adult child relationships are replete with tensions between positive and negative aspects. Connidis and McMullin (2002) further elaborate the concept of ambivalence to highlight how social structure and individual agency concerning family situations must be examined simultaneously to better understand the nature of family relations over the life course. For instance, intersecting hierarchies of class and gender may produce very different ambivalent situations for working women faced with caregiving responsibilities of a parent. Connidis and McMullin (2002) argue that while a woman with a professional job may have the option of hiring others to provide hands on care for her mother, a working class woman more often must take vacation time, cut back hours, or quit altogether to provide this care. The source of ambivalence may hence derive from very different places; in the case of the professional woman it may stem from acute challenges to her identity, in the case of the working class woman it instead impinges on her income. In other words, positive and negative aspects of relationships arise through the interplay of structural opportunities and constraints on individual action.

There is evidence of ambivalence or tension between expectations that children will care for older adults in times of need, and the hope that older adults will not burden children given the demands of life in America. Qualitative research revealed that Arab American elders hold ambivalent views regarding receiving care from their children and nursing home care. For example, while elders maintained the ideal that children are obliged to provide care to their parents, they simultaneously did not want to burden their children (Ajrouch, 2005).

In contemplating the framework of intergenerational solidarity and ambivalence among Arab Americans, it is important to highlight that this is a diverse group with respect to national origin, religion, and socioeconomic standing. Furthermore, the term Arab American encompasses the descendents of the first waves of immigrants to the USA, whose immigration experience falls within the European assimilation framework, and the new immigrants, some of whom come from war torn and economically disadvantaged backgrounds. Such factors may shape the parent–adult child relationships in significant ways, and draw attention to living arrangements of older adults, and the quantity and quality of care they can expect to receive from adult children.

One clear trend occurring in the USA over the last 50 years is the higher likelihood that elders live alone (Bureau of U.S. Census, 2010; Diwan & Coulton, 1994).

This living arrangement trend is less likely in Arab countries, though not uncommon (Sibai, Beydoun, &Tohme, 2009). Multigenerational household living in the Arab world varies by socioeconomic status (Farsoun & Farsoun, 1974). In other words, the tendency for multiple generations to live in one household often reflects economic need as opposed to cultural preference, a pattern that carries over upon immigration. Although the extended family does not typically live together in the USA, multiple generations are available to one another when needed. In ethnic enclaves close geographic proximity is also common. Faster methods of communication and travel also facilitate contact among family members who do not live in close proximity to each other. Indeed, it is not uncommon for immigrants from Arab-speaking countries to bring aging parents to stay in the USA for months at a time every year.

Sociological writings on Arab families continue to stress that elders receive respect and protection and can expect their adult children to care for them in old age (El-Kholy, 1988; Salari, 2002; Sengstock, 1996). Even though the family continues to serve as the main provider of care for older adults in Arab societies, changes in family structure suggest that new generations of aging parents may no longer have access to the protections and support that their parents accessed. This is primarily a result of economic pressures on young generations, outmigration, and increasing demands for women to work outside the home. This change has been highlighted in writings on Arab societies as early as the mid-1980s (Al-Thakebs, 1985) and in more recent scholarship (Olmsted, 2005).

The literature on the living and care arrangements of Arab American elderly is virtually nonexistent. The few writings available specifically address the experiences of Muslim, not Arab, immigrant families in the USA, and present two contrasting positions. The first argues that because the family unit serves as the main party responsible for care provision to older members, government-sponsored care, especially nursing home care at the end of life, will fail because it directly challenges cultural values (Al Heeti, 2007; Duffy, Jackson, Schim, Ronis, & Fowler, 2006). The second position suggests that, despite commitment to religious and cultural beliefs, in a context of shifting values and increasing economic pressures, Muslim immigrant families will find it increasingly challenging to care for their older adult members (Hasnain & Rana, 2010). Hasnain and Rana advance that, unlike other ethnic and immigrant groups, the Muslim community has yet to participate in developing care policies for older adults that have a US orientation, yet also take the religious and cultural values of the immigrant community into account.

While it is documented that greater proportions of elders live alone today, perceptions of lonely feelings appear to vary by culture (van Tilburg, de Jong Gierveld, Lecchini, & Marsiglia, 1998; Victor et al., 2002). A recent study found that not being married and reporting poor health explained a critical amount of variance in loneliness among older Arab Americans (Ajrouch, 2008). Moreover, neither positive relationship quality with a child or aspects of acculturation (number of years in the USA, language, cultural behaviors) influenced subjective rating of loneliness, suggesting that cultural and social characteristics play a less important role in experiences of loneliness among Arab Americans than do personal status characteristics such as health and marital status. Poor health and not being married, while found in the general literature to significantly affect loneliness, also hold critical importance for Arab Americans. Each influences the ability to engage in activities, the former due to physical limitations and the latter due to the absence of an appropriate social partner. Deficits in physical health and not having a life partner may constitute asset loss not easily compensated by social and cultural capital.

Successful Aging

Successful aging as a theoretical framework is attributed to the seminal work of John Rowe and Robert Kahn (1998) who proposed a model meant to challenge the notion that aging is a period of decline and loss. Instead, aging is presented in a preventive framework. The concept advocates modifications in individual behaviors as a pathway to success in old age. Successful aging signifies a time of potential health and well-being and is measured by objective indicators including the absence of disease, high physical and cognitive functioning, and active social engagement. Yet, cultural norms and values that vary from one society to the next make a universal definition of successful aging problematic. The "Western" cultural bias and assumption of homogeneity among older persons may be most aptly illustrated in the focus on the individual as an agent of change. Interestingly, attaching the term "successful" to aging connotes a Western, capitalistic individualism and has thus been a topic of some controversy. That is, success is attributable altogether to individual action. In collectivist cultures, well-being in old age is determined by a different set of criteria.

The concept of healthy or successful aging is culturally bound and requires a multidimensional definition (Phillips et al., 2010). Using mortality, disability, and health care access as indicators shows that whereas immigrants are living longer in the USA, they may not necessarily experience healthy or successful aging. As people age, they may value maintaining social connectedness or discovering new meanings in life as much as they value their ability to maintain physical functioning (Baltes & Carstensen, 1996). For example, among Latino elders, perceptions of emotional well-being were influenced by the quality of their social relations and ability to fulfill cultural expectations (Beyene, Becker, & Mayen, 2002). Other immigrant studies emphasized the importance of maintaining close familial relationships to healthy aging and the detrimental consequences of losing traditional roles within the family. In a study on Salvadoran immigrant families in the USA, for example, older adult members exhibited good mental health despite the fact that this group of immigrants experienced tremendous stress due to the context of their immigration and illegal status (Gelfand, 1989). The author hypothesized this to be the result of satisfactory relationships with adult children and the ability of elders to maintain support roles in the family, such as caring for grandchildren and transmitting cultural and religious values.

The successful aging framework assumes an equal playing field, where hard work and determination may produce an outcome deemed successful. Not addressed are obstacles beyond an individual's control shaped by social status and social structural factors such as gender, class, race, and ethnicity that may affect an individual's ability to cope with life circumstances, and hence impinge on the aging experience (Phillips et al., 2010). As Holstein and Minkler (2003) contend, access to resources, including healthy diets, good health care, and sufficient income, in great part shape an individual's ability to choose a healthy lifestyle. Ideals of success furthermore tend to discount natural processes, threatening to marginalize groups of older adults who already fall outside mainstream ideals. For instance, a woman with thinning hair and a wrinkling face or the wheelchair-bound man who spent his life working as a day laborer—each represents situations about which the individual has little control, yet at the same time comes to represent failure in the aging process. A call to broaden the successful aging perspective has occurred in recent years, specifically involving the need to incorporate subjective assessments of what it means to have aged successfully (Bowling & Dieppe, 2005; Holstein & Minkler, 2003). Successful aging is clearly multidimensional, the meaning of which varies depending on various factors.

We consider two ways in which successful aging may hold importance for Arab Americans. First, the idea of successful aging puts forth a commitment to redefining usual aging as decline. Emphasizing individual action (while acknowledging larger social constraints) as a pathway to ensuring optimal health and well-being in later life may provide an alternative outlook to viewing decline in later life as inevitable. A commitment to successful aging may empower Arab Americans, both young and old, in new ways. Second, what it means to age successfully must be better understood among Arab Americans. No studies have assessed meanings of successful aging within this ethnic group, but drawing from research on other immigrant groups (Beyene et al., 2002; Gelfand, 1989) and writings on the structure and function of Arab American families (Aswad, 1997; El-Kholy, 1988), the well-being of Arab Americans in old age may be shaped to a large degree by factors such as the existence and quality of social networks than by physical functioning. Moreover, because respect and veneration of elders is embedded in Arab culture, Arab Americans may expect enhanced social status as they age. Therefore, loss of social status as a result of immigration and the changing context and priorities in the USA may exert negative effects on their mental health. As with other immigrant groups, successful aging for Arab Americans may be strongly determined by their ability to maintain traditional roles in the family, as decision-makers and as transmitters of traditional culture, especially to grandchildren. Those who subscribe to a successful aging framework for understanding the aging process must balance the potential advantages of individual agency with the cultural and traditional expectations that some Arab Americans hold.

Implications for Future Research and Practice

Overall Americans are having fewer children and living longer. These demographic trends signify many changes for aging families including a tendency to view children as more of a responsibility as opposed to a resource, and hence a lower likelihood of investing in children and higher tendency to invest in retirement (Ekerdt, 2004). Greater life expectancy also has had a significant impact on family structure and relations. Living longer means lengthening the amount of time spent in particular familial relationships (Farkas & Hogan, 1995). Arab Americans, who are part of the American mosaic, are increasingly experiencing these trends. Yet, the issue of aging and well-being among Arab Americans is still in need of study and deeper examination. Based on our review of the literature, we propose a future research agenda below to fill in knowledge gaps on this important topic as well as delineate some implications for practice.

We begin with the identification and recognition of limitations that have impeded the study of older Arab Americans in general. First, access to representative data on this group is limited by the fact that persons of Arab ancestry in the USA are officially classified as White. As such, quantitative studies on Arab Americans in general are based on non-representative samples from one geographic location (such as the metropolitan Detroit area), one segment of the Arab American community (immigrants), the US Census data (which have its own host of methodological challenges, see Samhan, Chap. 2), or have employed convenience sampling. Comparative research that examines the aging experiences of Arab Americans by generational status and age at migration, for example, would require innovative designs to gather representative data among this difficult to reach population. The enormous cost of such studies represents a challenge to gathering representative data on Arab Americans. Such obstacles pose the most serious limitation to the development of knowledge about the diverse aging experiences within the Arab American community. Future studies must find ways to gather representative samples both on a community as well as a national level. Such an approach would enormously advance the understanding of Arab American aging.

In the context of limited empirical evidence, it is safe to state that commonly held cultural beliefs about the position of the elderly in Arab families may not be generalizable to all Arab Americans. Qualitative research which examines changes in meanings of aging as an outcome of immigration is needed. Based on the gaps identified in our review of the literature, we propose that two areas of research are in urgent need of exploration.

The first is on the meanings of healthy or successful aging among Arab Americans. Moving away from a biomedical model of what it means to be healthy in old age, qualitative studies can guide researchers in identifying the culturally embedded criteria Arab American elders employ to gauge their well-being. As research on other immigrant and ethnic groups has revealed, physical functioning or lack of physical illness may not be the most important determinants of subjective well-being in old age. Similarly, Arab culture may place heavier emphasis on the enhancement of social status with aging more than on maintaining physical functioning. Nevertheless, social status may well depend on physical well-being and mobility, e.g., having the ability to attend family gatherings or religious institutions. Attending to the meanings and beliefs of Arab Americans would help guide the development of culturally sanctioned approaches to advancing lifestyle behaviors to promote healthy choices over the life course.

The second area in need of inquiry relates to gaining a better understanding of the needs of Arab Americans with respect to care provision in old age. While the family continues to serve as a major source for support for elders, health care policy in the USA has spawned a change in the mix of home care services and family support. It still remains a fact, however, that those with the financial resources to access home care formal support use them, and hence no real increase in home care or long-term care services has occurred over the last decades (Konetzka & Werner, 2009). Moreover, ethnic minorities are less likely to use formal care services (Mui & Burnette, 1994), making the role of family, especially children, particularly critical in times of need. The dominant view in Arab culture is that the family remains the sole provider of care to aging members. However, as the limited available literature on Arab and Muslim American elders suggests (Ajrouch, 2005; Hasnain & Rana, 2010), the picture is more complex. With immigration and changes in family structure, older adults may request less care from their children and learn to expect more state-sponsored financial and social care. Furthermore, religious institutions may come to represent an accepted source of support for aging families. The view that Arab Americans will only accept care from their children or close family members should be confirmed with empirical evidence through rigorous sociological study, since often people express one culturally accepted view they believe is the norm, but experience and accept another which more realistically meets their needs and life experiences. Studies may explore how Arab American elders perceive state-sponsored versus religious institution organized versus family care. The benefit from an examination of elders' views on how programs can be developed and designed to complement and support family care provision will provide critical data for new directions in aging Arab American communities around the country.

The outcome of this research will have important implications for policies and practice. Adherence to cultural values such as familism or filial obligation (Herrera, Lee, Palos, & Torres-Vigil, 2008; Scharlach et al., 2006) plays a role in care practices and needs to be considered as programs and policies evolve to address the growing numbers of older adults. This is particularly relevant for the Arab American case, where cultural norms dictate the obligatory role of children to caregiving, yet changing realities of longer than ever life expectancies, fewer children, and work obligations pose competing demands that make older adults ambivalent about the role adult children are expected to play should the need arise (Ajrouch, 2005). With demographic shifts, economic pressures, and increasing mobility, Arab American families face challenges in being the sole providers of care for their aging members. Clearly, culturally appropriate programs and care are needed to complement that provided by family members. The parameters of this care must be based on sound empirical evidence. It is critical that care policies incorporate the views and needs of older Arab Americans, including those who can rely on family care as well as those who cannot. Future directions may indicate the need for a new theoretical framework to understand Arab Americans and the aging process.

References

Abdulrahim, S. (2008). "White" or "other": Racial subjectivity and the Arab immigrant experience in the United States. In A. Jamal & N. Naber (Eds.), *Race and Arab Americans before and after 9/11: From invisible citizens to visible subjects* (pp. 131–146). Syracuse, NY: Syracuse University Press.

Abdulrahim, S., & Baker, W. (2009). Differences in self-rated health by immigrant status and language preference among Arab Americans in the Detroit metropolitan area. *Social Science and Medicine, 68*(12), 2097–2103.

Abraído-Lanza, A. F., Dohrenwend, B. P., Ng-Mak, D. S., & Turner, J. B. (1999). The Latino mortality paradox: A test of the "salmon bias" and healthy migrant hypotheses. *American Journal of Public Health, 89*(10), 1543–1548.

Abu-Laban, S. M. (1991). Family and religion among Muslim immigrants and their descendents. In E. H. Waugh, S. M. Abu-Laban, & R. B. Qureshi (Eds.), *Muslim families in North America* (pp. 6–31). Edmonton, AB: The University of Alberta Press.

Ajrouch, K. J. (1997). *Ethnicity, gender and identity among second-generation Arab Americans: Growing up Arabic in America*. Ph.D. dissertation, Wayne State University, Detroit, MI.

Ajrouch, K. J. (2004). Gender, race, and symbolic boundaries: Contested spaces of identity among Arab-American adolescents. *Sociological Perspectives, 47*(4), 371–391.

Ajrouch, K. J. (2005). Arab-American immigrant elders' views about social support. *Ageing & Society, 25*(5), 655–673.

Ajrouch, K. J. (2007a). Resources and well-being among Arab-American elders. *Journal of Cross-Cultural Gerontology, 22*(2), 167–182.

Ajrouch, K. J. (2007b). Health disparities and Arab-American elders: Does intergenerational support buffer the inequality–health link? *Journal of Social Issues, 63*(4), 745–758.

Ajrouch, K. J. (2008). Social isolation and loneliness among Arab American elders: Cultural, social, and personal factors. *Research in Human Development, 5*(1), 44–59.

Ajrouch, K. J., Antonucci, T. C., & Janevic, M. R. (2001). Social networks among Blacks and Whites: The interaction between race and age. *The Journals of Gerontology Series B: Psychological Sciences and Social Sciences, 56*(2), S112–S118.

Ajrouch, K. J., & Jamal, A. (2007). Assimilating to a white identity: The case of Arab Americans. *International Migration Review, 41*(4), 860–879.

Al Heeti, R. M. (2007). Why nursing homes will not work: Caring for the needs of the aging Muslim American population. *The Elder Law Journal, 15*(1), 205–231.

Al-Thakeb, F. H. (1985). The Arab family and modernity: Evidence from Kuwait. *Current Anthropology, 26*(5), 575–580.

Antonucci, T. C. (1985). Social support: Theoretical advances, recent findings and pressing issues. In I. G. Sarason & B. R. Sarason (Eds.), *Social support: Theory, research and applications* (pp. 21–37). The Hague: Marinus Nijhof.

Arab American Institute Foundation. (2008). Arab Americans; demographics. Retrieved from August 14, 2013. http://www.aaiusa.org/arab-americans/22/demographics

Aswad, B. C. (1997). Arab American families. In M. K. DeGenova (Ed.), *Families in cultural context* (pp. 218–238). Mayfield, CA: Mayfield.

Baltes, P. B., & Baltes, M. M. (1990). Psychological perspectives on successful aging: The model of selective optimization with compensation. In P. B. Baltes & M. M. Baltes (Eds.), *Successful aging: Perspectives from the behavioral sciences* (pp. 1–34). New York: Cambridge University Press.

Baltes, M. M., & Carstensen, L. L. (1996). The process of successful ageing. *Ageing and Society, 16*(4), 397–422.

Barakat, H. (1985). Arab families. In E. Femea (Ed.), *Women and the family in the Middle East: New voices of change* (pp. 27–48). Austin, TX: University of Texas Press.
Bengtson, V. L., & Kuypers, J. A. (1971). Generation differences and the "developmental stake". *Aging & Human Development, 2*, 249–260.
Bengtson, V. L., & Schrader, S. S. (1982). Parent–child relations. In D. Mangen & W. Peterson (Eds.), *Handbook of research instruments in social gerontology* (pp. 115–185). Minneapolis, MN: University of Minnesota Press.
Berk, M. L., Schur, C. L., Chavez, L. R., & Frankel, M. (2000). Health care use among undocumented Latino immigrants. *Health Affairs, 19*(4), 51–64.
Beyene, Y., Becker, G., & Mayen, N. (2002). Perception of aging and sense of well-being among Latino elderly. *Journal of Cross-Cultural Gerontology, 17*(2), 155–172.
Bowling, A., & Dieppe, P. (2005). What is successful ageing and who should define it? *British Medical Journal, 331*(7531), 1548–1551.
Brittingham, A., & de la Cruz, G. P. (2005). *We the people of Arab ancestry in the United States. Current population reports*. Department of Commerce, Washington, DC. Retrieved May 18, 2006, from www.census.gov
Bureau of U.S. Census. (2010). America's families and living arrangements: 2010. U.S. Census Bureau, Housing and Household Economic Statistics Division, Fertility & Family Statistics Branch. Retrieved March 12, 2011, from http://www.census.gov/population/www/socdemo/hh-fam/cps2010.html
Connidis, I. A., & McMullin, J. A. (2002). Sociological ambivalence and family ties: A critical perspective. *Journal of Marriage and the Family, 64*(30), 558–567.
Cumming, E., Dean, L., Newell, D., & McCallfrey, I. (1960). Disengagement: A tentative theory of aging. *Sociometry, 23*, 23–35.
Cumming, E., & Henry, W. (1961). *Growing old*. New York, NY: Basic Books.
Dallo, F., Al-Snih, S., & Ajrouch, K. J. (2009). The prevalence of disability among US- and foreign-born Arab Americans: Results from the 2000 US Census. *Gerontology, 55*(2), 153–161.
Diwan, S., & Coulton, C. (1994). Period effects on the mix of formal and informal in-home care used by urban elderly. *Journal of Applied Gerontology, 13*(3), 316–330.
Duffy, S. A., Jackson, F. C., Schim, S. M., Ronis, D. L., & Fowler, K. E. (2006). Racial/ethnic preferences, sex preferences, and perceived discrimination related to end-of-life care. *The American Geriatrics Society, 54*(1), 150–157.
Ekerdt, D. J. (2004). Born to retire: The foreshortened life course. *The Gerontologist, 44*(1), 3–9.
Elder, G. H. (1999). *Children of the great depression: Social change and life experience*. Boulder, CO: Westview Press. (Original work published 1974)
El-Kholy, A. A. (1988). The Arab American family. In C. H. Mindel & R. Habenstein (Eds.), *Ethnic families in America: Patterns and variations* (pp. 145–162). New York, NY: Elsevier.
Farkas, J. I., & Hogan, D. P. (1995). The demography of changing intergenerational relationships. In V. L. Bengtson, K. W. Schaie, & L. Burton (Eds.), *Adult intergenerational relations: Effects of social change* (pp. 1–18). New York, NY: Springer.
Farsoun, S., & Farsoun, K. (1974). Class and patterns of association among kinsmen in contemporary Lebanon. *Anthropological Quarterly, 47*(1), 93–111.
Frisbie, W. P., Cho, Y., & Hummer, R. A. (2001). Immigration and the health of Asian and Pacific Islander adults in the United States. *American Journal of Epidemiology, 153*(4), 372–380.
Gelfand, D. E. (1989). Immigration, aging, and intergenerational relationships. *The Gerontologist, 29*(3), 366–372.
Giarrusso, R., Feng, D., & Bengtson, V. L. (2004). The inter-generational stake phenomenon over 20 years. In M. Silverstein (Ed.), *Annual review of gerontology and geriatrics* (pp. 55–76). New York, NY: Springer.
Gualtieri, S. M. (2001). Becoming "White": Race, religion, and the formation of Syrian/Lebanese ethnicity in the United States. *Journal of American Ethnic History, 20*(4), 29–58.
Harevan, T. K. (2001). Historical perspectives on aging and family relations. In R. H. Binstock & L. K. George (Eds.), *Handbook of aging and the social sciences* (pp. 141–159). San Diego, CA: Academic.

Hasnain, R., & Rana, S. (2010). Unveiling Muslim voices. Aging parents with disabilities and their adult children and family caregivers in the United States. *Topics in Geriatric Rehabilitation, 26*(1), 46–61.

Havighurst, R. J., Neugarten, B. L., & Tobin, S. S. (1968). Disengagement and patterns of aging. In B. Neugarten (Ed.), *Middle age and aging: A reader in social psychology* (pp. 161–172). Chicago, IL: University of Chicago Press.

Herrera, A. P., Lee, J., Palos, G., & Torres-Vigil, I. (2008). Cultural influences in the patterns of long-term care use among Mexican American family caregivers. *Journal of Applied Gerontology, 27*(2), 141–165.

Hill, T. D., Angel, J. L., Balistreri, K. S., & Angel, R. J. (2010). Nativity, immigration, and the cognitive functioning trajectories of older Mexican Americans. Retrieved January 27, 2012, from http://www.utexas.edu/lbj/caa/2010/presentations/HillT.pdf

Holstein, M. B., & Minkler, M. (2003). Self, society, and the "new gerontology". *The Gerontologist, 43*(6), 787–796.

Hummer, R. A., Benjamins, M. R., & Rogers, R. C. (2004). Racial and ethnic disparities in health and mortality among U.S. elderly populations. In N. B. Anderson, R. A. Bulatao, & B. Cohen (Eds.), *Critical perspective on racial and ethnic differences in health in late life* (pp. 53–94). Washington, DC: National Research Council and National Academic Press.

Jackson, J. S. (2002). Conceptual and methodological linkages in cross-cultural groups and cross-national aging research. *Journal of Social Issues, 58*(4), 825–835.

Jenkins, C. N., Le, T., McPhee, S. J., Stewart, S., & Ha, N. T. (1996). Health care access and preventive care among Vietnamese immigrants: Do traditional beliefs and practices pose barriers? *Social Science Medicine, 43*(7), 1049–1056.

Joseph, S. (2000). Gender and citizenship in the Middle East: Introduction. In S. Joseph (Ed.), *Gender and citizenship in the Middle East* (pp. 3–32). Syracuse, NY: Syracuse University Press.

Kahn, R. L., & Antonucci, T. C. (1980). Convoys over the life course: Attachment, roles, and social support. In P. B. Baltes & O. Brim (Eds.), *Lifespan development and behavior* (Vol. 3, pp. 253–286). New York, NY: Academic.

Kandiyoti, D. (1998). Bargaining with patriarchy. *Gender and Society, 2*(1), 274–290.

Konetzka, R. T., & Werner, R. M. (2009). Review: Disparities in long-term care: Building equity into market-based reforms. *Medical Care Research and Review, 66*(5), 491–521.

Kusow, A. M., & Ajrouch, K. J. (2011). *Conceptualizing immigrant replenishment: Patterns of assimilation among Arab immigrants in the United States*. Paper presented at contemporary research in Arab American studies: New trends and critical perspectives: A conference in honor of Michael Suleiman, November 4–6, Detroit, MI.

Lara, M., Gamboa, C. M., Kahramanian, I., Morales, L. S., & Bautista, D. E. (2005). *Acculturation and Latino health in the United States: A review of the literature and its sociopolitical context*. Santa Monica, CA: RAND Corporation.

Lucas, J. W., Barr-Anderson, D. J., & Kington, R. S. (2003). Health status, health insurance, and health care utilization pattern of immigrant black men. *American Journal of Public Health, 93*(10), 1740–1747.

Luscher, K., & Pillemer, K. (1998). Intergenerational ambivalence: A new approach to the study of parent–child relations in later life. *Journal of Marriage and the Family, 60*, 413–425.

Markides, K. S., Salinas, J., & Sheffield, K. (2009). The health of older immigrants. *Generations, 32*(4), 46–52.

Markides, K. S., & Wallace, S. P. (2007). Minority elders in the United States: Implications for public policy. In R. A. Pruchno & M. A. Smyer (Eds.), *Challenges of an aging society: Ethical dilemmas, political issues* (pp. 193–216). Baltimore, MD: The John Hopkins University Press.

Meyer, J. (2001). *Age: 2000. Census 2000 brief.* Washington, DC: U.S. Department of Commerce. Retrieved 18 February, 2011, from http://www.census.gov/prod/2001pubs/c2kbr01-12.pdf

Mui, A. C., & Burnette, D. (1994). Long-term care service use by frail elders: Is ethnicity a factor? *The Gerontologist, 34*(2), 190–198.

Naff, A. (1985). *Becoming American: The early Arab immigrant experience*. Carbondale, IL: Southern Illinois University Press.

Olmsted, J. C. (2005). Gender, aging, and the evolving Arab patriarchal contract. *Feminist Economics, 11*(2), 53–78.

Orfalea, G. M. (1988). *Before the flames: A quest for the history of Arab Americans*. Austin, TX: University of Texas Press.

Parrott, T. M., & Bengtson, V. L. (1999). The effects of earlier intergenerational affection normative expectations, and family conflict on contemporary exchanges of help and support. *Research on Aging, 21*, 73–105.

Phillips, J., Ajrouch, K. J., & Hillcoat-Nalletamby, S. (2010). *Key concepts in social gerontology*. London, UK: Sage.

Read, J. G., Emerson, M. O., & Tarlov, M. (2005). Implications of Black immigrant health for US. Racial disparities in health. *Journal of Immigrant Health, 7*(3), 205–212.

Riley, M. W., Kahn, R. L., & Foner, A. (1994). *Age and structural lag: Society's failure to provide meaningful opportunities for work, family and leisure*. New York, NY: Wiley.

Rook, K. S. (1992). Detrimental aspects of social relationships: Taking stock of an emerging literature. In H. O. F. Veiel & U. Baumann (Eds.), *The meaning and measurement of social support* (pp. 157–169). New York, NY: Hemisphere.

Rowe, J. W., & Kahn, R. L. (1998). *Successful aging*. New York, NY: Dell.

Salari, S. (2002). Invisible in aging research: Arab Americans, Middle Eastern immigrants, and Muslims in the United States. *The Gerontologist, 42*(5), 580–588.

Schaie, K. W., & Strother, C. R. (1968). The effect of time and cohort differences on the interpretation of age changes in cognitive behavior. *Multivariate Research, 3*, 259–294.

Scharlach, A. E., Kellam, R., Ong, N., Baskin, A., Goldstein, C., & Fox, P. J. (2006). Cultural attitudes and caregiver service use: Lessons for focus groups with racially and ethnically diverse family caregivers. *Journal of Gerontological Social Work, 47*(1/2), 133–156.

Sengstock, M. C. (1996). Care of the elderly within Muslim families. In B. C. Aswad & B. Bilgé (Eds.), *Family and gender among American Muslims: Issues facing Middle Eastern immigrants and their descendents* (pp. 271–295). Philadelphia, PA: Temple University Press.

Sibai, A. M., Beydoun, M. A., & Tohme, R. A. (2009). Living arrangements in ever-married older Lebanese women: Is living with married children advantageous? *Journal of Cross-Cultural Gerontology, 24*(1), 5–17.

Silverstein, M., Gans, D., Lowenstein, A., Giarusso, R., & Bengtson, V. L. (2010). Older parent–child relationships in six developed nations: Comparisons at the intersection of affection and conflict. *Journal of Marriage and the Family, 72*(4), 1006–1021.

Sirkeci, I. (2005). War in Iraq: Environment of insecurity and international migration. *International Migration, 43*(4), 197–214.

The Zogby Study. (1997). *Detroit MSA ethnic census*. Dearborn, MI: ACCESS Marketing.

Van Tilburg, T., de Jong Gierveld, J., Lecchini, L., & Marsiglia, D. (1998). Social integration and loneliness: A comparative study among older adults in the Netherlands and Tuscany, Italy. *Journal of Social and Personality Relationships, 15*(6), 740–754.

Victor, C. R., Scambler, S. J., Shah, S., Cook, D. G., Harris, T., Rink, E., et al. (2002). Has loneliness amongst older people increased? An investigation into variations between cohorts. *Ageing & Society, 22*, 585–597.

Wrobel, N. H., Farrag, M. F., & Hymes, R. W. (2009). Acculturative stress and depression in an elderly Arabic sample. *Journal of Cross-Cultural Gerontology, 24*(3), 273–290.

Yee, B. K. (1994). The social and cultural context of adaptive aging by Southeast Asian elders. In J. Sokolovsky (Ed.), *The cultural context of aging: Worldwide perspectives* (pp. 293–303). Westport, CT: Bergin and Garvey.

Yount, K. M. (2005). The patriarchal bargain and intergenerational co residence in Egypt. *The Sociological Quarterly, 46*, 137–164.

Yount, K. M., & Sibai, A. (2009). The demography of aging in Arab countries. In P. Uhlenberg (Ed.), *International handbook of population aging* (pp. 227–315). Dordrecht, The Netherlands: Springer.

Zogby, J. (1990). *Arab America today: A demographic profile of Arab Americans*. Washington, DC: Arab American Institute.

Chapter 7
Using Convoys of Social Relations to Understand Culture and Forgiveness from an Arab American Perspective

Kristine J. Ajrouch and Toni C. Antonucci

Introduction

In the complex world in which we live, we are unfortunately often confronted by difficult, hurtful, and harmful situations. The ability to forgive is likely to help people be least harmed by such circumstances, but people often find it difficult to forgive others or even themselves. The topic of forgiveness has traditionally been understood within the realm of religion, yet new developments in the social sciences demonstrate forgiveness to be an important area in need of research. Evidence is emerging to suggest that the ability to forgive influences emotional and physiological health (Berry & Worthington, 2001; Lawler et al., 2005; Lawler-Row, Karremans, Scott, Edlis-Matityahou, & Edwards, 2008; Maltby, Day, & Barber, 2004; Maltby, Macaskill, & Day, 2001; McFarland, Smith, Touissaint, & Thomas, 2012; Toussaint, Williams, Musick, & Everson, 2001; Witvliet, Ludwig, & Vander Laan, 2001). One explanation for why forgiveness may be beneficial for health is that it deepens and promotes positive interpersonal relationships (Harris & Thoresen, 2005; Worthington & Scherer, 2004). It may also be that positive interpersonal relationships can promote forgiveness. We know little, moreover, about how ethnicity and culture shape understandings of forgiveness.

K.J. Ajrouch (✉)
Sociology, Anthropology, Criminology, Eastern Michigan University, 712 Pray-Harrold, Ypsilanti, MI 48197, USA
e-mail: kajrouch@emich.edu

T.C. Antonucci
Institute for Social Research, University of Michigan, 426 Thompson Street, Ann Arbor, MI 48104, USA
e-mail: tca@umich.edu

S.C. Nassar-McMillan et al. (eds.), *Biopsychosocial Perspectives on Arab Americans: Culture, Development, and Health*, DOI 10.1007/978-1-4614-8238-3_7,

Forgiveness is defined as a pro-social response in which there is a change in one's thoughts, emotions, and behaviors toward a transgressor (McCullough & Witvliet, 2002). In this chapter, we highlight how social relations inform the experiences of potentially hurtful interactions and situations by examining what forgiveness means in everyday life for Arab American college students. Going to college signifies a developmental period in which people regularly encounter, often for the first time, others of a different race or culture. With this in mind, we set out to identify cultural characteristics that inform attitudes about social relations and forgiveness. In so doing, we address the multiple ways in which social relations are experienced, including community ties, close family relations, as well as distant, less intimate relationships. We also include the college context of these Arab American students, speculating that college contexts might be associated with both differential exposure to experiences that require forgiveness as well as differing levels of perceived support. We focus on Arab Americans and forgiveness because of their distinctive cultural and political context. Their experiences are especially unique both as a minority group and as a frequent target of discrimination. We begin by presenting the theoretical perspective that guides this line of research.

Theoretical Perspective

Our program of research revolves around the study of social relations (Antonucci, Birditt, & Ajrouch, 2011). Much of our work has followed in the tradition of such classic thinking as George Herbert Mead, who proposed that social relationships are the basis of human existence. Social relations are, according to Mead, considered the source from which emerges the development of a self. In our work, social relations are considered multidimensional. For instance, we acknowledge that relationships vary in their levels of closeness to the individual and include both positive and negative attributes. Identifying such nuance provides a means by which to examine the complexity that encompasses everyday social relations. Moreover, we recognize that social relations that "go bad," i.e., are hurtful or harmful, have far reaching effects on psychological and physical well-being. Finally, we acknowledge the dynamic nature of social relations, which are known to change over the life course. This theoretical framework is known as the convoy model of social relations (Antonucci, 2001; Kahn & Antonucci, 1980). The convoy model advances that personal (age, gender, ethnicity, etc.) and situational (role, community, values, etc.) factors influence one another, as well as the structure, type, and quality of social relations and well-being. We use this framework to better understand how personal, situational, and social relations characteristics influence attitudes and acts of forgiveness, all of which link to well-being and health (see Fig. 7.1).

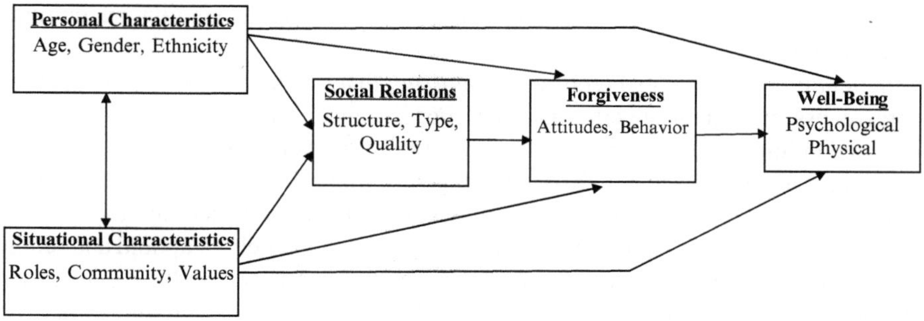

Fig. 7.1 Expanded convoy model of social relations and forgiveness

Culture, Convoys, and Forgiveness

It is increasingly recognized that culture plays an important role in the meanings that people attribute to various situations and experiences. Cultural approaches to the study of social relations often introduce specific values and norms. The accumulating literature identifies several value dimensions to elaborate cultural variations in the structure and quality of social relationships. Some of those most widely accepted include individualism/collectivism, relatedness/separateness, traditional/secular, and self-expression/survival (Hofstede, 1980; Inglehart & Welzel, 2005; Markus & Kitayama, 1991; Triandis, Bontempo, Villareal, Asai, & Lucca, 1988). For example, cultures that are individualistic/separate and value self-expression are said to focus on maintaining relationships that are beneficial for personal goals; include parents' investments in children that are more psychological than economic; have people who feel obligated to family but perceive it as voluntary; feel at ease interacting with strangers; and consider people as separate, nonoverlapping entities. Individualism is also associated with more direct goal oriented conversation styles (Kağitçibaşi, 1996; Oyserman, Kemmelmeier, & Coon, 2002). On the other hand, cultures ascribing to collectivism, relatedness, and/or survival tend to believe that group membership is unchangeable and in-group exchanges are based on principles of equality and generosity (Oyserman et al., 2002; Takahashi, Ohara, Antonucci, & Akiyama, 2002). They tend to have extended families in which young people provide direct financial help to the elderly; there is greater preference for sons, higher fertility rates, and an old age security value of children. These cultures are more likely to have social interactions with in-group members, engage in indirect communication styles, and be more concerned with partner's feelings. Arab culture has been described as falling more within the collectivist cultural orientation (Buda & Elsayed-Elkhouly, 1998), and the family unit identified as key to identity, status, and security (Barakat, 1993). Indeed, the centrality of family to Arab American life has been well-documented (Ajrouch, 1999; Aswad, 1997; Read, 2004; Read & Oselin, 2008). Family comprises a key presence in convoys of social relations over the life course (Antonucci & Akiyama, 1995). Convoys of social relations, therefore, are likely to develop and function differently depending on cultural orientations.

Attention to culture also requires recognizing that the practice and expression of forgiveness may incur specific qualities. For instance, forgiveness in collectivist-oriented cultures promotes reconciliation between the hurt or injured party and the perpetrator (Von Feigenblatt, 2010). Such goals emphasize making a rational decision to forgive as opposed to emotional incentives for inner peace; in other words, forgiveness in collectivist-oriented cultures is motivated largely to uphold and retain group harmony (Hook, Worthington, & Utsey, 2009). As such, culture may shape the conditions under which one tends to forgive and has direct implications for social relations and well-being.

The importance of social relations to overall health and well-being has prompted many scholars to inquire into the mechanisms by which social relations operates and has influential effects. It is clear that anger, conflict, hostility, insults, and other hurtful behaviors can have significant negative effects on health. At the same time, it is increasingly recognized that being able to forgive may help the individual cope with such negativity. Research has documented that the ability to forgive increases as people get older (Enright, Santos, & Al-Mabuk, 1989; McCullough & Witvliet, 2002; Toussaint et al., 2001). Nevertheless, examination of factors that underpin forgiveness at earlier points in the life course can provide useful information to guide the development of interventions to help young adults cope emotionally with stressful and/or traumatizing events (e.g., displaying forgiveness about hostile events). Those who experience such situations may use social relations as a motivation to learn how to forgive. Motivation may come from the desire to have close others think well of them, or an attempt to emulate attitudes and behaviors of close others who experienced similar situations. As a result, the tendency to forgive may result in better quality relationships; while those with better quality relationships may be more positive, have a better sense of self-worth and have the generosity of spirit that would facilitate forgiving.

The study of forgiveness among Arab Americans is both unique and illustrative. First, the nature of social relations within Arab American culture, particularly the high value placed on family relations, draws attention to the ways that close and important relationships inform attitudes and behaviors around the act of forgiveness. Second, the growing sentiment of "otherness" that is both projected on to Arab Americans by mainstream U.S. society (Shaheen, 2001), as well as internalized by recent cohorts of Arab American youth (Ajrouch, 2000; Ajrouch & Jamal, 2007) hold potential insights into relations between Arab Americans and other racial/ethnic groups. In this chapter, we focus on forgiveness as a potential window into understanding the increasing complexity of social relations and their pervasive influence on health and well-being. We note also that context (i.e., situation) is important both with regard to expectations about social relations and the experience of circumstances, behaviors, or events that might warrant forgiveness (McFarland et al., 2012). In the multifaceted world in which we live, we are unfortunately often confronted by difficult, hurtful, and harmful situations. We specifically focus on the concepts of culture, social relations, and forgiveness by presenting data from a recently completed focus group study in the metro-Detroit area.

Arab American Focus Groups in Metro-Detroit

We explored the concept of forgiveness among young Arab Americans in the greater Detroit area. Metro-Detroit is home to the largest, most visible concentration of Arab Americans outside of the Middle East (Brittingham & de la Cruz, 2005) and is, therefore, an ideal place to examine forgiveness among Arab Americans. Three focus groups that comprise 6–9 students were conducted with both Muslim and Christian Arab American college students. Participants were recruited from student organizations at three public universities in southeast Michigan. The universities varied in size, diversity, and scope, referenced here with pseudonyms. The largest university, University of X, has over 40,000 students, most of whom live on campus. It is considered a Research I university, and attracts students nationally, but has lower levels of ethnic diversity than the other two. University of Y is the smallest university of the three, with a little less than 9,000 students enrolled. It is considered a commuter university, attracts students regionally, and of the three has the largest Arab American student body. It is located in close proximity to large Arab American communities. University of Z has over 20,000 students, and is considered one of the most diverse campuses in the mid-west United States where students are equally likely to live on campus and/or commute. Although University of Z is racially/ethnically diverse, Arab Americans comprise a tiny fraction of the student body.

Discussions were facilitated by the first author, herself of Arab American descent, and lasted 1–2 h. The data presented were collected between November 2011 and March 2012. Semi-structured questions were asked around the following themes: General Strategies to Cope with Problems/Conflict in Relationships; Family Strategies to Cope with Problems in Relationships; Racial/Ethnic-Specific Insults; Forgiveness—What it means to You.

The method described in this chapter has both strengths and limitations. Qualitative investigations, and particularly focus group discussions, are well suited to capture the meaning of lived experience, and make visible ideas and issues about which there is little knowledge. Contributions of focus group members reveal participants' thoughts and the language they use to structure their experiences; the group setting encourages the participants to tell detailed stories (Agar & MacDonald, 1995; Hughes & DuMont, 1993; Morgan, 1988). As such, they provide a powerful tool by which to discern the intricacies of culture, social relations, and forgiveness. They provide clues about group dynamics and allow us to come closer to uncovering how participants make sense of their world (Martinez, 2002). Yet, limitations must also be noted. Given the convenience nature and small size of the sample, findings may not be generalizable to all Arab Americans. Instead this method provides an opportunity to uncover initial insights into the topic of study, with a focus on conceptual rigor (Marvasti, 2004), as well as access to "rich and informative insights" into a "specific environment or culture" (Jarrett & Burton, 1999: 177).

The focus group interviews were audio-taped and then transcribed verbatim. The coding of the focus group discussions followed the accepted procedures of grounded theory as elaborated by Strauss (1987). Analysis began by reviewing the transcribed text to identify regularly occurring phrases, as well as for those phrases that were counterintuitive or surprising (Miles & Huberman, 1994). As the coding is elaborated, its relationship to other categories or themes increasingly appeared. In analyzing the transcriptions, we uncovered attitudes and experiences of forgiveness in social relations, with three major themes that emerged across groups: (1) Culture and Social Relations; (2) Perception of Arabs from Outside; and (3) Forgiveness.

Culture and Social Relations

Discussions among focus group participants uncovered understandings that college students have of their own ethnic culture. This self-defining process is important for several reasons. First, it provides a lens with which to view how members of an ethnic culture describe themselves. Feelings and attitudes as told by in-group members provide a unique means by which culture can be understood by those who live and experience it on a daily basis. This type of subjectivity provides a powerful tool for humanizing "others." This is a particularly important exercise in the case of Arab Americans since the average non Arab-American knows relatively little about Arab Americans, and what is known is ascertained almost exclusively via relatively negative media portrayals (Shaheen, 2001). Second, by privileging a self-definition, intra-group social experiences of an ethnic group are voiced, providing key insights into how and why social relations are enacted, particularly in the context of hurtful events. Defining aspects of Arab culture that emerged in the focus groups included references to place, family honor, and gender relations.

Place arose as important especially to participants from the University of Y, and illustrates how a situational factor, such as community living, influences culture and social relations. The University of Y is located in the heart of an ethnic enclave, and is a university with a visible Arab American presence. Participants discussed an appreciation of the way it facilities close relationships with others.

> Zahra: …I mean, when you find out someone is Arabic, you kind of have a more closeness to that person. You feel like they're more like you…
>
> Nina: …That's why you see, like a bunch of Arabs hanging out. Like a bunch of Blacks hanging out. You know, like they're always together, like secluded really. And, if you see someone—if you see someone who's Black with someone who's White, you're, like, what's he trying to do…
>
> Ali: It's really hard to find someone that's really diversified. I rarely—I rarely find someone like that.
>
> (University of Y)

Zahra and Nina elaborate on the tendency for Arab Americans to prefer one another's company, and equate such action as similar to self-segregating practices of other groups on campus, e.g., Blacks and Whites. When Ali states the challenge in finding someone "diversified," he introduces the notion that having friends who are not Arab is a rare occurrence. Reasons for this sense of community range from perceptions of being raised with similar morals (e.g., do not drink alcohol), to losing friends from other cultural groups because of prejudiced attitudes toward Arabs. Yet, the tendency to congregate together, especially living in an ethnic community, raises a concern that it prohibits wider understanding of those outside their culture.

> Joseph: --well, I don't want to say raised, but, you know John—they moved to North Carolina, like, twelve years ago. He goes to Michigan State now, and, you know, to be honest, he's still tied to the religion. They are living now in the south, so—and they're the only ones, so, it's like, hey, you guys are Arab? They never even heard (chuckles) of Arab or Ali-- they can call him Ali or Ollie, you know--
>
> (Laughter)
>
> Joseph: ... they had a hard time, as far as when 9/11 happened, but they were respected. And when he comes here now, he's at Michigan State, he doesn't even like coming to Dearborn, because he's like, you guys live in this bubble, you don't know what the heck is going on around you. You have no other experiences besides living here, so you don't know what it's like living in North Carolina, or Arizona, or anywhere around the world. You know, but I could see exactly where he is coming from.
>
> (University of Y)

Living in a bubble is akin to being sheltered and unaware of what life is like outside of the cultural spaces through which residents of Dearborn move. On the one hand, it creates feelings of warmth, belonging, and community. Stemming from immigrant traditionalism, this source of positive community living simultaneously produces negative attributes in the form of gossip or "all eyes on you" that result in an enormous level of control and sanctioning (Ajrouch, 2000). Gossip, of course, constitutes one scenario where hurtful situations may arise. But more to the point of the observation of living in a bubble, the implicit message is that those who stay behind limit their opportunities to interact with and develop relationships outside of the community which may potentially narrow understandings of larger social worlds (Aswad, 1974; Gans, 1962). Success and failure among immigrants and their descendants living in ethnic enclaves occur through the social relationships that exist within families, between families, and how the ethnic community fits into the local area as well as larger American society (Zhou & Bankston, 1998). Ali later relays his situation of having moved out of Dearborn, and how that led him to have a new, difficult to name, perspective on those who remained.

> Ali: I went to Plymouth High School, and there were actually three high schools in one, we would have classes sort of like a college campus, and there were six thousand kids, and there are not many Arabs and, you know, a good diversity, it's so different there. I was in Dearborn my whole life. I moved there [Canton] for my high school years, and coming back here, I feel like-- I don't want to say people are more closed minded, but they are more, I don't know how to explain it—
>
> (University of Y)

Unable to verbalize his new perspective, he nevertheless sees a difference between being Arab when one lives within an ethnic enclave contrasted to living in an area where the number of Arabs is small. Though a community aspect to Arab culture was identified, where "place" mattered, aspects that transcended place also emerged, including the notion of family honor and gender.

Family honor referred to a sense that family name and reputation was highly significant and integral to the cultural outlook of Arab Americans. As such, instances where potential conflict may arise included a reference to Arab or Middle Eastern culture embodying family honor, and men, in particular, charged with defending it.

Lutfi: Well, I mean—in Middle Eastern life—I mean, when I went to the Middle East, it was very—it's a very male driven society, and it's so,—feeling like – How dare you insult my family, I'm gonna attack you. You know, it's just—it's so--

Samira: It's tied into anger, pride, all of that.

(University of Z)

The prominence of honor and men's responsibility to defend it is a well-known social fact in many cultures. For instance, it has been linked to fluctuating violent crime rates in different places and across time periods in the United States and Europe (Nisbett & Cohen, 1996; Roth, 2009). Indeed, defending honor has historically been seen as a means to gain respect and hence deter attacks from others, especially when no central government exists, or is too weak, to ensure protection and order. The fact that men must protect honor, however, highlights links between honor and masculinity. In Arab societies, family historically held ultimate responsibility for member well-being across the life course, with its patrilineal structure indicting men with enormous responsibility in the role of protector (Aswad, 1997). Identifying this aspect of their own culture, and understanding it as key to the enactment of social relations, particularly hurtful situations where one feels possibly wronged, provides some insight into how self-defined cultural attributes shape attitudes, feelings, and potentially behavior.

The significance of gender as key to cultural aspects of being Arab also emerged with references to family social relations. Mirroring previous work conducted in this area (Ajrouch, 1999, 2000, 2004) focus group participants noted different expectations depending on whether one was a man/boy or a woman/girl.

Reem: I think that's in our culture though, because I know my parents, it's ok for my brother to do something, but for my sister and I to do something, it's not ok. And it bugs me, and I tell them, but even with other families, it is the same in a sense…I don't know, if we were to be, like stay out past twelve o'clock, or go to a party or whatever, it's ok for him, but for the girls, there's more scrutiny upon it.

Roxanne: Also in gender, dating. My parents frown upon it. They do not directly frown upon me dating, but if I date, they feel it's a blow to my reputation as a woman in the community. But my brother, they think it's the funniest, cutest thing. If he has a girl over, "oh my God, look, Mac's got--" it's so funny to them. But for me, it's like, "Roxanne school comes first, don't, you know, boys." There's definitely a bias.

Facilitator: So do you feel mistreated then by your parents because of that?

Roxanne: I mean, I would if I didn't understand that this is, one theory, this is how their primed to think. So I do not think I am mistreated, but I, in essence I am being mistreated, but I know that they do not know any better.

Facilitator: Charley?

Charley: I agree that it's like that. I don't have any experience personally, because, I have, it's me and then four brothers, so I have no sisters to base it off of. But I do see that all the time, and I do agree that it's like that, and swayed toward uh, criticizing girls like that.

Roxanne: It's a big blessing for your Mom to have five boys. Everyone in the community smiles at that (Charley: (chuckles) yeah) right? That's a good thing.

(University of X)

The discrepancy focus group participants identify in how boys and girls are viewed and treated transcends religious affiliations in that Reem is Muslim while both Roxanne and Charley are Christian. Such data contribute to the notion that Arab culture/ethnicity, supersedes religious culture (Read & Oselin, 2008). It also emphasizes the dual worlds within which Arab American girls live. Girls who learn to navigate the two cultures, that of their parents and that of the dominant culture, will undoubtedly benefit from both worlds. However, the situation may arise where they embrace one culture over the other. Arab American girls, like girls from many immigrant cultures, occupy a unique position in that conforming to parental values constitutes a deviation from dominant cultural norms yet conforming to dominant cultural norms likely challenges parental values. Girls from Arab families living in the United States must negotiate between two worlds, and two sets of cultural values that often seem incompatible.

The three main aspects of culture identified, place (community), family honor, and gender relations inform social relations experiences where life is a family affair. Family, it should be noted, is broadly defined to include extended members and friends as core elements. Life events seldom occur outside of family scrutiny where family members are directly involved in one another's business.

> Lena: My Mom's side of the family, we are all in each other's business. If something happens, everyone is kind of a part of it, and I think that's kind of nice, in a way, because you're getting advice from several different people. But also it's annoying, because if you mess up then you're gonna get lectured by every single member.
>
> (Laughter)
>
> Mustapha: That's just so how my immediate family is. If I do something wrong, when I see my sister, she'll run to my parents. When I see my Mom, she'll yell at me, and then I see my Dad, he'll yell at me. Then I see my sisters, all three of them—they yell at me.
>
> (Laughter)
>
> Mustapha: You just get lectured at by everybody.
>
> (University of Y)

Moreover, family conflict varies from ignoring as a coping strategy to outright yelling and physical contact. The prominence of multiple ways to address hurtful situations within the family sphere showcases a diversity of reactions, but simultaneously suggests the emotional depth to the conflict and the means used to control or escape from the wrongful act/situation.

> Zahra: Well, with my family, I know not all, but most Arab families have problems within each other. Like uncles and aunts that don't talk to each other, brothers and brothers that-- there is that going on in my family, both with my Dad's side and my Mom's side of the family. And I noticed how they deal with it. They ignore. There have been years and years where they haven't talked to each other. My Dad and his brother, and my Mom's side, just recently, a lot of problems with her brother. And the way they deal with it, is ignoring, not, yeah that's it—just no contact...
>
> Alexandra: For me, I'm half white and half Arabic, so I've seen the extreme of both sides. For my Mom's side of the family, they're really, you know, civilized. They sit down and talk about things. But the Arabic side, they're more, like, screaming at each other. You said this, and he said this. And then, I always see my Grandma between the whole thing, because, you know, she's the mom of all the kids. And she's always, you find her screaming more than all the other people. And one time, she literally was really upset. She took off her slippers and started throwing them at everybody. And for—when it comes to Arabs fighting, it gets

really crazy, I think. I think for my Mom's side of the family, they're really—some of them, they hide things from—they don't confront each other about it. I think that's kind of a bad thing. But then for my Dad's side of the family, they do confront each other about it, but they get mad over the littlest things. So I guess there's pros and cons for both sides.

Mustapha: I think it's obvious that we have an aggressive way of dealing with--.

Lena: And we're very passionate about things—

Mustapha: Exactly. Yeah, about everything.

Lena: I know that it's wrong to generalize, but honestly it seems like it applies a lot. That we're just passionate—that we care so much, that we don't know how to express our needs and feelings.

Kemal: Yeah, we let our emotions get the best of us.

Joseph: Yeah, with everything.

Kemal: Probably what happens with my immediate family, we just like to go over it as a whole, and, usually when my Dad gets off work, or something, then we'll just all sit and talk about the issue, and try to resolve it in a way. But there are other problems with that, you know, sometimes yelling or something. (chuckle)

Joseph: It doesn't even have to be just in your immediate family. I mean, even if your friend is hurt by his parents or his other brother or something. You treat your friend you are really close to as your family, he's like your brother, and—but the bad part about that is you get brought into the middle of his family, and then you're gonna get yelled at, and stuff like that.

(University of Y)

The dichotomy introduced when Alexandra states she is "half white and half Arabic" illustrates an important view that Arab Americans have about their own culture. First, it clearly demarcates Arab identity as unique from white identity, an interesting situation given that Arab Americans are legally classified as white on all official government records (Ajrouch & Jamal, 2007; Samhan, 1999). Previous research has shown that perceptions of family closeness often define the ways members of various ethnic groups distinguish themselves from "Americans." For example, research dealing with the Polish (Lopata, 1994), Chaldeans (Sengstock, 1982) and various other European ethnic groups (Waters, 1990) have found that each think they have closer family ties than do "Americans." Interestingly, these data move beyond idealized notions of positive family relations to show that ways of dealing with family conflict have an ethnic character. It highlights a belief that Arab culture is uniquely expressive concerning family conflict.

The cultural norm to accept passionate expressions within family interactions does not extend to relations outside of family, however.

Asra: And then I think it's the cultural norm, like if I'm talking back at my sister, and I know it's normal in my family, but then somebody did it at work or somebody at school, I'd take it totally differently. I wouldn't talk back, you know, I would handle the situation, however that may be.

Facilitator: Yeah. What does that mean?

Asra: I don't know. I'd probably either shut them down with my words, or I don't know, walk away. You know, like okay, grow up, 'bye.'

Samira: I think it also depends on the person, because my sister is all about peace and love, and all that. But she'll kill you with just her words. She doesn't even need to touch me and I'm, like, Sis did you just say that?

(University of Z)

As the above narrative illustrates, within family reactions differ quite markedly from reaction with those outside the family. More restraint is the preferred approach when interacting with people outside the family. This approach usually is related to an awareness that to non-Arabs they are seen as representatives of all Arabs. These students make a conscientious effort to react with restraint so as to model ideal behaviors in their role as universal representatives of all Arabs. In other words, the focus group participants often referred to the fact that because they are visible as Arabs, they felt a need to conduct themselves in a respectful manner. Perceptions of how outsiders see Arabs are discussed below, but first, we highlight within group diversity.

Importantly, focus group participants introduced within group diversity. Though common cultural elements were shared by all as "Arab" Americans, there nevertheless existed a very real perception that not all Arab Americans are equal.

Shireen: Yeah, I feel like if there is respect there, then it's not as big of a deal. I have had Lebanese friends make Syria jokes, Syria-Lebanon jokes. And they are, [chuckles] if they are friends, that's no big deal. If its someone I just met them, then I take it personally, because it's like, who are you to, you do not know who I am, you do not know how I feel... so, it depends.

Amal: ...I think I would get more offended if it was somebody that I did not know, and I think it's just if it's like the time and the place to be making a joke about it, or I guess how they're saying it or what they're saying. Sometimes certain things really bug me more than other things. Some things that might not even affect...and you said specifically about if your culture or your heritage, sometimes those things won't bother me as much as someone said something else that does not really deal with my culture, but maybe about my gender or about an identity, another identity that I hold. But I think it's also, I don't mind making, sometimes I make a joke with a friend, that I know, if it's a friend, if we are making jokes back and forth, like she said Syria-Lebanese jokes, if I make a joke with someone that's let's say Lebanese, and they make a joke about me being Iraqi, I will take in a ok manner as long as I know that they are saying it in a way, I do not how put this—umm--

Facilitator: So are there tensions between the different Middle Eastern groups that you guys experience? I mean jokes that are based on national origins among or between yourselves?

Reem: I think every culture, every heritage, like me being Lebanese, Jordanian, Syrian whatever, they all want to show the world that they are the best, and so I think that it's competition to prove to the rest of the community that they are better than, and that's where these jokes come in. Again kind of like a way, to ease a problem or whatever.

Shireen: To some extent I disagree. Because I think because I am very proud of being Syrian, but I don't think that my culture is any better, or my nation is any better than any other. But I definitely think that it's just, I don't know, I mean, for example, Syrians don't make jokes about Lebanon and Syria as much as Lebanese do. And I think that's definitely because of what actually happened and stuff. And so for them that was something they grew up with, and that's something that was an issue with them. And for me that wasn't. And so I think it just really depends. I definitely think that there are tensions, but on the grander scheme of things, that's when we were together, but I feel if we were arguing with, like someone... that, for example ....pro-Israelis or something, we wouldn't start talking about (Reem: uh uhh) issues, like someone would not start stabbing me for being, (Roger: right) or making stabs at me for being Syrian, so--

(University of X)

Differences within the Arab American pan-ethnic category noted by focus group participants reveal important distinctions that not only influence social relations within the group, but hold special implications for outsiders who often view Arabs as homogeneous. Moreover the hierarchy identified where some national origin groups perceive themselves to be above others, calls attention to potential discomfort among and between Arab Americans. These points hold special significance for understanding how within-ethnic group social relations can inform perceptions of hurtful encounters or of being mistreated.

In sum, discussions point to key aspects of Arab culture identified by Arab Americans that inform ways in which social relations occur and how they will respond to minor transgressions such as ethnically targeted jokes. Clearly, some potentially hurtful statements or comments are easier to forgive than others and this partially depends on who is making them. Cultural elements described highlight areas where culture and social relations intersect. Such intersections hold significant implications for perceptions of Arab Americans by the general U.S. population.

Perception of Arabs from Outside

All participants acknowledged that perceptions of Arabs by others often include unflattering notions. As a result, participants identified ways of coping with the realization that one person's action represents all Arabs. Situations encountered vary by whether or not Arab Americans are identifiable as such. For instance, those who are visibly Muslim, e.g., wear the hijab, face situations that are more overt, and prompt a belief of having to model behaviors of an ideal human being.

> Sarah: …if you stand out, the proper way to go about this, is just act like an almost ideal person, or always know that your acting what your conduct is, reflects the whole population, the rest of the population, so just making sure that you are being the best person that you can be will clear up that misunderstanding.
>
> Marjan: I agree with her.
>
> Asra: Like, some people, they'll be really rude and they'll yell at you, like how that lady told you to go back to your country. You could snap back, or say something back that is even more hurtful, or you could just be calm and say something that will make them realize that they were wrong without kind of giving in to a Middle Eastern type stereotype, that they are violent and loud and angry. I think being calm in a situation is the best way to handle it.
>
> (University of Z)

Here, focus group participants identify a Middle Eastern negative stereotype and discuss how it informs relations with non-Arabs who mistreat them. Careful attention to how their own behavior contributes to a stereotype suggests the burden of being the exemplar for a diverse group. Recognizing this responsibility requires maturity and wisdom often acquired only later in life. Being a visible minority exposes people to negative experiences which create somewhat paradoxical circumstances. Repeated exposure, awareness of one's own minority status, ethnic identity, and one would assume, ethnic pride, enables these young people to think carefully about their experiences and their reactions. It is especially impressive that rather than focus on how to provide the facts or clarify specific untruths, they focus on how best to impress the misinformed with their model behavior. Rather than become angry or hostile, they aim to be forgiving and persuasive.

For others, whose "Arab" ethnicity was not so obvious, a struggle is identified where they are singled out as the exception, instead of the rule.

> Ali: Definitely, they should know. Someone should talk to them about, you know, tell them what they're thinking is wrong. That they can't judge a whole group, based on...ah, they're thinking in an ethnocentric manner. People see our culture is maybe different from others, and so because it's different, or any culture, not just ours. You know, they might think it's wrong, or strange.
>
> Lena: But the sad truth is that people don't like to change their minds, they assimilate more than they accommodate, and so they kind of look at you, like, oh, you are the exception... and then you're not like the rest of them, sort of thing.
>
> Ali: That's true, yeah.
>
> Kemal: And then you can talk about the fight, and you can compare it to 9/11, because as soon as that happened, all of a sudden the media is Muslim this, Muslim that. So, when people see that, and they're going to compare it to, you know, well all Muslims are like this guy, or like this group.
>
> Joseph: They classify you as a terrorist right away.
>
> (Laughter)
>
> Joseph: Regardless.
>
> Kemal: Whether they know you or not.
>
> Mustapha: It's like Lena said, and then when they meet you—
>
> Kemal: Yep.
>
> Mustapha: --and they see that you're different, all of a sudden they say, ok, you're an exception. You're not like the rest of them. As if the majority of them are the terrorists...
>
> Alexandra: Or like me, like when I meet people and I find out, you know, things about them, and they know who I am, I eventually tell them that I'm Arabic, at one point. And they're—and the look on their faces, it's really funny. They're, like, really? I'm, like, yeah. I'm really Arabic. And so, things slowly-- looking at that, things eventually change, for the good.
>
> Joseph: What she [Alexandra]said about being Arabic, that also affects the relationship, because if someone doesn't know what your background, or your culture, is, they're going to look at you totally differently once you tell them what you are. If they never knew you were Arabic, and they assumed just by, your looks, you were not Arabic—let's say you were Irish or Polish. Just by looks, they would look at you as if you are one of them. But once you tell them you're Arabic, they change their whole perspective about you.
>
> (University of Y)

Being the exception, as opposed to the rule, and struggling against such assessments, haunt those who are not readily identifiable as Arab. Though such scenarios indicate the presence of "ethnic options" (Waters, 1990) for some Arab Americans, most strive to announce themselves as Arab in the quest to directly combat negative stereotypes.

Educating others was also a theme introduced time and again as the participants talked about facing negativity.

> Nina: People didn't think I was Arab, and—that's another thing, because every class in high school, they have, there are a couple kids that are, the jerks. That are, you know, they're not going anywhere. You know...they're mean to everybody. And the guy was actually a friend of mine. And I was waiting. I was at my locker with one of my friends, and he's walking down the hallway, and he said, all I hear is, Yeah, Arabs, they don't do anything, they just—they smell, and they own gas stations. (chuckles) Something like that. So, I'm not a confrontational person, but that was the first time I actually heard somebody that was a friend of mine say something like that. So I stopped him in the hallway, and I turned to my friend, I'm just like, gee I don't smell, do I? He's just like, You're Arab? And I'm, like, yeah, I am Arab. Oh yeah, and my Dad doesn't own a gas station, in case you wanted to know. You know? I just think it's really funny, and he just went blank, the reaction is the funniest thing.
>
> Joseph: I feel like it's our job as Arabs to—
>
> Mustapha: Educate.
>
> Joseph: Educate-- be educated—yeah, to be able to tell them what's wrong with what they are saying...
>
> (University of Y)

The idea that knowledge is power guides the strategy to confront negativity with educating the transgressor. This approach mirrors coping strategies identified when Middle Eastern American adults encounter situations where they must face demeaning, hurtful, or dehumanizing acts (Marvasti, 2005). The fact that these young adults have embraced such an approach illustrates wisdom borne of experience and beyond most others of their own age.

> Marjan: I mean, I think it's also our job as Muslims to educate them if they don't know. Just give them the information in a kind of sly way, and be, like – Oh, and now I know, I didn't have to go through that uncomfortable—like having to ask them personally.
>
> Asra: Not even just as Muslims, but as Arab Americans, some people may get the wrong idea about us, just like everyone said, ignorance, lack of communication, they might just get the wrong idea.
>
> (University of Z)

Taking on the responsibility to pre-emptively educate before a hurtful comment/act can be made showcases the sophisticated understanding these young Arab Americans have of interethnic relations. Participants demonstrate the power of their own agency to alleviate conflict, tension, and mistreatment. Again, rather than react with anger to potential insults, they react proactively to create a more viable, less hostile circumstance that promotes positive social relations and prevents negativity.

In sum, discussions point to a recognition by participants that Arab Americans are perceived in a negative light by others. The social relations described highlight areas where culture and social relations intersect, as well as identify points where forgiveness may be needed. The application of forgiveness, however, was most salient in the realm of family relations.

Forgiveness

Forgiveness has been defined as a journey, not an act (Worthington, 2005). Worthington elaborates that true forgiveness requires a willingness to remember the transgression, and come to terms with it by facing it directly as a first step. Reaching an understanding of how and why it happened transforms the memory of the transgression, replacing negative emotions with empathy and understanding. The forgiving person thoughtfully considers why the act happened, and with that understanding transforms the memory of the transgression, though does not forget it. The ideal practice of forgiveness does not mean ending a relationship with the person who wronged, mistreated, or hurt another.

Though this ideal definition thoroughly illuminates the complexity of forgiving, it does not necessarily represent the pragmatic daily experiences of forgiveness. Religious teachings, both Christian and Muslim, contributed to the understanding of forgiveness among focus group participants, but its application and importance involved family relations and the expectation of close ties. Maintaining and/or breaking the close social relationship played a large role in the pragmatic understanding of forgiveness. We first illustrate how understandings of forgiveness inform a situation where close family ties break.

> Zahra: So I was thinking about my own family. Earlier, how I was saying my mom and her brother don't talk…So, it's been a long, long time since they haven't been talking, on and off, on and off. And a long time ago when they'd fight, he'd bring her flowers and say, I'm sorry, and my mom's his older sister, so she forgave him and we still had our connection with our uncle. But now recently, it's gotten really, really bad, and we haven't been seeing him, or going to his house, and my mom was thinking, religious-wise, she has to talk to him, this is her brother and not talking to a sibling is really bad. You know, what if something happens-- so she went to a Sheikh, you know? Okay. And she went to talk to him first, to see what my mom should do, and because this has been happening so many times—he says he is sorry, but he does the same stupid thing. He told her to—if it—because it causes her stress, and the Sheikh told her, if this causes you stress, and is hard—bothering to us, to even we don't want contact with him. So he just told her don't talk to him. And it came from him, so she has to—she's not gonna—yeah so religious wise she's not gonna talk to him.
>
> (University of Y)

The necessity of forgiveness was lodged in religious teachings, hence a religious leader, the Sheikh (similar to a Priest or Reverend) was consulted. Though the severing of a sibling tie is considered shameful, permission to end the relationship was seen as a means to retain well-being. If we define forgiveness as a process, it may be that ending a relationship when a wrong continues over time must occur in order to take the first step of directly facing, as opposed to forgetting, the mistreatment.

Though forgiving and forgetting were sometimes used interchangeably by focus group participants, the importance of family ties led to a sentiment of the necessity of forgiveness.

> Samira: No matter what you argue about, and no matter what you disagree about, the love is so strong, that it's not going to tear you apart. I mean, me and my brother fight all the time about… it gets bad but it never—well, it doesn't get physical between us with some walls, you know—

> and getting hit or something. But, I mean, it depends on the relationship with the people, too. If I'm fighting with a random person that I'm never going to see again, I'll probably give him a piece of my mind. Family….you know that they will always forgive you, always. I know in my house, at least each one of us has punched a hole in the wall, at least once it's happened. But, we just fix it. We all get the caulk and we all fix it together. And then you—and it's not even an hour later and you're laughing. It's like, okay now we have a hole in the wall…
>
> (University of Y)

Reference to situations of interpersonal forgiveness in the realm of family relations may hold special significance for Arab Americans because the family is so central to one's identity, security, and overall well-being. Indeed, a disposition toward forgiveness may help to maintain cohesive social relations, particularly those that have enormous benefits to overall well-being (McFarland et al., 2012). The links focus group participants made between forgiveness and family suggest that the issue of forgiveness is relevant to their daily lives, playing an important role in the maintenance and dissolution of relationships.

Implications

A focus on culture, social relations, and forgiveness among Arab American college students provides initial insights into the ways that Arab Americans cope with hurtful situations or a sense of being wronged. Using the convoy model of social relations to frame our observations, we found that personal characteristics, such as being Arab American, male or female, influenced the experience of situational characteristics, i.e., culture, which in turn shapes participants' social relations, both inside and outside of their ethnic group. It should also be noted that illustrative examples in this chapter presented the experiences of young adults. Age is a key personal characteristic, often indicative of role transitions and developmental trajectories over the life course that may uniquely inform social relations (Ajrouch, Antonucci, & Janevic, 2001). Furthermore, perceptions and examples of being "othered" are relayed, influencing their entire convoy, both contemporaneously and longitudinally, including their quality of life, health, and well-being. Finally, as noted earlier, we considered how personal characteristics, situational characteristics, and social relations influence individual perspectives concerning forgiveness of both nonfamily and family convoy members. The utility of the convoy model of social relations for thinking about how such elements have implications for health and well-being is discussed below.

Convoys of social relations are conceptualized as a structure of support that protects the individual across time and space (Antonucci, 2001; Kahn & Antonucci, 1980). The identification of place highlights the importance of ethnic community living to social relations, while family honor and gender relations draw attention to ideals of masculinity and femininity as influential in social relations. Each played a critical role in the experience of social relations, and hence the ways in which they link to health and well-being should be considered. Though self-identified, cultural elements provide important insights that sensitize practitioners to issues in need of attention, the wide range of diversity among Arab Americans requires that health practitioners not necessarily assume they understand the dilemma an Arab American faces. Importantly, the individuals and issues in need of attention may depend upon setting. For instance, the structure of social networks and the type and quality of support exchanged may differ depending on if one lives in an ethnic community and if one is a man or woman. Whether aspects of social relations conform to norms and expectations that accompany such personal and situational characteristics are very likely to influence both mental and physical health outcomes.

How an individual's convoy of social relations influence health may also be expressed in the kinds and quality of relations experienced with non-Arab Americans. Arab American college students appear to take on a minority status which exposes them to unique experiences. Whether visibly different or not, the goal to project a positive image is of central importance. Perceived discrimination, that is perceptions of unfairness or injustice, has been found to robustly predict psychological distress (Jackson, Williams, & Torres, 2003; Williams et al., 2012), self-rated health as well as physical health including high blood pressure, cholesterol, and obesity (Johnston & Lordan, 2012). Such experiences should be identified in future studies on Arab American health. The convoy model of social relations provides a heuristic framework for thinking about main effects of a stressor such as discrimination, and whether or not relationships may serve as a resource to alleviate effects on health.

Finally, the links between social relations and forgiveness are especially critical. Findings from this study provide preliminary insight into the meanings of forgiveness in an Arab American context. These cross-sectional data provide snapshots into the convoy and forgiveness experiences of a select group of Arab Americans, i.e., young college students. The data from these focus groups indicate that close ties represent relationships where forgiveness appears to be quite central for these young people. This arises as particularly salient given the central role family relations play in the well-being of Arab Americans. Discussions illustrate that participants clearly value family, but they recognize both the positive and negative aspects of relations within the family context. Convoys, like families, tend to include longitudinal relations which shape the structure and function of social relations and are then drawn upon when confronted with problematic or difficult circumstances in the present. These college students clearly indicated that their views of how social relations should be considered were shaped by their long-term family relations which in turn seemed to influence whether or not they were inclined to forgive hurtful, difficult, or conflictual circumstances they encountered.

Forgiveness is increasingly seen as a potential intervention for various situations including psychological therapy (Jacinto & Edwards, 2011) and youth violence in educational settings (Chubbuck, 2009–2010). Future directions should seek to more fully uncover the motives behind forgiveness among Arab Americans. Though we found that religious directives guided an understanding of forgiveness for both Muslim and Christian participants in our focus groups, motives may vary by religious affiliation or by country in which one lives (Ballester, Chatri, Sastre, Riviere, & Mullet, 2011; Mullet & Azar, 2009). Overall, this chapter shows that, as Enright et al. (1989) suggested in their study of forgiveness and adolescents, the tendency to forgive is very much influenced by (their convoy of) social relations.

Acknowledgement We are grateful to the Fetzer Institute for their support of this research.

References

Agar, M., & MacDonald, J. (1995). Focus groups and ethnography. *Human Organization, 54*, 78–86.

Ajrouch, K. J. (1999). Family and ethnic identity in an Arab American community. In M. Suleiman (Ed.), *Arabs in America: Building a new future* (pp. 129–139). Philadelphia: Temple University Press.

Ajrouch, K. J. (2000). Place, age, and culture: Community living and ethnic identity among Lebanese American adolescents. *Small Group Research, 31*, 447–469.

Ajrouch, K. J. (2004). Gender, race, and symbolic boundaries: Contested spaces of identity among Arab-American adolescents. *Sociological Perspectives, 47*, 371–391.

Ajrouch, K. J., Antonucci, T. C., & Janevic, M. R. (2001). Social networks among blacks and whites: The interaction between race and age. *The Journals of Gerontology. Series B, Psychological Sciences and Social Sciences, 56B*(2), S112–S118.

Ajrouch, K. J., & Jamal, A. (2007). Assimilating to a white identity: The case of Arab Americans. *International Migration Review, 41*(4), 860–879.

Antonucci, T. C. (2001). Social relations: An examination of social networks, social support, and sense of control. In J. E. Birren & K. Warner Schaie (Eds.), *Handbook of aging: Psychological sciences* (pp. 427–453). San Diego: Academic.

Antonucci, T. C., & Akiyama, H. (1995). Convoys of social relations: Family and friendships within a life span context. In R. Blieszner & V. H. Bedford (Eds.), *Handbook of aging and the family* (pp. 355–372). Westport, CT: Greenwood Press.

Antonucci, T. C., Birditt, K. S., & Ajrouch, K. J. (2011). Convoys of social relations: Past, present and future. In K. Fingerman, C. Berg, T. C. Antonucci, & J. Smith (Eds.), *Handbook of life span development* (pp. 161–182). New York: Springer.

Aswad, B. C. (1974). The southeast Dearborn Arab community struggles for survival against urban "renewal". In B. C. Aswad (Ed.), *Arabic speaking communities in American cities* (pp. 53–84). New York: Center for Migrations Studies.

Aswad, B. C. (1997). Arab American families. In M. K. DeGenova (Ed.), *Families in cultural context* (pp. 218–238). Mayfield, CA: Mayfield Publishing.

Ballester, S., Chatri, F., Sastre, M. T. M., Riviere, S., & Mullet, E. (2011). Forgiveness-related motives: A structural and cross-cultural approach. *Social Science Information, 50*(2), 178–200.

Barakat, H. (1993). *The Arab world: Society, culture, and state*. Berkeley, CA: University of California Press.

Berry, J. W., & Worthington, E. L., Jr. (2001). Forgivingness, relationship quality, stress while imagining relationship events, and physical and mental health. *Journal of Counseling Psychology, 48*, 447–455.

Brittingham, A., & de la Cruz, G. P. (2005). We the people of Arab ancestry in the United States. *Current Population Reports*. Washington, DC: Department of Commerce. Retrieved May 18, 2006, from, http://www.census.gov/prod/2005pubs/censr-21.pdf.

Buda, R., & Elsayed-Elkhouly, S. M. (1998). Cultural differences between Arabs and Americans: Individualism-collectivism revisited. *Journal of Cross-Cultural Psychology, 29*(3), 487–492.

Chubbuck, S. (2010). Forgiveness education: Urban youth's perception and collective narratives. *Journal for the Study of Peace and Conflict, Annual edition* (2009–2010), 77–88.

Enright, R. D., Santos, M. J. D., & Al-Mabuk, R. (1989). The adolescent as forgiver. *Journal of Adolescence, 12*(1), 99–110.

Gans, H. J. (1962). *Urban villagers: Group and class in the life of Italian-Americans*. New York: The Free Press.

Harris, A. H. S., & Thoresen, C. E. (2005). Forgiveness, unforgiveness, health, and disease. In E. L. Worthington Jr. (Ed.), *Handbook of forgiveness* (pp. 321–348). New York: Routledge.
Hofstede, G. H. (1980). *Culture's consequences, international differences in work-related values*. Beverly Hills, CA: Sage.
Hook, J. N., Worthington, E. L., & Utsey, S. O. (2009). Collectivism, forgiveness, and social harmony. *The Counseling Psychologist, 37*(6), 821–847.
Hughes, D., & DuMont, K. (1993). Using focus groups to facilitate culturally-anchored research. *American Journal of Community Psychology, 21*, 775–806.
Inglehart, R., & Welzel, C. (2005). *Modernization, culture change, and democracy*. New York: Cambridge University Press.
Jacinto, G. A., & Edwards, B. L. (2011). Therapeutic stages of forgiveness and self-forgiveness. *Journal of Human Behaviour in the Social Environment, 21*(4), 423–437.
Jackson, J. S., Williams, D. R., & Torres, M. (2003). Perceptions of discrimination, health and mental health: The social stress process. In A. Rockville & M. D. Maney (Eds.), *Social stressors, personal and social resources, and their mental health consequences* (pp. 86–146). Bethesda, MD: National Institute of Mental Health.
Jarrett, R. L., & Burton, L. M. (1999). Dynamic dimensions of family structure in low-income African American families: Emergent themes in qualitative research. *Journal of Comparative Family Studies, 30*, 177–187.
Johnston, D. W., & Lordan, G. (2012). Discrimination makes me sick! An examination of the discrimination-health relationship. *Journal of Health Economics, 31*(1), 99–111.
Kağitçibaşi, Ç. (1996). *Family and human development across cultures: A view from the other side*. Hillsdale, NJ: Lawrence Erlbaum Associates.
Kahn, R., & Antonucci, T. C. (1980). Convoys over the life course: Attachment, roles and social support. In P. Bates & O. Brim (Eds.), *Life span development and behaviour* (pp. 253–286). New York: Academic.
Lawler, K. A., Younger, J. W., Piferi, R. L., Jobe, R. L., Edmondson, K., & Jones, W. H. (2005). The unique effects of forgiveness on health: An exploration of pathways. *Journal of Behavioral Medicine, 28*, 157–167.
Lawler-Row, K. A., Karremans, J. C., Scott, C., Edlis-Matityahou, M., & Edwards, L. (2008). Forgiveness, physiological reactivity and health: The role of anger. *International Journal of Psychophysiology, 68*, 51–58.
Lopata, H. Z. (1994). *Polish Americans*. New Brunswick, NJ: Transaction.
Maltby, J., Day, L., & Barber, L. (2004). Forgiveness and mental health variables: Interpreting the relationship using an adaptational-continuum model of personality and coping. *Personality and Individual Differences, 37*, 1629–1641.
Maltby, J., Macaskill, A., & Day, L. (2001). Failure to forgive self and others: A replication and extension of the relationship between forgiveness, personality, social desirability and general health. *Personality and Individual Differences, 181*, 1–6.
Markus, H. R., & Kitayama, S. (1991). Culture and the self: Implications for cognition, emotion, and motivation. *Psychological Review, 98*(2), 224–253.
Martinez, I. L. (2002). The elder in the Cuban American family: Making sense of the real and ideal. *Journal of Comparative Family Studies, 33*, 359–375.
Marvasti, A. B. (2004). *Qualitative research in sociology*. Thousand Oaks, CA: Sage.
Marvasti, A. (2005). Being Middle Eastern American: Identity negotiation in the context of the war on terror. *Symbolic Interaction, 28*(4), 525–547.
McCullough, M. E., & Witvliet, C. V. O. (2002). The psychology of forgiveness. In C. R. Snyder & S. Lopez (Eds.), *Handbook of positive psychology* (pp. 446–458). New York: Oxford University Press.
McFarland, M. J., Smith, C. A., Touissaint, L., & Thomas, P. A. (2012). Forgiveness of others and health: Do race and neighborhood matter? *The Journals of Gerontology. Series B, Psychological Sciences and Social Sciences, 67*(1), 66–75.

Miles, M. B., & Huberman, A. M. (1994). *Qualitative data analysis* (2nd ed.). Thousand Oaks, CA: Sage.
Morgan, D. L. (1988). *Focus groups as qualitative research*. Newbury Park, CA: Sage.
Mullet, E., & Azar, F. (2009). Apologies, repentance, and forgiveness: A Muslim–Christian comparison. *The International Journal for the Psychology of Religion, 19*(4), 275–285.
Nisbett, R. E., & Cohen, D. (1996). *Culture of honor*. Boulder, CO: Westview Press.
Oyserman, D., Kemmelmeier, M., & Coon, H. M. (2002). Cultural psychology, a new look: Reply to Bond (2002), Fiske (2002), Kitayama (2002), and Miller (2002). *Psychological Bulletin, 128*(1), 110–117.
Read, J. G. (2004). *Culture, class, and work among Arab-American women*. New York: LFB Scholarly Publishing.
Read, J. G., & Oselin, S. (2008). Gender and the education-employment paradox in ethnic and religious contexts: The case of Arab Americans. *American Sociological Review, 73*, 296–313.
Roth, R. (2009). *American homicide*. Boston: Harvard University Press.
Samhan, H. H. (1999). Not quite white: Race classification and the Arab-American experience. In M. W. Suleiman (Ed.), *Arabs in America: Building a new future* (pp. 209–226). Philadelphia: Temple University Press.
Sengstock, M. C. (1982). *The Chaldean Americans: Changing conceptions of ethnic identity*. New York: Center for Migration Studies.
Shaheen, J. G. (2001). *Reel bad Arabs: How Hollywood vilifies a people*. Brooklyn, NY: Olive Branch Press.
Strauss, A. (1987). *Qualitative analysis for social scientists*. Cambridge, UK: Cambridge University Press.
Takahashi, K., Ohara, N., Antonucci, T. C., & Akiyama, H. (2002). Commonalities and differences in close relationships among the Americans and Japanese: A comparison by the individualism/collectivism concept. *International Journal of Behavioral Development, 26*(5), 453–465.
Toussaint, L. L., Williams, D. R., Musick, M. A., & Everson, S. A. (2001). Forgiveness and health: Age differences in a US probability sample. *Journal of Adult Development, 8*, 249–257.
Triandis, H. C., Bontempo, R., Villareal, M. J., Asai, M., & Lucca, N. (1988). Individualism and collectivism: Cross-cultural perspectives on self-ingroup relationships. *Journal of Personality and Social Psychology, 54*(2), 323–338.
Von Feigenblatt, O. F. (2010). Forgiveness and culture: An interdisciplinary dialogue. *Journal of History and Social Sciences, 1*(1), 1–9.
Waters, M. C. (1990). *Ethnic options: Choosing identities in America*. Berkeley, CA: University of California Press.
Williams, D. R., John, D. A., Oyserman, D., Sonnega, J., Mohammed, S. A., & Jackson, J. S. (2012). Research on discrimination and health: An exploratory study of unresolved conceptual and measurement issues. *American Journal of Public Health, 102*(5), 975–978.
Witvliet, C. V. O., Ludwig, T. E., & Vander Laan, K. (2001). Granting forgiveness or harboring grudges: Implications for emotion, physiology, and health. *Psychological Science, 12*, 117–123.
Worthington, E. L. (2005). *The power of forgiving*. West Conshohocken, PA: Templeton Foundation Press.
Worthington, E. L., Jr., & Scherer, M. (2004). Forgiveness is an emotion-focused coping strategy that can reduce health risks and promote health resilience: Theory, review, and hypotheses. *Psychology and Health, 19*, 385–405.
Zhou, M., & Bankston, C. L. (1998). *Growing up American: How Vietnamese children adapt to life in the United States*. New York: Russell Sage.

Part II
The Psychosocial Development of Arab Americans

Julie Hakim-Larson

There are no graves here. These mountains and plains are a cradle and a stepping-stone. Whenever you pass by the field where you have laid your ancestors look well thereupon, and you shall see yourselves and your children dancing hand in hand. Verily you often make merry without knowing. (K. Gibran, 1978/1923, The Prophet, pp.87–88).

Introduction

Ancestral ties to the Arab world provide the foundation for the psychosocial development of Arab Americans. Psychosocial development can be construed as involving three core developmental tasks: developing a sense of *trust* in others, developing an achieved *identity* and well-rounded sense of self in relation to others, and attaining a mastery of *ego integrity* whereby a person looks upon the past with emotional acceptance (Sneed, Whitbourne, & Culang, 2006). The chapters in this part address such psychosocial development in Arab Americans in the context of their acculturation, ethnic identity, history of traumatic experiences, mental health risks and resilience, educational and work experiences, and overall health within their home environments and communities.

As will be addressed throughout the chapters of this part, the psychosocial development of Arab Americans has been affected by a variety of normative history-graded and age-graded influences as well as nonnormative life events (Baltes, Reese, & Lipsitt, 1980). *Normative history-graded* influences are historical events, such as wars, famine, natural or economic disasters, which tend to have a similar

J. Hakim-Larson (✉)
Department of Psychology, University of Windsor,
Windsor, ON, Canada N9B 3P4
e-mail: hakim@uwindsor.ca

impact on an entire generation or birth cohort of a population such as the children of the Great Depression or their baby boomer children. The psychosocial development of Arab Americans has been affected by a host of worldwide events from the wars in the Middle East to the aftermath and backlash of attitudes in the United States after the tragedy of the attacks of 9/11. *Normative age-graded* influences affect people of the same age in a similar manner; Arab Americans face the same developmental tasks as other Americans when it comes to expectations by age—learning to drive a car as an adolescent, finishing high school by age 18 years, deciding on a career and making higher education choices in young adulthood, childbearing and child-rearing in adulthood, and facing retirement and eventually death in old age. *Non-normative life events* have an impact but differ uniquely from person to person and family to family. Given that Arab Americans represent such a diverse group of countries-of-origin and multiple generations, it is perhaps with nonnormative life events that we see some of the most unique psychosocial influences; for example, while an immigrant from Iraq and an immigrant from Lebanon may share a history of conflict and war in their homelands, the nature of their experiences could be quite different depending on when they lived in the Middle East and just who was involved in the conflict.

The Arab world has witnessed many normative history-graded influences extending from ancient history and these events form part of the long-term collective memory of the people (Zebian & Brown, 2013). This extended timeline of conflicts and political changes occurs even now and includes the youth movements in the Middle East during the Arab Spring of 2011. Thus, there is currently a juxtaposition of ancient conflicts with youthful innovation, edginess, and motivation for change. While the effects of the Arab Spring are yet to be fully realized, a public opinion survey in Arab countries and Iran late in 2011 showed that political issues involving democratic reforms and human rights were now top level priorities in comparison to public opinion rankings in 2009 (Arab American Institute, 2011). The effects of the history of economic problems, war, and conflicts on the younger generation appear to have reverberated throughout the older generation as well in the Middle East.

As noted throughout this book, the reasons for immigration from the Arab world to other countries in Europe and the Americas are varied, and include refuge from war and/or famine, freedom from oppression, the search for economic prosperity, and a spirit of adventure seeking (e.g., Suleiman, 1999). Many of the very issues that are related to ongoing protests and youth movements in the Middle East also formed the underlying basis for the immigration of some Arabs to North American over the past century.

In her chapter on acculturation and ethnic identity in Arab immigrants to North America, Mona Amer highlights the many protective and risk factors that have been shown to be related to their acculturation and psychological outcomes. Protective factors discussed include having a strong ethnic identity, using religion, family, and other forms of social support to cope, and having an available community network. On the other hand, risks include familial conflict over acculturation, assimilation pressures, public hostility after 9/11, discrimination, marginalization, and isolation from potential sources of support. While refugees from the Arab world have been shown to be vulnerable to mental health problems such as depression, anxiety, and posttraumatic stress disorder given their history of disrupted developmental tasks, adaptive psychosocial adjustment is also a potential outcome. From a developmental psychopathology perspective, adaptive psychosocial development has the opportunity to occur when both genetics and the environment interact in ways that protect individuals from risks; thus, some people are able to display resilience even in the face of the adverse effects of the exposure to war and discrimination (e.g., Masten, 2007). Resilience may be displayed by the ability to develop healthy attachments and trust in others, achieve a secure identity, and successfully integrate the events of one's past, difficult though it may be, into a resolved feeling of acceptance.

As described in the chapter on trauma, resilience, and recovery by Ibrahim Kira, Mona Amer, and Nancy Wrobel, it is a challenge for family members and health professionals alike in working to overcome the cumulative severe traumas embedded in the psychological histories of some Arab American refugees. *Collective identity traumas* incorporate the collective suffering of the peoples of the Middle East, including torture, oppression, autocratic government rule, and a succession of direct and neighboring wars. In addition, gender discrimination for women and the non-normative trauma of domestic violence experienced by some intensify the types of post-migration stressors encountered with acculturation, discrimination, and post 9/11 backlash. The experience of refugees varies as well by which period of the life span was most affected. For example, children and adolescents may be affected by a disruption to the attachment system, while refugee elders may face having to learn a new language and new way of everyday life. As reviewed by Kira et al., there are a number of models of recovery designed to help trauma survivors, but among these multi-systemic perspectives, ecological models seem to hold the most promise as they are quite comprehensive and incorporate various relevant contexts including the use of community agencies and the legal system.

Issues relevant to the mental health and well-being of Arab Americans across the life-span are further delineated in the chapter by Nancy Wrobel and Ashley Paterson. In particular, they describe studies that show how level of acculturation, religious affiliation, and education level among other factors have been linked to mental health outcomes including depressive and anxiety disorders. Taking a developmental view by looking at the age-graded tasks of Arab American children, adolescents, and adults from youth to old age, Wrobel and Paterson highlight the variety of stressors that can put individuals at risk for psychopathology. Guidelines for practitioners are provided in this chapter with the aim of fostering the culturally sensitive assessment and treatment of Arab Americans in need of mental health services.

Critical to the adaptive psychosocial development of Arab Americans are their achievements at school and work. Karen Haboush and Nicole Barakat describe in their chapter how resilience is based on the successful navigation of individuals in educational and employment contexts. In the Arab world as in the United States, both educational and occupational successes are highly regarded. Haboush and Barakat document how historical trends in education and employment in Arab American immigrants are related to various government policies, labor practices and needs, and sociopolitical contexts or "zeitgeist." The chapter authors further delineate the importance of the school and work environments for healthy identity development in children, adolescents, and adults, including individuals with disabilities and those who are learning English as a second language. Unfortunately, at times prejudicial attitudes and discriminatory practices are still challenges to be overcome by Arab American students, employees, and those advocating on their behalf. Haboush and Barakat highlight the importance of future research trends in assisting in the progress for Arab Americans at school and work in the wide range of communities in which they live.

This part of the book concludes with a chapter by Hikmet Jamil on environmental health in Arab American community settings. As noted by Jamil, various countries in the Middle East are now attempting to make progress in setting social and environmental public health policies to benefit the people affected. However, this was not historically the case. Throughout the history of immigration to the United States, for example, the lack of government attention to public health and well-being in many Middle Eastern countries-of-origin led to deficiencies in public health education and services. Thus, Arab American immigrants often brought health problems with them that may have been exacerbated by the social and physical environments in which they settled. Jamil discusses issues such as lead poisoning, air pollution, workplace safety issues, and smoking and their impact on chronic diseases from a public and environmental health perspective.

The bio-ecological systems framework of Urie Bronfenbrenner (1994) and Swick and Williams (2006) seems to be an especially appropriate way to organize the complex interplay of persons and environments that are involved in the stresses and everyday experiences of Arab Americans as described in the chapters of this part on psychosocial development. Bronfenbrenner's theory incorporates a series of nesting influences on the development of individuals. At the *microsystem* level of analysis, the child, adolescent, or adult interacts directly with others in the social network of family, school, and work, while the *mesosystem* involves the next higher level of analysis whereby the various microsystems interact with each other (e.g., the parent–child system interacts with the parent–child-teacher system). An example of a mesosystem would be an immigrant mother having conflicts with her adolescent daughter about going on an overnight field trip with her class from school; the dynamic interaction between the mother-daughter pair and the daughter's teacher would be considered a mesosystem. The developing daughter is directly involved in the processes both at home and at school with the teacher. The *exosystem* incorporates the interaction of two or more systems, at least one of which only indirectly involves the person of interest; nonetheless, the interaction has an important influence on the individual's development; an example would be an interaction between the home setting, where a parent and developing child interact, and the parent's place of employment (where the influence on the developing child is indirect). *Macrosystems* incorporate all three of the above in a broad and comprehensive way organized by subcultural or cultural systems of belief, social roles, and psychological understanding. Finally, the *chronosystem* refers to the stability and changes that occur over time in both the developing person and the environments in which he or she functions. In Bronfenbrenner's approach, the importance of genetics cannot be overlooked as the bio-ecological model predicts that gene–environment interactions are pervasive and dynamic, and that the underlying genetic potential of many humans is not as yet fully realized due to environmental constraints. Indeed, consistent with Bronfenbrenner's hypothesis, the chapter authors in this part of the book on psychosocial development place emphasis on the many ways in which the social and physical environments of Arab Americans can be improved to help optimize their adaptation, health, and well-being.

References

Arab American Institute (AAI). (2011). The "Arab Spring" effect. Retrieved from http://www.aaiusa.org/dr-zogby/entry/the-arab-spring-effect/

Baltes, P. B., Reese, H. W., & Lipsitt, L. P. (1980). Life-span developmental psychology. *Annual Review of Psychology, 31*, 65–110.

Bronfenbrenner, U. (1994). *Ecological models of human development* (International encyclopedia of education 2nd ed., Vol. 3, pp. 1643–1647). Oxford: Elsevier.

Gibran, K. (1978/1923). *The prophet*. New York: Knopf.

Masten, A. (2007). Resilience in developing systems: Progress and promise as the fourth wave rises. *Development and Psychopathology, 19*, 921–930. doi:10.1017/S0954519407000442.

Sneed, J. R., Whitbourne, S. K., & Culang, M. E. (2006). Trust, identity, and ego integrity: Modeling Erikson's core stages over 34 years. *Journal of Adult Development, 13*, 148–157. doi:10.1007/s10804-007-9026-3.

Suleiman, M. (1999). *Arabs in America: Building a new future*. Philadelphia: Temple University Press.

Swick, K. J., & Williams, R. D. (2006). An analysis of Bronfenbrenner's bio-ecological perspective for early childhood educators: Implications for working with families experiencing stress. *Early Childhood Education Journal, 33*, 371–378. doi:10.1007/s10643-006-0078-y.

Zebian, S., & Brown, N. (2013). Living in History in Lebanon: How the civil war and other historical events affect the organization of autobiographical memory. *Memory*. doi:10.1080/09658211.2013.775310.

Chapter 8
Arab American Acculturation and Ethnic Identity Across the Lifespan: Sociodemographic Correlates and Psychological Outcomes

Mona M. Amer

> *Even when the language hurdle is overcome and foreign accents are barely discernible; when tastes and manners of the larger society have been imbibed in large drafts; when the Old World customs are scorned as visible tags of foreignness or hindrances not only to acceptance in American society but to feeling—to being—American; and even when, many native values are, no matter how reluctantly, compromised or dropped, assimilation need not have been achieved. It is a continuous process in the lifetime of the first generation... whether it can be achieved in the lifetime of the next generation is an open question.*
>
> (Naff, 1985, p. 8)

Arabs in America are situated within a remarkably unique combination of paradoxes that affect their cultural identities and attachment to American society. They are racially categorized as "White" although their skin colors can vary across the spectrum and they are perceived by others to be "not quite White" (Samhan, 1999). Whereas their legal classification places them alongside the majority, they experience life in the USA as a minority group, including forced marginalization and discrimination. Although these contradictions render them an invisible minority (Naber, 2000), they have gained increasing visibility especially in the post-9/11[1] sociopolitical world. In this decade after 9/11, the stereotypes regarding Arabs have grown overly simplified and conflated with "Muslim," although during this same period the Arab American community increased significantly in diversity of national origin, histories, reasons for immigrating, socioeconomic factors, and acculturation patterns.

[1] Throughout this chapter the abbreviation "9/11" will be used to refer to the September 11, 2001, World Trade Center attacks.

M.M. Amer (✉)
Psychology Unit, The American University in Cairo,
P.O. Box 74, Fifth District, New Cairo 11835, Egypt
e-mail: monaamer@aucegypt.edu

S.C. Nassar-McMillan et al. (eds.), *Biopsychosocial Perspectives on Arab Americans: Culture, Development, and Health*, DOI 10.1007/978-1-4614-8238-3_8,

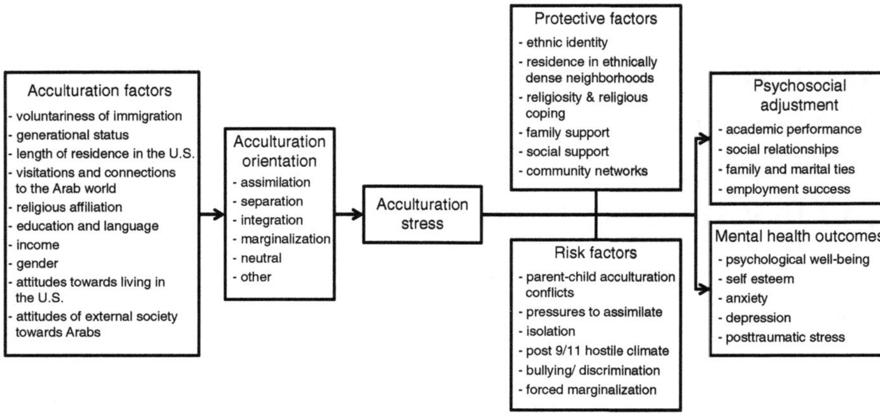

Fig. 8.1 Factors identified in research related to Arab American acculturation and psychological outcomes

Perhaps the most compelling acculturation paradox is that as an immigrant minority group, Arabs in America have the task of adapting to the host "White" culture, of which they are already classified as being members! Yet the White classification is in itself a historical point of contention for Arab people in the USA. This chapter traces these historical roots as well as contemporary acculturation patterns among Arabs living in the USA. There is a particular focus on sociodemographic factors that contribute to higher Arab ethnic immersion and increased adoption of American culture, as well as how these acculturation indicators in turn influence psychological well-being. Many of the findings in the research literature are illustrated in Fig. 8.1. These patterns may differ across the lifespan, and as such the chapter includes a focus on the experiences of youth and elderly, as well as how traditional gender roles are interwoven in Arab American culture. Finally, previous literature is critiqued with an eye for future research and community programming that can facilitate the immigration and acculturation of Arab Americans.

History of Arab Acculturation to America

Arab immigration to the USA occurred in three phases, each characterized with distinct strategies of adapting to American society. The first phase took place from the late 1800s to World War II, with most immigrants coming from Greater Syria (now, Syria and Lebanon). The majority of these immigrants were Christians who voluntarily immigrated seeking economic betterment (Naff, 1985). They worked as farmers, peddlers, and small store owners (Suleiman, 1999) and were typically uneducated and spoke little English (Samhan, 1987). These early Arabs perceived their residence in America to be a temporary state and thus continued to maintain primary allegiance to their homeland in terms of language, customs, and even political affiliations (Naff, 1985; Suleiman, 1999). Their identity was more deeply attached to their family lineage, religious sect, or home village, rather than the American community or a pan-Arab identity that had not yet emerged (Samhan, 1987; Suleiman, 1999).

The early settlers were relatively separated from American society, and then during World War I they additionally faced forced isolation from their homeland. This resulted in both a heightened sense of communal solidarity and an increased preference to assimilate in American society (Suleiman, 1999). These early primarily Christian Syrians rapidly assimilated into the educational, economic, political, and cultural landscapes of American life (Samhan, 1987). This process was facilitated by their second-generation children who had already been raised without the linguistic and ethnic traditions of their parents (Naff, 1985; Suleiman, 1999). By World War II, many of the early settlers and their children had successfully melted into the fabric of American society (Naff, 1985; Suleiman, 1999).

Arab immigration was constricted in the first half of the twentieth century due to the two World Wars as well as shifting immigration policies and a quota system that favored Northern Europeans (Samhan, 1987, 1999; Suleiman, 1999). After World War II, the Arabs who arrived to America brought with them higher levels of nationalism and Arab ethnic pride compared to their predecessors. Heightened Arab identity corresponded with the independence of Arab nations from colonial powers and the growth of a nationalistic and pan-Arab movement in the mid-1900s (Naff, 1985; Samhan, 1987). This second wave of immigrants included a higher proportion of women, young adults, Muslims, and Palestinian refugees displaced by the establishment of Israel in 1948 (Naber, 2000).

Subsequently, a third wave of immigration began in the 1960s in response to less restrictive immigration policies. Unlike the previous waves, these new immigrants were more diverse in national origin, the majority coming from Syria, Lebanon, Palestine, Egypt, and Iraq (Samhan, 1999). More recently the USA has seen immigrants from Yemen, Somalia, Gulf countries, and North Africa. Although many in the third wave came voluntarily for educational and economic opportunities (Wrobel, Farrag, & Hymes, 2009), significant numbers arrived fleeing wars, sectarian violence, and religious persecution, including significant populations of refugees. The majority were Muslims for whom religion was an important component of their ethnic identity (Suleiman, 1999).

The more recent communities of Arabs comprising the third wave are more keen to maintain their ethnic and religious traditions, are more nationalistic, and are more vocal in their disapproval of US foreign policy (Naber, 2000), thereby showing less assimilation than their predecessors (Samhan, 1999). Some are even culturally isolated in their own ethnic and religious communities with minimal interaction with the larger society (Shain, 1996). These trends towards cultural marginalization were further reinforced by America's stalwart support for Israel—and thus against Arab nations—in the 1967 war. Such foreign policies kindled prejudice and hostility towards Arabs (Naber, 2000; Shain, 1996). Parallel to these trends was the cultivation and politicization of a distinct pan-Arab "Arab American" identity to which the Arab community showed increasingly strong allegiance (Naber, 2000; Shain, 1996).

Throughout the history of Arab immigration and adaptation to American society, a controversial question regarding their racial identity has repeatedly emerged (Samhan, 1999). During the first 30 years of their presence in significant numbers, persons from Syria were assumed to be White; however, the government often classified them as "Turks" because their homeland was under rule of the Ottoman Empire (Suleiman, 1999). The American public also showed confusion regarding these immigrants, referring to them as Turks, Armenians, Assyrians, and Arabians (Naff, 1985). In the early 1900s, public opinion became increasingly antagonistic towards Syrians and other persons who were perceived to be almost-White such as Italians and Greeks. At that time the government declared that Syrians were classified as "Asian" or from "Turkey in Asia." In one case a judge conceded that Syrians were Caucasian but decided that they were not White (i.e., European) enough to meet the benchmark for citizenship. As such they were denied naturalization and citizenship rights. Subsequently these immigrants launched a series of petitions to be considered for citizenship with arguments about their Caucasian roots and close relation to Europeans; the government continued to respond with contradictory and unclear assessments of these immigrants' racial status (Samhan, 1999; Suleiman, 1999).

Currently the US government designates peoples from Middle Eastern and North African origin in the categories of White or Caucasian (Naber, 2000). However, there are diverse preferences among Arab communities regarding their identification with different racial statuses (Ajrouch & Jamal, 2007). Some feel protected by the "White" classification, some advocate for a special ethnic status such as "Hispanic," others prefer to be viewed as a minority of color, some select the "Other" status, and still others prefer to be identified specifically as "Arab" or "Middle Eastern" (Naber, 2000; Samhan, 1999; Suleiman, 1999). Arab Americans who do not identify with the "White" category tend to be recent immigrants, Muslims, and those who endorse their "Arab American" identity (Ajrouch & Jamal, 2007). These diverse racial/ethnic identities illustrate the heterogeneity of the Arab community and their diverse acculturation patterns.

Acculturation Theory and Research Findings

Acculturation as discussed in this chapter refers to the process of adapting to a dominant host culture that differs from the ethnic or national culture of origin. During this process immigrants and their descendants are challenged with the task of negotiating aspects of both cultures while developing a coherent sense of self. There are several theoretical models of acculturation, each with underlying assumptions regarding which acculturation strategies are more advantageous to psychological well-being. These models focus on psychological acculturation, or the individual-level adaptation process, rather than a sociological view of group acculturation. Researchers have built upon these theoretical frameworks when studying factors associated with different acculturation orientations among Arab Americans.

Models of Acculturation

Early approaches to studying acculturation focused on the *assimilation* model, which proposed that as immigrants adapt to a new host culture, they are increasingly internalizing characteristics of the host culture while simultaneously shedding aspects of their culture of origin (Castro, 2003; Richardson, 1967). According to Richardson (1967), for assimilation to occur, immigrants need to first experience satisfaction with the host culture, next begin to identify with it, and then they "acculturate," or gradually approximate the attitudes, beliefs, and behaviors of those from the host culture. An assumption of this linear model was that increased assimilation corresponded with positive adaptation (Rumbaut, 1997).

Over time theorists began to question the validity of the unidirectional linear model and its underlying premise that the traditional culture decreases in an inverse relationship to the host culture (Rumbaut, 1997). Instead, they argued that both host and traditional cultures fall on separate or orthogonal continuums and any person can demonstrate varying levels of both (Castro, 2003). The term *biculturalism*, which previously indicated the midpoint on the assimilation continuum (Castro, 2003), now began to refer to significant engagement with both host and traditional cultures under the bidimensional models (Berry, 1997).

Perhaps the most well known of the bidimensional models was proposed by John Berry (1997). He argued that individuals determine the extent to which they will adopt the new host culture and/or maintain the old. Those who gain high immersion in the host culture with low retention of the traditional culture are labeled *assimilated*. The opposite pattern of maintaining high levels of traditional culture and resisting the adoption of the host culture is called *separation* or isolation. Some people, however, select the strategy of fostering both the host and traditional cultures, which is called *integration*. Finally, persons who eschew both the host and traditional cultures experience *marginalization*.

Previous writers have argued that integration is associated with the most positive psychological adaptation, followed by assimilation and separation, while marginalization is linked with problematic outcomes such as emotional distress and identity confusion (Berry, 1997; Castro, 2003). Positive adaptation is reflected in a clear sense of self, high self-esteem, and good mental health (Castro, 2003). Berry's conceptual model has come under criticism, with empirical evidence showing inconsistent results regarding the salutary effects of the different acculturation orientations (Rudmin, 2003). As such, many acculturation theorists have found it more useful to focus on *acculturation stress* as a predictor of psychological adaptation rather than acculturation orientation per se. Acculturation stress refers to significant tensions and demands experienced by the acculturating individual in the process of adapting to the new society, and this construct aligns with stress and coping models (Berry, 1997).

Because acculturation stress emerges in response to frictions between the acculturating individual and his/her new host country, it can be assumed that persons with higher levels of traditional culture identification may face more acculturation stress. This self-identification with the traditional culture is often referred to as *ethnic identity* and incorporates a sense of emotional attachment and belonging towards the ethnic group, a desire to learn about the ethnicity, and adoption of ethnic values and beliefs (Phinney & Ong, 2007). Adult immigrants arrive with an already developed—although dynamically shifting—sense of ethnic identity that may increase or decrease in strength over time (Phinney & Ong, 2007). However, youth who are raised in the host culture must be socialized into adopting knowledge, attitudes, and behaviors of their traditional ethnic culture (Castro, 2003). The process of retaining and nurturing ethnic identity (for immigrants) or socializing into the ethnic culture (for those born in the host country) is called *enculturation* (Yoon, Langrehr, & Ong, 2011). Enculturation provides a natural mechanism for transmitting the ethnic culture across generations (Castro, 2003).

Ethnic Identity Among Arab Americans

For generations of Arab immigrants to America, religion and family have remained essential components of their Arab ethnic identity. Research shows that religiosity is intricately interwoven in the ethnic consciousness and is used as a benchmark for helping immigrants determine what aspects of American society to adopt or reject. This is so much so that immigrants may make reference to religious issues when asked to discuss ethnic issues (Ajrouch, 1999). In addition to religion, community culture and family are also deeply interconnected with the framework of Arab identity (Beitin & Allen, 2005), with family and social networks serving as the foundation upon which ethnic identity is shaped (Ajrouch, 2000).

For those from the second and later generations, Arab ethnic identity is nurtured primarily in the home environment, which may include extended family members and a neighborhood Arab enclave in some regions of the U.S. Family members, particularly parents, socialize children from a young age to identify with their Arab origins. Some of this enculturation occurs through explicit instruction, whereas a significant portion is through more subtle demonstrations of the Arab culture such as maintenance of the Arab patrilineal system. Purposeful instruction in religiously and culturally acceptable behavioral practices was not necessary in the home country because such behaviors were part of the natural way of life (Ajrouch, 1999). Living in America on the other hand challenges these Arab Americans to negotiate their ethnic and American identities and emerge from the encounters with a cohesive sense of self (Beitin & Allen, 2005). Furthermore, Arab Americans combine both their Arab and American identities in a unique pattern that produces a distinct identity that is different from the original Arab and American cultures (Mango, 2010).

Factors Influencing Arab American Acculturation

Researchers have identified several factors that influence Arab Americans' acculturation and the relative strength of their ethnic and American identities. One predictive factor is amount of exposure to American culture, as reflected in number of years residing in the USA as well as generational status. *Longer length of residence in the USA* is associated with greater immersion and identification with American culture (Amer, 2005; Faragallah, Schumm, & Webb, 1997). Likewise, fewer and less frequent visits to the Arab homeland are associated with greater adoption of American culture (Faragallah et al., 1997), whereas more frequent visitations are associated with separation from American society (Amer & Hovey, 2007).

With respect to *generational status*, children who were born or raised in the USA may find a natural ease in embracing American beliefs and practices compared to their parents, and adult immigrants become increasingly immersed in American culture as their residence continues (Faragallah et al., 1997). Compared to immigrants, second-generation Arab Americans report higher levels of engagement with American culture and lower levels of traditional Arab beliefs, customs, language, and social networks (Amin, 2000; Read, 2004). With each subsequent generation, adoption of American culture increases (Amer, 2005) and maintenance of the traditional culture and language fades (Amer, 2005; Seymour-Jorn, 2004).

Although both common sense and research have shown that amount of exposure to the USA leads to greater adoption of American culture and shedding of Arab ethnic identity, the relationship is more complex as attitudes of individuals can play a role. For example, a study of male Saudi Arabian sojourner university students found that those with more positive attitudes towards Americans were more likely to desire social contact with them and in turn engage in such ongoing contact with Americans (Alreshoud & Koeske, 1997). Similarly, Arab ethnic identity can be nurtured by communities that purposefully teach and transmit the Arabic language, aiming at maintaining the traditional culture and religion, and Arab youth who wish to become closer to their national heritage and Islamic religion may voluntarily choose to enhance their Arabic language skills (Seymour-Jorn, 2004).

Attitudes or perceptions of American culture may be influenced by the extent to which the Arab individuals' own religious and cultural backgrounds diverge or converge with American culture. One of the key determinants is *religion*, a fundamental component of Arab collective identity and culture. Both Christian and Muslim Arab Americans use religion as a guidebook for what aspects of American culture to adopt or reject (Eid, 2003; Read, 2004). In that respect, religion is often utilized as a source of strength in withstanding pressures from American society to adopt values and behaviors that contradict ethnic traditions. For instance, a study of Canadian Arab young adults found that religious identity was associated with strength of ethnic identity and traditional gender roles (Eid, 2003).

In addition to religiosity, *religious affiliation* can itself predict acculturation patterns, with previous literature highlighting differences between Arab Christians and Muslims. Compared to Christians, Muslims tend to score lower on indicators of immersion in American society (Ajrouch & Jamal, 2007; Amer, 2005; Awad, 2010; Faragallah et al., 1997) and higher on indicators of Arab ethnic identity (Amer & Hovey, 2007; Awad, 2010; Faragallah et al., 1997; Marshall & Read, 2003; Read, 2002, 2004). Aside from Arab values and beliefs, indicators of ethnic identity include maintaining Arab friendship networks, participating in ethnic organizations, and marrying within the ethnic group (Read, 2002).

The differences between Christians and Muslims may be conflated with the trend of a large proportion of recent Muslim immigrants who arrived with high levels of Arab nationalism and have had a shorter length of residence in the USA (Marshall & Read, 2003). However, other reasons have been suggested for why Christians report higher adoption of American culture while Muslims report higher ethnic identity. Christians may find the acculturation process less taxing because they share the same religion as the dominant culture (Ajrouch, 2007; Ajrouch & Jamal, 2007; Awad, 2010; Faragallah et al., 1997). They may have also left their nation of origin in search of greater religious freedom or to escape minority status, so positive attitudes towards the new culture facilitate greater American culture immersion (Faragallah et al., 1997). For Muslims on the other hand, acculturation is further compounded by hostile prejudices and discriminatory behavior targeting specifically Islam and Muslims (Ajrouch, 2007); they are more likely to be seen as outsiders (Naber, 2000). As such, Muslims may face more stressors adapting to American culture including discrimination (Amer, 2005; Awad, 2010; Padela & Heisler, 2010).

Discrimination serves as a risk factor in the acculturation process because it can lead to segregation of Arab Americans (Hassouneh & Kulwicki, 2009). Arabs have faced discrimination since their early arrival to the USA, long before 9/11 (Faragallah et al., 1997; Samhan, 1987). In recent years research has documented substantial experiences of discrimination among Arab Americans post 9/11 ranging from ethnic slurs to assaults on self and property (Abu-Ras & Abu-Bader, 2009; Awad, 2010; Beitin & Allen, 2005; Hassouneh & Kulwicki, 2007, 2009; Moradi & Hasan, 2004; Padela & Heisler, 2010). Persons who immigrate at older ages (and thus appear to be more foreign) report more discrimination (Faragalla et al., 1997). Paradoxically, those of the second generation have reported more discrimination compared to the first, which can be attributed to greater level of interactions with the wider American society (Gaudet, Clément, & Deuzeman, 2005). Similarly, higher immersion in American culture can increase opportunities for Muslims to experience discrimination, although their Christian counterparts may face less (Awad, 2010).

Finally, higher *socioeconomic status* including income and education has been associated with greater adoption of American culture (Amer, 2005). Two studies (Amer, 2005; Amer & Hovey, 2007) found that higher education was associated with less participation in Arab ethnic practices. Education is often associated with language. Facility with the English language is a factor that helps facilitate acculturation to American society and is therefore subsequently associated with positive psychological well-being (Ajrouch, 2007; Beitin & Allen, 2005; Wrobel et al., 2009). A study of Arab American elderly found that English skills were worse for refugees and sojourners compared to those with lengthier or more permanent legal status in the USA (Wrobel et al., 2009). This suggests that language may actually be a proxy for amount of exposure to the USA rather than a factor that directly impacts acculturation and well-being.

Acculturation and Psychological Well-Being

Consistent with acculturation theory, a few studies have found that higher host culture immersion—especially with a bicultural approach—is predictive of better psychosocial well-being among Arab Americans. Greater interaction with American culture (e.g., making American friends) and adoption of American beliefs and practices have been associated with higher satisfaction with US life (Faragallah et al., 1997) and less acculturation stress and depression (Amer, 2005). For example, Arab American couples that made a concerted effort to immerse in American society believed that this strategy helped facilitate their coping with acculturation and post-9/11 stressors (Beitin & Allen, 2005). This pattern was also seen for bicultural individuals who had high levels of both American and Arab identities (Amer, 2005).

On the other hand, and contrary to acculturation theory, some studies have found a strategy of exclusively maintaining traditional Arab ethnic culture to be more predictive of positive psychosocial well-being compared to assimilating or integrating both Arab and American cultures (Amin, 2000). Studies have shown that greater adoption of the host culture is associated with more depression and lower self-esteem (Gaudet et al., 2005) and less family satisfaction (Faragallah et al., 1997). Likewise, Arab Americans with high biculturalism demonstrate lower personal self-esteem (Barry, 2005) and lower personal and emotional adjustment (Amin, 2000). Potential explanations for why Arabs who attempt to integrate or assimilate in American culture report lower psychosocial well-being include greater exposure to prejudice and discriminatory behavior from the host culture and feelings of inferior group status when surrounded by those from the dominant culture (Barry, 2005), as well as cultural and social isolation from their ethnic group (Gaudet et al., 2005).

It is moreover evident that maintaining Arab ethnic identity has salubrious effects on psychological well-being. Arab ethnic identity has been associated with better college adjustment and social adjustment (Amin, 2000), higher collective self-esteem (Barry, 2005), and less acculturation stress (Britto & Amer, 2007). A study by Gaudet et al. (2005) found that higher Lebanese ethnic identity was associated with fewer acculturation daily hassles, which in turn decreased risk for depression which was subsequently related to better self-esteem. Even simply being of Arab ethnic background is associated with positive mental health. For example, in a study in Michigan, per official death records Arab Americans had significantly lower rates of suicide compared to nonethnic Whites. This was hypothesized by the authors to be related to higher ethnic identity, living in an ethnic enclave, religiosity, religious coping, strong community networks, and social support (El-Sayed, Tracy, Scarborough, & Galea, 2011).

Acculturation Stress

In light of contradictory findings regarding acculturation strategies, acculturation stress may be a more sensitive predictor of psychological adjustment. Factors that predict higher acculturation stress for Arab Americans include less competence in

English, lower education, involuntary immigration, and shorter length of residence in the USA (Wrobel et al., 2009). In turn, experiences of acculturation stress are linked with psychological distress among Arab Americans (Hassouneh & Kulwicki, 2007) including depression (Amer, 2005; Wrobel et al., 2009). Related to the concept of acculturation stress is that of acculturation daily hassles, which have been found to mediate the relations between acculturation factors (ethnic identity, Canadian identity, discrimination) and mental health (depression and self-esteem) (Gaudet et al., 2005).

Salient acculturation stressors for Arab Americans include discrimination and perceived marginalization from American society, which can increase worries and potential emotional distress (Hassouneh & Kulwicki, 2009) and decrease satisfaction with living in the USA (Faragallah et al., 1997). Post-9/11 backlash in particular has been linked to increased stress and psychological distress (Abu-Ras & Abu-Bader, 2009). For example, a representative survey of 1,016 Arabs and Chaldeans in Michigan found that experiences of discrimination were linked to higher emotional distress and less happiness (Padela & Heisler, 2010). In their study of Arab Americans in Florida, Moradi and Hasan (2004) found a significant association between perceived ethnic–racial discrimination and worsened mental health symptoms, with sense of personal mastery over one's life partially mediating this relationship. Thus, having a higher sense of personal control served as a protective factor in buffering the stressful consequences of discrimination.

Culturally Embedded Protective Factors

Some protective factors have been found to buffer the stressful acculturation process for Arab Americans. Families, including extended families, form the backbone of the Arab culture and are as such a valued source of social and tangible support (Naber, 2006; Read, 2004). For example, Beitin and Allen (2005) discovered that spousal support served as a resource for resilience for Arab American couples coping with the post-9/11 anti-Arab context. In other studies, Arab Americans who had stronger family support and more cohesive family ties reported lower levels of depression (Abu-Ras & Abu-Bader, 2009; Amer, 2005) and anxiety (Amer, 2005). Immigrant communities that are predominantly professional and have arrived in the absence of chain migration may experience less family support (Keck, 1989). For such isolated nuclear families, friends often assume the roles that extended family would have had back home such as assistance in child-rearing.

Friendships, social networks, and community networks can be sources of support in the acculturation process. Arabs come from communities that value collectivism and interdependence and thus they are accustomed to receiving emotional and tangible supports from others (Abu-Ras & Abu-Bader, 2009). A previous study found that social support was associated with less acculturative stress, less depression, and less anxiety (Amer, 2005). In their study of Arab and Muslim Americans, Abu-Ras and Abu-Bader (2009) documented that availability of community support was related to lower levels of depression and posttraumatic stress and likewise Beitin and Allen (2005) found community support to be a factor in enhancing resilience.

Religiosity has also been proposed as a source of support for Arab Americans, particularly since religion is an important component of the Arab culture. Previous research has found that Arab Americans utilize religious beliefs, supports, and coping strategies to help manage acculturation and post-9/11 stressors (Beitin & Allen, 2005). However, interestingly, other studies have not found religion or religious coping to be associated with acculturation stress or mental health status (Abu-Ras & Abu-Bader, 2009; Amer, Hovey, Fox, & Rezcallah, 2008). Therefore, further research is needed to examine the role of religiosity as a coping strategy for Arab American adults and youth.

Arab American Acculturation Across the Lifespan

Age of immigration and ages at which acculturative stressors are faced can influence acculturation and identity formation. For example, teenage Arab Americans who lived through the post-9/11 backlash may in response have felt marginalized and thus may have developed an identity that eschewed American culture, whereas older Arab Americans may have an already established cultural identity that was somewhat protected from these events (Ajrouch & Jamal, 2007). Even a decade after 9/11 the sociopolitical climate continues to be hostile towards Arabs, thereby continuing to impact the acculturation of Arab American adults and youth.

Youth

The development of an integrated personal identity is a natural developmental challenge for all youth, yet this process is more complicated for Arab youth who are juggling ethnic and American identities. The process is influenced by several external systems, including parents, peers, school, community, and media, each of which can serve as sources of stress or support. For example, Arab youth may face school stressors such as invisibility in the curriculum and antagonism from peers and school personnel (Ayish, 2003). Since 9/11 these types of stressors such as bullying and other forms of discrimination have increased and have led to Arab children feeling marginalized (Britto, 2008). In response, these youth may develop greater attachment to their ethnic identity and ethnic community (Ayish, 2003), which in turn has been linked with higher self-esteem (Mansour, 2000). Arab youth ethnic identity is nurtured by family socialization and the family continues to serve as a primary resource for ethnic identity development (Ajrouch, 2004).

As with adults, religion plays a role in Arab ethnic identity development, particularly in providing guidelines for which behaviors are acceptable (Ajrouch, 2000). Unlike their parents, however, for whom religious creed and rituals are genuinely and deeply interwoven with ethnic identity, among the second-generation religious affiliation is experienced differently. It is instead often utilized as a proxy for ethnic identity even if underlying religious beliefs and rituals are not observed (Eid, 2003).

In other words, religion may be used symbolically as a way to define the boundaries of ethnic identity and publicize commitment to the ethnic community, and as such these youth may apply religion in a flexible manner depending on situational contexts.

Previous literature has noted that Arab youth may negotiate and prioritize their religious and cultural identities by using various self-labels such as "Palestinian," "Arab American," and "Muslim American" (Christison, 1989). They may also classify or distance themselves from other labels such as "boater" (referring to immigrants with poor English, cultural awkwardness, and lower social status) and "White" (associated with privilege, education, but also excessive freedom and lack of responsibility) (Ajrouch, 2000, 2004). These variations in labels and hyphenated identities continue into adulthood and provide an indicator of their immersion in Arab versus American cultures (Mango, 2010; Read, 2004).

Arab youth are acutely aware of differences between Arab and American cultures, particularly in regard to the acceptability of behavioral practices, and a central task in their development is to negotiate these differences. Perhaps the most striking example is that of dating: having a boyfriend/girlfriend is part of normal development in the USA but is frowned upon by Arab culture and religious values (Ajrouch, 1999). The disparities between ethnic and American cultures are experienced more profoundly for Arab American girls compared to boys. Arab youth perceive Arab girls to be respectful and honorable, while American girls are perceived to be immodest, immoral, but with a desirable independence (Ajrouch, 1999, 2004; Naber, 2006).

As such, gender serves as a focal point with respect to Arab American youth development, with cultural standards differing for boys and girls (Keck, 1989) and boys sometimes receiving preferential treatment (Abudabbeh, 2005). Studies have reported dissatisfaction and complaints from adolescent girls regarding double standards (Ajrouch, 1999, 2004; Keck, 1989). The girls describe restrictions in entertainment, dating, and working that boys do not face; girls often need to return home earlier and face more limitations in places they can visit. Girls experience pressure to conform to ethnic standards of behaviors to preserve the family honor (Ajrouch, 1999, 2004). The brothers themselves are often involved in controlling and chastising their sisters if their sisters' behaviors transgress in ways that could sully the family reputation; boys are socialized into such behaviors by modeling adult males and parents in the community (Ajrouch, 1999, 2004).

Parent–Child Relationships

Cultural differences between US-born youth and their immigrant parents can result in intergenerational and intercultural conflicts. Parents come from traditional Arab cultures where elders are respected and heeded, the worldview is focused on the past, and stability and conformity are valued. On the other hand the youth are raised in an individualistic, industrialist society in which the worldview emphasizes the future (Ajrouch, 1999). These cultural differences may produce tensions within the youths who are continuously navigating among cultures, as well as between the youth and their parents.

Parents who adhere more strongly to their traditional culture face difficulties in raising their children to meet these cultural guidelines (Christison, 1989). Many Arab American adults parent with an authoritarian style (Abudabbeh, 2005) and use religion as a foundation for cultural instruction (Ajrouch, 1999). Parental involvement may range from selecting Arab friends for their children (Ajrouch, 1999), to censoring sexual content from television and reading materials for their adolescents (Hattar-Pollara & Meleis, 1995), to recommending marriage partners for older youth (Christison, 1989). While Arab American parents may acknowledge the importance of their children's independence and interactions with American society (Christison, 1989; Read, 2004), the question of where to draw boundaries of what is appropriate presents ongoing challenges. Both parents and children report that as a result of anxieties over potential adoption of culturally unacceptable American practices, some parents may become overly restrictive especially with their daughters or at least may be perceived as such (Ajrouch, 1999; Keck, 1989). The local Arab community may influence this parenting process by collectively contributing to the child-rearing (Keck, 1989) and indirectly monitoring and restricting undesirable behaviors with the use of community gossip (Ajrouch, 2000).

Youth perceptions of their parents' acculturation and parenting control can moreover affect their psychological well-being. For example, university students who perceived their parents to be more immersed in American culture showed better well-being, particularly if the parents had a more open style of parenting. Parental maintenance of traditional ethnic culture was similarly associated with better well-being for children with less controlling parents (Henry, Stiles, Biran, & Hinkle, 2008). Likewise, a study of Arab American university students found that those who shared a similar acculturation strategy to their own parents demonstrated better psychosocial adjustment (Amin, 2000).

Gender Roles During Adulthood

Child-rearing practices among Arabs in the USA are especially cautious in enforcing traditional gendered codes of conduct throughout adulthood (Eid, 2003). The maintenance of traditional gender roles is a marker of adherence to the collective Arab ethnic identity, and women observe these traditional gender roles as a sign of the family's ethno-religious identity (Eid, 2003; Read, 2004). The Arab family is generally patrilineal, patriarchal, and hierarchical (Abudabbeh, 2005; Read, 2004). Marriage is valued as a sacred institution, parents and elders are expected to be respected, and the father (or eldest male) has the highest authority (Abudabbeh, 2005). Women are viewed with high status with respect to their child-rearing and domestic functions, while their engagement in the public sphere may be relatively limited or valued less (Read, 2002, 2004). On the other hand, men adopt the primary economic responsibility of the family (Ajrouch, 1999).

Because actions of individual family members can reflect upon the reputation of the whole family (Ajrouch, 1999; Hassouneh & Kulwicki, 2009), serious violations of these gender roles—such as premarital sex among young women—can tarnish the family's honor and status within the community. In a sense, such violations weaken the barriers with Western culture and thus dilute the purity of the ethno-religious heritage (Eid, 2003; Naber, 2006). Moreover, women themselves are viewed as vehicles for transmitting ethnic beliefs and traditions to subsequent generations and for ensuring that these beliefs and traditions are maintained and nurtured in the family context (Eid, 2003; Read, 2004).

On the other hand, some authors have speculated that Arab American women—particularly from the second generation and those with higher education—may question or openly revolt against the traditional gender roles that have been foisted upon them (e.g., Eid, 2003; Suleiman, 1999). This opposition to traditional gender roles may be stimulated by resentment against the double standards, what they perceive to be offensive beliefs about women and cultural restrictions, as well as pressures from mainstream society to shed aspects of the conservative traditions. Moreover, Arab immigrant women, especially among those who have higher socio-economic status, may be less likely to adhere to traditional patriarchal gender roles compared to women in the Arab world (Marshall & Read, 2003).

Based on the emphasis of female gender roles within the family's ethno-religious identity, it is reasonable to assume that Arab men would be more likely to assimilate to American culture compared to their female peers. Men have greater social freedom as youth and more opportunity to engage with the host culture through their work settings. Women also often arrive to America with less education, English language skills, driving skills, and comprehension of the American culture (Suleiman, 1999). Indeed, one study found that female Arab Americans showed higher levels of ethnic identity and intrinsic religiosity compared to males (Amer & Hovey, 2007). On the other hand, other research found no significant differences between male and female participants on measures of acculturation and ethnic identity (Gaudet et al., 2005) and acculturation stress (Amer, 2005; Wrobel, et al., 2009). One study of college students even found greater female assimilation to American culture and English language compared to males (Amin, 2000), which is in line with the theory that more educated second-generation women would be less likely to retain traditional gender roles (Read, 2004).

Elderly

As the family life cycle progresses, family roles reverse as young adults are expected to care for their elderly parents. The concept of having parents reside in nursing homes is an affront to traditional Arab values (Abudabbeh, 2005; Salari, 2002). Therefore, families play an important role for Arab American elders who often live near family members and ethnic social/community networks (Ajrouch, 2005). Despite family and community supports, Arab elderly face acculturative stressors such as pressures to gain competence in English language, to assimilate, and to maintain ethnic practices; all these pressures are associated with higher levels of depression (Wrobel et al., 2009).

Such acculturation tensions may be heightened for elderly Arab American parents who arrive to the USA to live with their adult children. They often remain isolated in their home environment; their freedoms and engagement with American society are restricted by lack of English language skills, transportation, and employment or other formal engagement (Christison, 1989). However, those who live in ethnic enclaves with other Arabic-speaking residents may not suffer as much from acculturative stress because the pressures to learn English and shed ethnic beliefs and practices would be reduced (Wrobel et al., 2009).

Arab American elders who were born and raised in the USA show greater acculturation and better mental health compared to their immigrant counterparts. For example, US-born Arab elderly are more likely to speak English and less likely to engage in Arab behavioral practices compared to immigrants (Ajrouch, 2008). They report larger and more diverse social networks (Ajrouch, 2005), with acculturation mediating this relationship between immigration status and social networks (Ajrouch, 2008). US-born elders also demonstrate better mental health including less loneliness (Ajrouch, 2008), less depression, and more life satisfaction, relationships that appear mediated by higher education and facility with English (Ajrouch, 2007).

Discrimination continues to be an acculturative stressor throughout the lifespan. It has been theorized that immigrant Arab elderly could potentially face more discrimination than the US-born Arab Americans because they would be more easily recognized as Arab based on their dress, accent, and cultural practices (Salari, 2002). On the other hand, one research study found that elderly who are born in the USA report significantly more perceived discrimination compared to immigrants, especially after September 11 (Ajrouch, 2005). This is consistent with the research presented above that indicated that persons who are more embedded in American society may be more likely to have opportunities to encounter discrimination.

Methodological Approaches

Most research with Arab American acculturation has been with adults, with fewer studies focusing on children or elderly. One of the primary challenges in Arab American research is recruiting participants, especially due to the geographically dispersed nature of the Arab American community. Moreover, because persons from the Middle East and North Africa are classified as "White," they are an invisible minority and difficult to identify from sampling frames. To address this challenge, there have been two main methods of data collection. The first is through college campuses: advertising through student clubs, international student offices, and mass e-mailing (e.g., Barry, Elliott, & Evans, 2000). The second is community sampling, using key informants, religious institutions, and community centers as resources to recruit participants. Only a couple of studies have used traditional mailing methods (e.g., Alreshoud & Koeske, 1997; Faragallah et al., 1997). A more recently utilized strategy is Internet-based research (e.g., Amer & Hovey, 2007;

Barry et al., 2000). This method is cheaper and less time-consuming, offers greater anonymity, and facilitates access to participants who reside in other cities. However, such studies are typically in English and thus exclude significant portions of the Arab American community who are less educated or affluent or are not as facile with the computer and Internet (e.g., the elderly).

Because there has been an emphasis on Berry's acculturation model, many studies (e.g., Amer, 2005; Amer & Hovey, 2007; Amin, 2000; Barry, 2005) take the tack of classifying participants into acculturation orientations based on their self-reported endorsement of American and Arab cultures. This is usually measured with a question assessing desired (or actual) ethnic versus American cultural adoption. While this approach overlays nicely with theoretical perspectives because it categorizes participants into four groups, it is somewhat clumsy in statistical analyses that are reduced to group comparisons. Other researchers prefer to use more complex questionnaires to measure variability in cultural adoption. However, unfortunately there is a paucity of psychometrically sound and culturally sensitive instruments available. While many researchers choose to use widely available measures such as Phinney's Multigroup Ethnic Identity Measure, some questionnaires have been developed specifically for the Arab American population such as the Male Arab Ethnic Identity Measure (Barry et al., 2000).

Critique

Most of the research related to Arab American acculturation discussed above has been based on quantitative survey designs using questionnaires, or qualitative approaches. This has produced a substantial body of knowledge, particularly regarding Arab American immigration experiences and sociodemographic characteristics. However, risk and protective factors for the acculturation process have yet to be examined with more depth, and most studies use small sample sizes. As a result, the studies limit potential within-group comparisons (Faragallah et al., 1997), have produced contradictory findings that have not been resolved, and limit generalizability of the results.

Small-sample research tends to treat Arab Americans as a homogeneous group, which defies the reality of their heterogeneity. For example, Read (2004) discussed how Arab Americans are so diverse in terms of immigration status, demographics, religion, nation of origin, traditionalism, etc., that it is difficult to make generalizations or theories regarding the reasons for female labor force participation. Additionally, authors often do not frame or interpret their findings within the context of the ethnic density of the location where the sample was obtained. Living in an ethnic enclave can be a very different experience and may come with stronger social and community networks and less pressure to assimilate (Ajrouch, 2000).

There are concerns regarding the way Arab acculturation and assimilation to America has been presented in the literature. Many previous writers have depicted the Arab identity as a static experience that conflicts with American culture. The underlying assumption is that acculturation begins with point of arrival at the shores of the USA. However, it is important to remember that most Arab countries were colonized by European nations up to the mid-twentieth century, followed by decades of modernization and international exchange of ideas, products, and technologies (Eid, 2003). So in reality, those living in the Arab world have faced long-standing exposure to Western concepts and traditions, and many have assimilated these cultural imports while others have struggled against them and cultivated greater nationalism and Islamization to counteract them (Eid, 2003). Therefore, the relationship between Arab and Western cultures is complex and the process of acculturation begins prior to immigration.

The classification of Arab Americans into distinct acculturative strategies is also too simplistic to truly represent the diversity and complexity of their hyphenated identities. For example, Christison (1989) juxtaposed Palestinians who feel strong affiliation to their American identity but restrict their socialization to others from their ethnic group, to Palestinians who consider their residence in the USA to be transient and thus refuse the American citizenship but at the same time are immersed in American society with mostly American friends. Two studies (Amin, 2000; Britto & Amer, 2007) discovered a distinct subgroup of participants who endorsed "neutral" or midpoint levels of Arab and American identities; this group does not neatly fit in Berry's four main strategies. In a study of Arab American women, Mango (2010) discussed how participants changed how they labeled their identity (e.g., American, Middle Eastern, Iraqi, Christian) based on the context of what they were discussing, indicating an identity that is complex and ever fluctuating. The author also suggested that the women faced a challenge finding wording that could embrace all their various identities.

Although Berry's (1997) initial acculturation model took into account the influence of the host culture, research has generally overlooked the impact of the surrounding society on determining Arab Americans' acculturation. An example of this contextual impact was seen in Beitin and Allen's (2005) study of Arab American couples. Many of the couples experienced the construction of their identities as being determined or influenced by society's own interpretation and negative messages about Arabs and Muslims. Ayish's (2003) research on Arab youth found that over recent years, the youths' specific self-labels have been replaced by internalization of more general labels (e.g., Arab, Muslim) that were imposed on them by post-9/11 societal stereotypes transmitted through media and peers.

Finally, the extant literature often views Arab Americans as a group that is suffering or in need; a narrative of resilience is generally unnoticed. In a departure from this problem-focused literature, a study of Arab American couples showed how they gained strength from overcoming traumas and stressors both in the homeland and in the USA and how they built upon multiple sources of family, community, and religious resources (Beitin & Allen, 2005). Similarly, a study of Arab American children found that they reported higher self-concept in multiple components (including physical appearance, academic skills, social relationships) compared to children living in Lebanon (Alkhateeb, 2010).

Implications for Community Practice and Research

Previous research has documented several risk factors and stressors for acculturating Arab Americans. Future research will need to bring greater visibility to voices of resilience and to identify protective factors that can be enhanced and emphasized in community-based programming. These programs can be developed by local ethnic-based community organizations such as the Arab Community Center for Economic and Social Services (ACCESS) and Arab American and Chaldean Council, both located in Detroit, Michigan. Protective factors can be fostered in interventions that target community members who are at risk for acculturative stressors (e.g., recent immigrants, Muslims, those with lower socioeconomic resources). For example, programs can aim to help orient immigrants to American culture, enhance English language skills, improve social networks, and negotiate between ethnic and host cultural demands. Because discrimination has emerged in the research as a salient acculturation stressor for Arab Americans, it is recommended that Arab communities collaborate with their local communities to develop interventions to address this issue. Efforts can focus on prejudice reduction within the local host community, enhanced coping skills among Arab recipients of discrimination, and policy aimed at protecting the Arab community.

Published literature can serve as a guidebook in developing priorities for program development. For example, it is evident that among youth, issues of bullying, school discrimination, and identity confusion may need to be addressed particularly in the school context and that nurturing ethnic identity can have salutary effects. However, further research is needed in several areas related to Arab acculturation such as more closely examining the contradictory findings on psychological outcomes of different acculturation orientations, identifying other acculturation stressors and protective factors, better understanding the experiences of younger children, and clarifying distinctions among more refined subgroups (e.g., based on nationality of origin, age at immigration). Moreover, it is preferable to not depend solely on scholarly literature but rather to develop interventions based on assessment of local community needs. In this way, programs can be tailored to meet the needs and strengths of specific subgroups (e.g., "female young adults seeking employment"). Such specifically tailored programming may diverge from currently available programs that serve more general groups such as "Arab immigrants." All interventions should consider the acculturation status of participants such as language and literacy. Finally, program evaluation should be conducted to evaluate the effectiveness of the interventions and results should preferably be published in the scholarly literature so that other communities can access and build upon previous successes.

References

Abudabbeh, N. (2005). Arab families: An overview. In M. McGoldrick, J. Giordano, & N. Garcia-Preto (Eds.), *Ethnicity and family therapy* (3rd ed., pp. 423–436). New York: The Guilford.

Abu-Ras, W., & Abu-Bader, S. H. (2009). Risk factors for depression and posttraumatic stress disorder (PTSD): The case of Arab and Muslim Americans post-9/11. *Journal of Immigrant & Refugee Studies, 7*, 393–418.

Ajrouch, K. (1999). Family and ethnic identity in an Arab-American community. In M. W. Suleiman (Ed.), *Arab-Americans: Continuity and change* (pp. 129–139). Philadelphia: Temple University Press.

Ajrouch, K. J. (2000). Place, age, and culture: Community living and ethnic identity among Lebanese American adolescents. *Small Group Research, 31*, 447–469.

Ajrouch, K. J. (2004). Gender, race, and symbolic boundaries: Contested spaces of identity among Arab American adolescents. *Sociological Perspectives, 47*(4), 371–391.

Ajrouch, K. J. (2005). Arab American elders: Network structure, perceptions of relationship quality, and discrimination. *Research in Human Development, 2*(4), 213–228.

Ajrouch, K. J. (2007). Resources and well-being among Arab-American elders. *Journal of Cross Cultural Gerontology, 22*, 167–182.

Ajrouch, K. J. (2008). Social isolation and loneliness among Arab American elders: Cultural, social, and personal factors. *Research in Human Development, 5*(1), 44–59.

Ajrouch, K. J., & Jamal, A. (2007). Assimilating to a White identity: The case of Arab Americans. *International Migration Review, 41*, 860–879.

Alkhateeb, H. M. (2010). Self-concept in Lebanese and Arab-American pre-adolescents. *Psychological Reports, 106*, 435–447.

Alreshoud, A., & Koeske, G. F. (1997). Arab students' attitudes toward and amount of social contact with Americans: A causal process analysis of cross-sectional data. *The Journal of Social Psychology, 137*, 235–245.

Amer, M. M. (2005). *Arab American mental health in the post September 11 era: Acculturation, stress, and coping*. Unpublished doctoral dissertation, The University of Toledo, Ohio.

Amer, M. M., & Hovey, J. D. (2007). Socio-demographic differences in acculturation and mental health for a sample of 2nd generation/early immigrant Arab Americans. *Journal of Immigrant and Minority Health, 9*, 335–347.

Amer, M. M., Hovey, J. D., Fox, C. M., & Rezcallah, A. (2008). Initial development of the Brief Arab Religious Coping Scale (BARCS). *Journal of Muslim Mental Health, 3*, 69–88.

Amin, A. H. (2000). *Cultural adaptation and psychosocial adjustment among Arab American college students*. Unpublished doctoral dissertation, Northwestern University, Evanston, IL.

Awad, G. H. (2010). The impact of acculturation and religious identification on perceived discrimination for Arab/Middle Eastern Americans. *Cultural Diversity and Ethnic Minority Psychology, 16*, 59–67.

Ayish, N. (2003). *Stereotypes and Arab American Muslim high school students: A misunderstood group*. Unpublished doctoral dissertation, George Mason University, Fairfax, VA.

Barry, D. T. (2005). Measuring acculturation among male Arab immigrants in the United States: An exploratory study. *Journal of Immigrant Health, 7*(3), 179–184.

Barry, D., Elliott, R., & Evans, E. M. (2000). Foreigners in a strange land: Self-construal and ethnic identity in male Arabic immigrants. *Journal of Immigrant Health, 2*(3), 133–144.

Beitin, B. K., & Allen, K. R. (2005). Resilience in Arab American couples after September 11, 2001: A systems perspective. *Journal of Marital and Family Therapy, 31*(3), 251–267.

Berry, J. W. (1997). Immigration, acculturation, and adaptation. *Applied Psychology: An International Review, 46*(1), 5–34.

Britto, P. R. (2008). Who am I? Ethnic identity formation of Arab Muslim children in contemporary U.S. society. *Journal of the American Academy of Child and Adolescent Psychiatry, 47*, 853–857.

Britto, P. R., & Amer, M. M. (2007). An exploration of cultural identity patterns and the family context among Arab Muslim young adults in America. *Applied Development Science, 11*(3), 137–150.

Castro, V. S. (2003). *Acculturation and psychological adaptation*. Westport, CT: Greenwood.

Christison, K. (1989). The American experience: Palestinians in the U.S. *Journal of Palestine Studies, 18*(4), 18–36.

Eid, P. (2003). The interplay between ethnicity, religion, and gender among second-generation Christian and Muslim Arabs in Montreal. *Canadian Ethnic Studies, 35*(2), 30–60.

El-Sayed, A. M., Tracy, M., Scarborough, P., & Galea, S. (2011). Suicide among Arab-Americans. *PLoS ONE, 6*(2), e14704. doi:10.1371/journal.pone.0014704.

Faragallah, M. H., Schumm, W. R., & Webb, F. J. (1997). Acculturation of Arab-American immigrants: An exploratory study. *Journal of Comparative Family Studies, 28*(3), 182–203.

Gaudet, S., Clément, R., & Deuzeman, K. (2005). Daily hassles, ethnic identity and psychological adjustment among Lebanese-Canadians. *International Journal of Psychology, 40*(3), 157–168.

Hassouneh, D. M., & Kulwicki, A. (2007). Mental health, discrimination, and trauma in Arab Muslim women living in the US: A pilot study. *Mental Health, Religion and Culture, 10*(3), 257–262.

Hassouneh, D., & Kulwicki, A. (2009). Family privacy as protection: A qualitative pilot study of mental illness in Arab-American Muslim women. *Research in the Social Scientific Study of Religion, 20*, 195–215.

Hattar-Pollara, M., & Meleis, A. I. (1995). Parenting their adolescents: The experiences of Jordanian immigrant women in California. *Health Care for Women International, 16*(3), 195–211.

Henry, H. M., Stiles, W. B., Biran, M. W., & Hinkle, S. (2008). Perceived parental acculturation behaviors and control as predictors of subjective well-being in Arab American college students. *The Family Journal: Counseling and Therapy for Couples and Families, 16*, 28–34.

Keck, L. T. (1989). Egyptian Americans in the Washington, D.C. area. In B. Abu-Laban & M. W. Suleiman (Eds.), *Arab-Americans: Continuity and change* (pp. 103–126). Belmont: Association of Arab-American University Graduates.

Mango, O. (2010). Enacting solidarity and ambivalence: Positional identities of Arab American women. *Discourse Studies, 12*, 649–664.

Mansour, S. S. (2000). *The correlation between ethnic identity and self-esteem among Arab American Muslim adolescents*. Unpublished Master's thesis, West Virginia University, Morgantown, WV.

Marshall, S. E., & Read, J. (2003). Identity politics among Arab-American women. *Social Science Quarterly, 84*, 875–891.

Moradi, B., & Hasan, N. T. (2004). Arab American persons' reported experiences of discrimination and mental health: The mediating role of personal control. *Journal of Counseling Psychology, 51*, 418–428.

Naber, N. (2000). Ambiguous insiders: An investigation of Arab American invisibility. *Ethnic and Racial Studies, 23*(1), 37–61.

Naber, N. (2006). Arab American femininities: Beyond Arab virgin/American(ized) whore. *Feminist Studies, 32*(1), 87–111.

Naff, A. (1985). *Becoming American: The early Arab immigrant experience*. Carbondale, IL: Southern Illinois University Press.

Padela, A. I., & Heisler, M. (2010). The association of perceived abuse and discrimination after September 11, 2001, with psychological distress, level of happiness, and health status among Arab Americans. *American Journal of Public Health, 100*, 284–291.

Phinney, J. S., & Ong, A. D. (2007). Conceptualization and measurement of ethnic identity: Current status and future directions. *Journal of Counseling Psychology, 54*(3), 271–281.

Read, J. G. (2002). Challenging myths of Muslim women: The influence of Islam on Arab-American women's labor force activity. *The Muslim World, 92*, 19–37.

Read, J. G. (2004). *Culture, class, and work among Arab-American women*. New York: LFB.

Richardson, A. (1967). A theory and a method for the psychological study of assimilation. *International Migration Review, 2*(1), 3–30.

Rudmin, F. W. (2003). Critical history of the acculturation psychology of assimilation, separation, integration, and marginalization. *Review of General Psychology, 7*(1), 3–37.

Rumbaut, R. G. (1997). Assimilation and its discontents: Between rhetoric and reality. *International Migration Review, 31*, 923–960.

Salari, S. (2002). Invisible in aging research: Arab Americans, Middle Eastern immigrants, and Muslims in the United States. *The Gerontologist, 42*, 580–588.

Samhan, H. H. (1987). Politics and exclusion: The Arab American experience. *Journal of Palestine Studies, 16*(2), 11–28.

Samhan, H. H. (1999). Not quite white: Race classification and the Arab-American experience. In M. W. Suleiman (Ed.), *Arabs in America: Building a new future* (pp. 209–226). Philadelphia: Temple University Press.

Seymour-Jorn, C. (2004). Arabic language learning among Arab immigrants in Milwaukee, Wisconsin: A study of attitudes and motivations. *Journal of Muslim Minority Affairs, 24*(1), 109–122.

Shain, Y. (1996). Arab-Americans at a crossroads. *Journal of Palestine Studies, 25*(3), 46–59.

Suleiman, M. W. (1999). Introduction: The Arab immigrant experience. In M. W. Suleiman (Ed.), *Arabs in America: Building a new future* (pp. 1–21). Philadelphia: Temple University Press.

Wrobel, N. H., Farrag, M. F., & Hymes, R. W. (2009). Acculturative stress and depression in an elderly Arabic sample. *Journal of Cross Cultural Gerontology, 24*, 273–290.

Yoon, E., Langrehr, K., & Ong, L. Z. (2011). Content analysis of acculturation research in counseling and counseling psychology: A 22-year review. *Journal of Counseling Psychology, 58*, 83–96.

Chapter 9
Arab Refugees: Trauma, Resilience, and Recovery

Ibrahim Aref Kira, Mona M. Amer, and Nancy Howells Wrobel

History of Arab Refugees in the USA

While Arab immigration to America started around 1870 with the first wave from Lebanon, significant numbers of Arab refugees fled oppression and conflict in the aftermath of the Arab–Israeli conflict wars in 1948 and 1967. More continued to arrive after the Lebanese civil war in 1975, the Iraq–Iran war and the Israeli invasion of Lebanon in 1982. Significant populations of Iraqi refugees came in response to the first Gulf War of 1991 and the subsequent oppression of Shiites. The second Gulf War of 2002, with the American invasion of Iraq and Shiite–Sunni civil conflict brought more refugees from Iraq. Other waves came in response to the Sudan and Somali civil wars in the 1920s (e.g., Kayyali, 2006).

According to data posted by the US Office of Refugee Resettlement (2010), Somali and Iraqi refugees are among the largest groups of recent Arabic refugee arrivals to the USA. Over 60,000 Somali and 40,800 Iraqi refugees were admitted to the USA between 2000 and 2009. Additionally, nearly 20,000 Sudanese refugees mostly fleeing the genocide in Darfur. The majority of Arab refugees are either

I.A. Kira (✉)
Center for Cumulative Trauma Studies, 4906 Woodhurst Way,
Stone Mountain, GA 30088, USA
e-mail: kiraaref@aol.com

M.M. Amer
Department of SAPE/Psychology, The American University in Cairo,
420 Fifth Avenue, 3rd floor, New York, NY 10018, USA
e-mail: monaamer75@gmail.com

N.H. Wrobel
Department of Behavioral Sciences, University of Michigan-Dearborn,
Dearborn, MI 48128, USA
e-mail: nwrobel@umd.umich.edu

S.C. Nassar-McMillan et al. (eds.), *Biopsychosocial Perspectives on Arab Americans: Culture, Development, and Health*, DOI 10.1007/978-1-4614-8238-3_9,

Muslim or Christian. They live in almost all US states; however, the largest groups initially arrived in Texas, Michigan, Illinois, California, Minnesota, and Ohio. While most of the refugees from the Arab world came to permanently resettle in the USA, some, especially Palestinians, view themselves as in exile rather than as refugees, and this perception likely has an effect on both their attitudes and behaviors (Stockton, 1985).

Trauma and Mental Health: Theoretical Constructs and Research Results

The Development-Based Traumatology Framework

The development-based traumatology framework (DBTF) (e.g., Kira, 2001, 2010; Kira et al., 2008; Kira, Templin, et al., 2011; Kira, Fawzi & Fawzi, 2012; Kira et al., 2013) is a useful guide for the assessment of traumatic experiences that Arab refugees endured, and the associated developmental psychopathology for children, youth, adults and elderly of both genders. DBTF identifies four main traumas: (1) attachment traumas in early childhood; (2) identity traumas in adolescence and adulthood that can be divided into (a) personal, (b) interpersonal, (c) intergroup or collective, and (d) role identity traumas; (3) survival traumas; and (4) secondary (or interdependence) traumas. Further, DBTF differentiates between four types of traumas, Type I, (e.g., car accident) that happened once, Type II which may be more complex as it happened and continued in the past but stopped (e.g., child abuse, torture), and Type III, which is continuous, ongoing, and involves direct and indirect micro and macro aggressions (e.g., discrimination and racism). Type IV is the cumulative trauma dynamics for those who are multiply traumatized and or poly-victimized. Arab refugees, compared to most immigrants and the mainstream, have suffered more from the intergroup identity trauma of oppression; in addition, some suffered torture or witnessed genocide. Many Arab refugees experienced unique traumatic adversities before leaving their own countries, during the transition into other countries, and upon arrival and during resettlement in the USA. Although war, oppression and torture-related traumatic events are the initial causes of refugees' hardships, findings suggest that the day-to-day challenges and concerns in the country of resettlement, as well as the discrimination and backlash post September 11, 2001, mediate psychological distress associated with the original traumas (Kira, Lewandowski, et al., 2010; Rasmussen et al., 2010). The following sections will elaborate on some of the main traumas that Arab refugees to the USA have endured, including oppression, gender discrimination, discrimination and backlash post September 11, and acculturation stressors.

Trauma-Related Factors and Collective Identity Traumas

To better help Arab refugees, it is important to consider the personal and ecological factors that contributed to their suffering. The effects of collective intergroup trauma dynamics, with its ecological dimensions, are different from the effects and dynamics of personal single traumas that are targeted in the designs of most interventions (e.g., Kira, 2010; Kira et al., 2008). As described later in this chapter, multi-systemic models that are based on Bronfenbrenner's (1986) social–ecological model are promising.

Collective Traumas: Oppression and Torture in Country of Origin

In contrast to personal identity traumas such as sexual abuse, collective identity traumas are traumatic events such as oppression and torture that target the group(s) that the individual strongly identify with. This distinction is important because most of the evidence based interventions are designed rather to address personal and interpersonal traumas. A series of collective identity traumas in the Arab world has generated several waves of collective suffering (e.g., Abi-Hashem, 2008). These include the autocratic Arab political systems—both secular and religious—that practiced oppression, torture and even genocide (for example in Darfur) of their citizens. Other kinds of collective traumas endured by Arabs include the first and second Gulf Wars, the American invasion of Iraq, and the lingering Arab–Israeli conflict. Such collective identity traumas, in addition to other historical traumas, have contributed to suffering while at the same time enhancing collectivist ties among the victims of the suffering (Kira, 2010).

Uprooting, cultural dislocation, and displacement further compound the traumas experienced by Arab American refugees. Many were forcibly uprooted from their social support networks and displaced into a new environment, which profoundly disrupted their sense of relational connectedness and contributed to psychological distress. Of special concern are Arab women, for whom the family connection is especially valued (e.g., Dwairy, Achoui, Abouserie, & Farah, 2006); therefore, relational disconnection may be even more profound for female refugees.

Gender Discrimination and Domestic Violence

Female refugees may face unique traumas related to gender inequality that affect their mental health. Gender discrimination is a Type III ongoing trauma for females that mediates or moderates the effects of other life traumas (Kira et al., 2008; Kira, Smith,

Lewandowski, & Templin, 2010). While present in American culture, gender discrimination is more profoundly observed in the Arab refugee cultures. Depending on the particular national and socio-cultural subgroups, discrimination against girls and women may include domestic violence (Kulwicki & Miller, 1998), early and forced marriage, female genital mutilation, honor killings, rape in conflict situations, sexual exploitation, trafficking (for labor or sexual exploitation), and disparities in education, labor and even in food allocation within the household (e.g., Hynes & Cardozo, 2000).

Recent research has shown that gender discrimination can have significant mental health effects on refugee women after controlling for all their other life traumas. Gender discrimination was found to be associated with increases in dissociation, PTSD symptoms, suicidality, and deficits in executive function (Kira, Smith, et al., 2010).

Acculturation Stressors

In addition to the stressors of war, dislocation, oppression, torture, and gender discrimination, many Arab refugees face other stressful challenges such as economic hardships and the process of adapting to a new culture. Many Arab refugees may have held professional occupations in their home countries but they are unable to gain employment that matches their previous professional status. This loss in status can be associated with increased risk for depression and other symptoms (e.g., Kira et al., 2007). Some traditional women may be more isolated from the wider American society than their male counterparts because they do not work or engage in social activities in mainstream society. Compared to men, acculturative stressors are disproportionately higher for refugee women with less education and English fluency, and they experience more social isolation (e.g., Halcón et al., 2004). This kind of isolation is one of the factors that can precipitate depressive illness.

Further, cumulative acculturative stress can negatively affect the mental health of Arab refugees. Previous studies of non-refugee Arabs in the USA have shown higher levels of acculturative stress to be positively associated with increased prevalence of polysubstance abuse (Arfken, Kubiak, & Farrag, 2009) and anxiety and depression (Amer, 2005; Amer & Hovey, 2007). These results are likely to be relevant to Arab refugees as well. In a meta-analytic study of refugees worldwide, including Arab refugees, Porter and Haslam (2005) found that acculturative stress was associated with negative mental health outcomes.

Discrimination and Backlash Post 9/11

One of the major acculturative stressors and a traumatogenic factor that affects Arab refugees' adjustment and integration to their new society is the discrimination and backlash against them. These stressors have increased especially after the tragic events of September 11, 2001 (subsequently referred to as "9/11" in this chapter). Discrimination, stereotype, and prejudice against Arab Americans existed before

9/11 (e.g., Shaheen, 2003). However, in the aftermath of 9/11, three types of backlash traumas, including different micro and macro aggressions, significantly increased. First, many Arab American refugees became recipients of hostile interpersonal exchanges with members of the mainstream society, ranging from subtle insults to more violent hate crimes. Second, the media and other institutions have spread anti-Arab rhetoric and negative stereotypes, which has been a source of ongoing stress for these Arab refugees. A third source of stress has been discriminatory institutional practices such as racial profiling and other government policies such as portions of the Patriot Act (e.g., Ibish, 2003; Kira, Lewandowski, et al., 2010).

There is empirical evidence that post 9/11 backlash and perceived discrimination has negatively impacted the wider Arab American community (e.g., Abu-Ras & Suarez, 2009; Kira, Lewandowski, et al., 2010; Moradi & Hassan, 2004). For example, studies of Arab Americans have found a significant relationship between perceived post 9/11 discrimination and increased psychological distress, reduced happiness levels, in addition to more health problems (Padela & Heisler, 2010; Panagopoulos, 2006). With respect to Arab refugees, empirical studies have found that discrimination and oppression explain the highest variance in Iraqi refugee's mental health symptoms after controlling for all previous traumas (Kira et al., 2008; Kira, Lewandowski, et al., 2010). Similar results were found for Somali refugees (Ellis, MacDonald, Lincoln, & Cabral, 2008). Further, Kira, Lewandowski and colleagues (2010) found discrimination was correlated significantly with neurological, cardiovascular, respiratory, and digestive disorders among Iraqi refugees.

Arab Muslims and Christians have suffered from discrimination with different degrees. Arab American Muslims reported a higher level of discrimination and distress than their Christians counterpart (Awad, 2010) and this pattern may be applicable to Arab refugees. Possible reasons are that Christians are entering the USA with the same dominant religion, while the Muslims are entering the USA with a different minority religion. This makes the transition less difficult for the Christians, so their overall satisfaction with life therefore stays higher. The Muslim refugees may experience discrimination both because they are Arab, and for being Muslims. It may be easier for Christians to support their spirituality than for Muslims because their religious preferences are not attacked. While we addressed some major traumatic events that Arab refugees endured, the following section addresses the cumulative mental health consequences of such traumas, and the role of mental health stigma in further complicating the negative consequences.

Cumulative Trauma-Related Disorders

The Effects of Cumulative Trauma Dynamics

Cumulative trauma can yield consequences such as cumulative trauma related disorders (CTD) that are more serious than PTSD. These may include executive function deficits, dissociation, psychotic symptoms, and psychiatric comorbidities

(Kira, 2010; Kira, Templin, et al., 2006). The cumulative effects of all traumas (including personal, interpersonal, intergroup, and others) have been found to explain unique variance in these mental health outcomes beyond that which is accounted for by the aggregate sum of all trauma and victimization types (e.g., Kira, 2010; Kira et al., 2008; Richmond, Elliott, Pierce, Aspelmeier, & Alexander, 2009). For these reasons, Arab refugees show significantly higher physical and mental health symptoms compared to the general population (Jamil et al., 2007).

Some refugees experience a gradual, chronic syndrome with each successive trauma exacerbating the person's condition. On the other hand, others may experience successive traumas without any observable response, until one final trauma serves as the precipitating factor that produces an acute and severe symptomatic response. The following clinical case example illustrates the acute sudden response to cumulative trauma in Arab American refugee populations.

Fatima (a pseudonym) is a 55-year-old Iraqi refugee. She has lived in Michigan for 6 years. She has nine living children, four boys and five girls, ranging in age from 10 to 25 years. In Iraq, she lost two brothers and two sons who had been killed by the Iraqi regime. She witnessed the killing of one of her sons and the other family members who were killed and were brought soaked in blood into the house. Each had to be buried without a funeral per instructions from the authorities, and the family had to pay the government for the bullets that executed them. After the failure of the uprising against the regime in 1991, Fatima had to flee, walking in the desert for days with her immediate family to Saudi Arabia where she spent 4 years in a refugee camp in the desert. She remembers the suicides in the camp and the violent killings of those who rose up against the repressive authorities who ran the camp. She remembers the isolation and desert tornado-like sand storms. When she came with her family to the USA, she had to deal with a different set of traumas; among them were her husband's infidelity and physical abuse. She divorced him. All her family members described Fatima as the heroine of the family whose personal resilience helped her and her family survive. Her functioning remained intact and she presented no symptoms for a long time.

After the first author had been treating her son for 2 years, her daughter was driving a car in which Fatima was a passenger. The daughter got involved in a moderate car accident that resulted in some mild bruises for Fatima. After the accident, Fatima started to develop serious symptoms of fears, panic attacks, auditory hallucinations, and nightmares congruent and sometimes noncongruent with the terrors she had experienced before, but not the car accident. Further, Fatima called her ex-husband to apologize and beg for forgiveness for divorcing him and violating his rights as man.

In this clinical vignette, the client survived a series of severe traumas, and the last, which probably may have been the least severe, acted as "the straw that broke the camel's back." Further, her resistance to gender discrimination and the role of males in a traditional culture collapsed in the decompensation process. We can see in this case that there are core traumas, a triggering trauma, and resilience thresholds. The core traumas and triggering traumas' profile can be charted and analyzed for each case and for each refugee community. Trauma profile analysis, rather than exploring only the single or triggering trauma, is important to assess in such victims.

Stigma of Mental Illness

Fatima's case exemplifies the effects of cumulative trauma on mental health symptoms among Arab refugees, and the need for mental health services to support the healing process. However, many Arab refugees may avoid such services due to stigma, further prolonging the negative mental health impacts. According to the traumatology perspective, this mental illness stigma is another Type III identity trauma that is continuously endured by clients and has negative impacts on mental health (Kira et al., 2008). Type III trauma is ongoing, and tends to be internalized or resisted by affected individuals. Individuals from collectivistic cultures experience greater self-stigma compared to those from individualistic cultures (e.g., Goldston et al., 2008). In Arab cultures, individual and family mental health problems may violate individual and family honor, and often brings shame to the person and his/her family. Arab Americans internalize the social and family prejudices around seeking help that may bring shame on oneself and the disgrace to their family (e.g., Soheilian & Inman, 2009). Further, Vogel, Heimerdinger-Edwards, Hammer, and Hubbard (2011) found evidence that dominant masculine ideals, which are *inherent in such cultures*, are related to higher levels of self-stigma. This is an identified barrier that contributes to disparities in accessing mental health services and results in overall negative attitudes toward counseling (e.g., Nassar-McMillan & Hakim-Larson, 2003). Thus, there is strong empirical evidence of the added deleterious mental health effects of stigma in some Arab American communities (Kira, Lewandowski, Templin, Mohanesh, & Abdulkhalek, 2011).

Methodological Approaches: The Effects of Arab Refugees' Trauma Across the Lifespan

A variety of cross-sectional—and to a lesser degree longitudinal—research methodologies have been used to study the mental health effects of traumas for Arab refugees. Some studies used qualitative approaches, with mixed methods approaches being less common. There is a need to increase the use of longitudinal and mixed methods studies in studying Arab refugees. In the following sections we review the various methodological approaches that have been used in trauma studies with Arab refugees, the topics that have been covered, and the findings concerning the effects of refugee traumas among youth and elderly.

The Effects of Refugee Traumas on Children and Adolescents

One of the most traumatic events that child refugees may face is loss of parents and family. Research has found that separation from family is consistently associated with negative health and mental health status for refugee children (Berman, 2001). In the USA, there is a program that places Sudanese refugee unaccompanied minors in foster care. The Unaccompanied Refugee Minors Program (URMP) of the Office of Refugees Resettlement manages over 300 unaccompanied refugee minors from different areas of Sudan. However, a longitudinal study of their mental health found that mental health counseling did not impact either positively or negatively on their mental health status (Geltman, Grant-Knight, Ellis, & Landgraf, 2008). Treating attachment traumas in affected refugee children is challenging.

A quantitative study of Somali refugee adolescents found worse mental health and PTSD symptoms for those who showed less acculturation and more discrimination (Ellis et al., 2008). Retaining Somali culture was found to be associated with better mental health for girls, whereas American acculturation was associated with better mental health for boys. Another study of Arab American adolescents using structural equation modeling (SEM) found that acculturation stress and discrimination were associated with psychological distress defined as externalizing and internalizing symptoms, anxiety, and depression (Ahmed, Kia-Keating, & Tsai, 2011). About one-third of this sample had parents of refugee status.

Cross-sectional and SEM studies of Iraqi refugee adolescents in Michigan found that cumulative trauma suppressed their cognitive abilities and I.Q., and was associated with increased discrepancy between verbal and perceptual reasoning toward decreased perceptual reasoning. Such suppression of cognitive abilities may be associated with underachievement and high drop-out rates in refugee adolescents (Kira, Lewandowski, Somers, Yoon, & Chiodo, 2012; Kira, Lewandowski, Yoon, Somers, & Chiodo, 2012).

The Effects of Refugee Traumas on the Elderly

Cross-sectional quantitative and qualitative studies found that the negative effects of cumulative stressors across the life span on the mental health of elderly Arab Americans were moderated by cultural factors and aging. Research findings on Arab American elders indicated that their stress levels were higher compared to other age groups. Perceived acculturative stress, especially challenges such as learning the English language, contributed to depression (Wrobel, Farrag, & Hymes, 2009). These patterns are likely to occur among elderly Arab refugees as well.

On the other hand, the elders in the Arabic refugees' communities are regularly regarded with deep respect. This is because within the Arab culture, care of the elderly is regarded as religious and cultural duty for children. Whether they live together with their children or separately, parents are usually consulted in important decisions. Despite their positive value, Arab elders continue to be at risk for loneliness and lower social support, and health problems (Ajrouch, 2008). Although there are to date few published studies on elderly within the refugee community in particular, it is likely that the same patterns occur among Arab refugee elderly. Moreover, these elderly may be even more at risk for social isolation and mental health problems due to uprootedness at a later age and disruption of lifelong social networks. Due to strong community ties in the Arab culture, these social support networks previously served as important sources of support and protection against stressors, so disruption of such bonds can be devastating.

Resilience and Protective Factors

Notwithstanding the cumulative traumas and mental health stressors discussed earlier, Arab refugees of all age and gender groups show resilience in successfully adapting to life in the USA. Their strong collective culture, their struggle for just causes and their culturally built intact families give them additional strengths. Further, a study of stigma of mental health in Arab refugees clients found that 40 % resist the stigma imposed on them (Kira, Lewandowski, et al., 2011).

Further, a study of Iraqi refugees who had survived torture reported that victims of other kinds of trauma showed less adjustment, less resilience, and less posttraumatic growth compared to the torture victims (Kira, Templin, et al., 2006). This finding was shown even though the tortured refugees had a significantly higher trauma dose. The Iraqi refugees in the study were more tolerant of religious and cultural differences and felt more supported by their community. It is important to build upon such resilience factors as part of multi-systemic ecological interventions. As discussed further below, the protective factors associated with higher resilience include family ties and religion.

Intact Family as a Protective Factor

Generally speaking, Arabs came from more intact families with less attachment disruptions and this make them more resilient to subsequent adversities (Dwairy et al., 2006). The family bond is central to the lives of Arab American refugees; as a result, social and financial obligations to family members who were left behind in the home country may be a source of stress, as resettled refugees may feel obligated to financially assist them. Studies of the trauma profiles of Iraqi refugee adolescents, compared to African American adolescents, found Iraqi adolescents experienced multiple war traumas, uprootedness, acculturation challenges, and political oppression in their homeland, and discrimination and post 9/11 backlash in their country of resettlement, while African American adolescents experienced more socially and family made traumas such as more attachment disruptions (Kira, Lewandowski, Somers, et al., 2012; Kira, Lewandowski, Yoon, et al., 2012).

Religion and Religious/Community Leaders as Protective Factors

Refugees from Arab backgrounds (Muslims and Christians alike) tend to value religion and are likely to use religious practices to cope with cumulative and ongoing stress (Kira, Templin, et al., 2006). This is consistent with Arab Americans in general, for whom religion and culture are significant sources of strength for both individual and social healing (Jackson & Lee, 1997). Arab religious leaders like Christian pastors and priests, Muslim imams, and sheikhs and other community leaders have an enormous amount of influence among their communities and can play a vital role in community outreach. Their role is important as part of the ecological approach for health and healing. They may get involved in mediating family conflicts, solving social problems or promoting positive community healing practices. They can integrate important issues into their weekly sermons and public lectures, as well as through interpersonal interactions with their followers. Orienting religious leaders to be community champions for improving physical and mental health can help reduce gender-based violence, female genital mutilation, and gender discrimination. They can also contribute to increased parental involvement with their children in schools, and to promote or organize community mobilization/education events among their followers (e.g., Herstad, 2009). The role of the religious institution may differ with regard to whether the institution is part of the majority or minority culture. Muslim refugees use the mosque for "bonding" (i.e., enhancing interpersonal and cultural traditions and connections), whereas Christian refugees use the church for bonding as well as "bridging" to the larger American society (Allen, 2010).

Implications for Clinical and Community Research and Practice

Unfortunately there is a paucity of empirical literature examining the effectiveness of different counseling interventions with Arab Americans (Hakim-Larson, Kamoo, Nassar-McMillan, & Porcerelli, 2007). There is an increased concern about the relevance and effectiveness of current mental health programs and interventions that are derived from individualistic and biomedical paradigms, and based mostly on addressing single personal identity trauma (e.g., Bracken, Giller, & Summerfield, 1997).

It has been suggested that adding cultural and ecological considerations will help in reducing the limitations of the individual model of recovery and countering the confines of the medical model of services in such populations (e.g., Summerfield, 2004). In this chapter, we argue that there is a need to develop or adopt new and more effective integrative service and intervention models for Arab refugees that integrate the individual and ecological models of recovery in multi-systemic, multi-component, multi-modal interventions (e.g., Kira, 2002, 2010). Such interventions should be appropriate for the unique experiences and needs of diverse Arab refugee subgroups (Keyes, 2000). Further, working with complex and cumulative traumas and related comorbidities needs new frameworks for transdiagnostic approaches (e.g., McEvoy, Nathan, & Norton, 2009) and recovery from complex traumas (e.g., Courtois, Ford, Herman, & van der Kolk, 2009). The sections that follow will include discussion of models to guide research as well as sections on clinical practice, outreach advocacy and law.

Individual and Ecological Models of Recovery

Each refugee's recovery process is unique, a deeply personal process, and is intertwined with his/her relationships with family, community, and society. Arab refugee individuals or families may come from different or even the same countries and cultures, but they can have different perceptions of their own culture, which make each individual or family unique. They may represent diverse sub-cultures, religious and sub-religious affiliations, social classes, levels of education, and political attitudes. Culturally competent clinicians should adopt "multifocal conceptual lenses" that show wider empathetic understanding of the socio-political and cultural context in the therapeutic encounter with each refugee client. Therapists should be trained to be flexible and open to different construals, and continue to be ready to address intercultural difficulties when they emerge (e.g., Bala & Kramer, 2010). On the other hand, there are some commonalities among Arab refugees such as family values, the role of women, and the importance of marriage (e.g., Abudabbeh & Nydell, 1993). As such, therapists should educate themselves in the historical, cultural, and socio-political dynamics of their refugee client's circumstances and gain greater awareness of their own biases, misperceptions, and negative countertransferences (e.g., Ahmed & Aboul-Fotouh, 2012).

Individual models of recovery focus on providing the individual, as a single system, with targeted interventions either to address a single diagnostic category, or to address comorbidity based on transdiagnostic approach. Transdiagnostic or unified treatments are those that are simultaneously tailored for multiple disorders based on commonalities among disorders including similar etiologies and functional relationships that tend to maintain the disorders (e.g., McEvoy et al., 2009). Such transdiagnostic protocols may be suitable for cumulative and complex trauma and resulted comorbid conditions. Ecological approaches, on the other hand, focus on the individual as a system within layers of different systems. The treatment should address all the influential systems that the individual is part of (e.g., Bronfenbrenner, 1986).

Individual Models of Recovery

To date, there are no empirical studies on the effectiveness of different psychotherapeutic diagnostic or transdiagnostic modalities with Arab American refugees. However, there are growing numbers of clinicians and scholars that increasingly suggest the effectiveness of cognitive behavioral approach with Arab Americans (Abudabbeh & Hays, 2006; Dwairy et al., 2006; Nassar-McMillan &

Hakim-Larson, 2003). Systemic family therapy has also been recommended (Al-Krenawi & Graham, 2005). Reviews of treatment modalities for PTSD in other refugee populations have not identified a particular treatment modality to be of superior effectiveness. However, there is some indication that cognitive-behavioral therapy and narrative exposure therapy may be effective (Crumlish & O'Rourke, 2010; Kruse, Joksimovic, Cavka, Wöller, & Schmitz, 2009).

However, it is important to caution that in using such interventions, talking about the traumatic details of torture can produce many uncontrolled emotions (e.g., Ford, Courtois, van der Hart, Nijenhuis, & Steele, 2005; Kira, Templin, et al., 2006). Traditional exposure therapy can be counterproductive and can decrease compliance and increase drop-out rates. On the other hand, modified exposure therapies such as narrative exposure therapy and testimony therapy, have shown to be effective with refugees (e.g., Crumlish & O'Rourke, 2010; Neuner, Schauer, Klaschik, Karunakara, & Elbert, 2004). Exercises to enhance relaxation and the activation of resources for coping with symptoms can be effective (Bemak, Chung, & Pedersen, 2003). Other writers have suggested more directive problem-solving approaches that provide specific and concrete solutions (e.g., Cerhan, 1990). Psycho-educational group therapy approaches have been found to be useful for persons who experienced multiple traumas (Lubin, Loris, Burt, & Johnson, 1998), and such groups may be effective for refugees as well. The psycho-educational program can include teaching about the effects of different kinds of traumas, the cross-generation transmission, the developmental course of post-trauma symptoms, and the rehabilitation process.

With respect to specific issues to work through during the course of treatment, interventions with Arab American refugees can address the context of ongoing acculturation and resettlement in addition to coping with the traumatic past. Past and present experiences of discrimination should not be overlooked. In fact, it should become a routine component of the clinical assessment and treatment planning in light of the impact of discrimination on refugees' emotional distress and collective self-esteem. In the earlier phase of treatment, it may be useful to focus interventions on problem solving skills, social support, and assertiveness training. Subsequently the therapist can facilitate a shift to exploring their past traumas (Kira, Ahmed, Mahmoud, & Wassim, 2010; Kira, Ahmed, et al., 2012). The overall goals in treatment include helping clients transcend their traumatic experiences so that they are eventually able to experience a sense of safety and security and rebuild their supportive social networks (Herman, 1997). The last stage may be uniquely important for uprooted refugees and an important factor in considering the development of integrated multi-systemic or ecological approaches for recovery.

Ecological Models of Recovery

A multi-systemic ecological model may help with the unique intergroup traumas that characterize refugee experiences. As discussed earlier, cumulative and collective identity inter-group trauma dynamics are unique in comparison to single personal identity and interpersonal traumas (Kira, 2010; Kira et al., 2008). Refugees have experienced uprootedness from their homelands, communities, and social support networks. Therapeutic approaches should therefore work on helping refugees to reestablish social connections and reduce the barriers towards doing so. As a result of the oppression and traumas they faced, refugees may have moreover experienced disruption not only their sense of personal agency, but also to their collective and social identities as agents of change in their communities. The therapeutic approach can facilitate enhancement of this sense of collective agency, especially within the context of the refugees' political struggles for just causes.

Multi-systemic ecological models of recovery that have been suggested for interpersonal traumas (e.g., Bronfenbrenner, 1986; Harvey, 1996; Neville & Heppner, 1999) need to be adapted for work with refugees (e.g., Kira, 2002, 2010). This socio-ecological framework suggests that the individual functions as part of social web of networks. Resumption of social roles and enhancing collective self-efficacy through reengagement with social institutions can prove effective, especially for uprooted refugees. Adaptations of ecological models for refugees and Arab Americans are evolving; for example, use of the wraparound approach for psychosocial rehabilitation of torture survivors (Kira, 2002, 2010), ecological model for treatment of Arabic women (Mourad & Carolan, 2010), ecological group therapy models that add community healing and establishing new advocacy organizations (Kira et al., 2012; Kira, Ahmed, Mahmoud, & Wassim, 2010) trauma systems therapy (TST) (Saxe, Ellis, Fogler, Hanson, & Sorkin, 2005; Saxe, Ellis, & Kaplow, 2007), and the post-disaster ecological recovery model (Abramson, Stehling-Ariza, Park, Walsh, & Culp, 2010). These models have ecological validity. Additionally, recent studies provide strong empirical evidence for the effectiveness of some of their variants (e.g., Abramson et al., 2010). For example, there is some empirical evidence of the effectiveness of multi-systemic wraparound torture rehabilitation approach (McColl et al., 2010).

In collectivistic cultures, healing usually takes place within the group context. For example, in the Arab culture it is common for families and community elders or religious or political leaders to be among the first sources of support for personal problems and/or health concerns. Therefore, when people are persecuted because of their group membership, a therapy approach that targets group self-esteem and efficacy among its goals seems logical and has greater therapeutic potential. Ecological models are even more advantageous because they are flexible in using adjustable criteria to focus on clients' priorities.

Clinical Practice Considerations for Subgroups

Irrespective of the individual and ecological models that are used to service Arab refugees, there are numerous clinical issues that providers should consider. The following sections describe clinical considerations for specific subgroups: Iraqi refugees, women, and youth.

Considerations and Lessons from Working with Iraqi Refugees

Recent studies show that Iraqi refugee torture survivors identify the reasons for surviving their torture as their political and religious beliefs (Kira et al., 2008; Kira, Templin, et al., 2006). Capitalizing on the refugees' identified natural survival strategies and strengths using appropriate cognitive attribution, reframing, and empowerment techniques can be helpful. The first author's clinical experience with Arab refugee victims of torture and political oppression confirms these research findings. One cannot avoid talking about religion and/or politics when treating victims of torture and political oppression.

For these Iraqi victims of torture and political oppression, therapists are encouraged to normalize their anger against the oppressor and facilitate the clients' resistance against oppression and seeking retributive justice. Studies of the effects of eliminating the oppressive regime in Iraq and accomplishing redress and retributive justice for Iraqi refugees found that such perceived retributive justice helps the victim to decrease depression and anxiety, increase feeling of peace with self and others, regain memory capacity and executive functions, and increase self-control. The perceived regaining of self-control was found to be central and significant in reducing depression and anxiety, as well as enhancing post-trauma growth and futuristic optimistic orientation for these refugees (c.f., Başoğlu et al., 2005; Kira, Lewandowski, et al., 2006; Kira et al., 2009). However, teaching forgiveness of those who collaborate with the system (not the dictators and major oppressors) can be helpful as it is associated with decreased PTSD and better health conditions (Kira et al., 2009).

Considerations When Working with Women

Research findings, discussed earlier, highlight the relevance of uprootedness, as well as gender discrimination in women's and girls' lives. When working with female Arab refugee clients, it is important to assess for internalized gender discrimination and gender-based violence, its effects on gender esteem, and its interaction with other discriminations and past and the current traumas (James, 2010; Kira, Smith, et al., 2010). While such discrimination may be internalized by some clients as the accepted norms, therapists can challenge aspects of culture that promote gendered violence and violations of women's human rights with a focus on empowerment, self-efficacy, and a sense of control (e.g., Kira, 2010; Kira, Smith, et al., 2010). However, clinicians should show sensitivity when assessing for history of domestic and sexual violence, as experiences of rape may be highly stigmatized. Revealing such experiences may be shameful and traumatic for female refugees. Moreover, intervention models should be tailored to the unique experiences of women, and build on their cultural strengths such as their central role in maintaining the family structure and caring for family members including parenting the youth.

Considerations When Working with Youth and Families: Multi-systemic, Multi-modal Interventions

The refuge processes exposes children and youth to different adversities including potential attachment disruptions, severe uprootedness and cumulative traumas. This may affect their psychosocial development and precipitate different internalizing and externalizing symptoms. Discrimination that overlaps with bullying in schools and communities are especially prevalent and may have deleterious mental health and cognitive effects (e.g., Kira, Yoon, Lewandowski, Somers, & Chiodo, 2011). A study of Somali and Oromo refugee youth in the USA found that their strategies for coping with distress included praying, sleeping, reading, watching TV, and talking with friends (Halcón et al., 2004). Clinicians can integrate the youth's preferred coping strategies when planning services to best meet the youths' mental health needs.

Some authors have recommended the cognitive-behavioral modality for refugee youth, although multifaceted integrated services may be more effective (Murray, Cohen, Ellis, & Mannarino, 2008). Two of the promising treatment approaches to addressing the multiple layers of refugees' youth's cumulative trauma are multisystemic therapy (MST; Henggeler, Schoenwald, Borduin, Rowland, & Cunningham, 1998) and Structural Ecosystems Theory (SET; Szapocznik & Coatsworth, 1999). Both treatment approaches are based on Bronfenbrenner's (1986) social-ecological model. This model views the individual as nested within multiple layers of systems such as family, school, and the wider community. Behavioral problems are activated and maintained by multiple factors that interact across the different ecological layers. Multimodal therapies that take into account the child's social ecology can be effective for refugees, especially because they incorporate intensive individual, family, and community levels of healing while being flexible in targeting the child's developmental stage and the presenting problems. Empirical research has found MST to be superior in comparison to traditional therapies for children with severe emotional and behavioral disturbances; however, its use for refugee children has yet to be examined.

Outreach, Advocacy and Law

In line with the ecological model for recovery, outreach, advocacy, and legal redress can be important for recovery. As victims of oppression, discrimination and cumulative trauma, Arab refugees need and deserve important resources and efforts to stop and alleviate their sufferings. Organizations that offer services to refugees are encouraged to engage in active outreach strategies such as workshops, support groups, and community forums. Programs can focus on orienting refugees to American society, providing psycho-education, and supporting resettlement such as in housing and employment. Community outreach efforts can circumvent the barriers towards seeking services such as mental illness stigma, use of alternative coping strategies, low awareness of mental health services, and logistical challenges (Ahmed & Aboul-Fotouh, 2012).

In addition to health and mental health services, agencies and organizations can offer refugees support in the resettlement process by advocating for refugee rights. Adult refugees may need support advocating for housing and employment opportunities, as well as in issues related to their legal status as residents in the USA. Refugee parents may need assistance in advocating for their children's rights in the school setting, especially in addressing marginalization in the curriculum and bullying (Ahmed & Aboul-Fotouh, 2012).

Legal supports may also be needed for refugees; for example, in cases of discrimination. In addition to efforts to support refugees with their individual cases as victims of discrimination, broader efforts need to be made to clarify and modify legal standards to better provide justice in these types of cases. One challenge is that although the mental health impacts of discrimination have been discussed in numerous studies, unfortunately the current psychiatric classification systems do not explicitly recognize the role of discrimination in producing distinct psychiatric conditions. Therefore, there is limited scientific evidence for lawyers and psychologists to use when assessing and arguing injury caused by discrimination. This leads to more latitude in the courtroom for different assessments and conclusions on the plaintiffs' cases. Another area where changes need to be made relates to gender discrimination and gendered oppression. These experiences are considered Type III trauma and can precipitate mental health concerns. It is important for the legal system to reframe legal standards as such, and to acknowledge domestic violence and gender based violence to be human rights violations and public criminal acts rather than private or personal acts (Burman & Chantler, 2005). Such paradigm shifts can enhance advocacy for gender equality, and facilitate reduction of gender disparities in the families, institutions, and cultures that presently maintain these disparities.

Conclusions

Arab American refugees have experienced a legacy of oppression, culturally embedded gender discrimination, torture and cumulative trauma in their homelands. During relocation and upon arrival to the USA they continue to experience acculturation stressors, uprootedness, stigmatization, and discrimination. The core traumas in their trauma profile are intergroup traumas which are different from the personal and interpersonal traumas that most mainstream counselors are trained to deal with and most of the evidence-based interventions are designed to treat. Improved supports and integrative ecological approaches for healing and adjustment may better help them to succeed in their new country of refuge. This will allow them to fully benefit from the second chance for freedom, democracy and healthy living opportunities, which this new refuge may grant them.

References

Abi-Hashem, N. (2008). Arab Americans: Understanding their challenges, needs, and struggles. In A. J. Marsella, J. L. Johnson, P. Watson, & J. Gryczynski (Eds.), *Ethnocultural perspectives on disaster and trauma* (pp. 115–174). New York, NY: Springer.

Abramson, D. M., Stehling-Ariza, T., Park, Y. S., Walsh, L., & Culp, D. (2010). Measuring individual disaster recovery: A socioecological framework. *Disaster Medicine and Public Health Preparedness, 4*, 46–54.

Abudabbeh, N., & Hays, P. A. (2006). Cognitive-behavioral therapy with people of Arab heritage. In P. A. Hays (Ed.), *Culturally responsive cognitive-behavioral therapy: Assessment, practice and supervision* (pp. 141–159). Washington, DC: APA.

Abudabbeh, N., & Nydell, M. K. (1993). Transcultural counseling and Arab Americans. In J. McFadden (Ed.), *Transcultural counseling: Bilateral and international perspectives* (2nd ed., pp. 261–284). Alexandria, VA: American Counseling Association.

Abu-Ras, W. M., & Suarez, Z. E. (2009). Muslim men and women's perception of discrimination, hate crimes, and PTSD symptoms post 9/11. *Traumatology, 15*, 48–63.

Ahmed, S., & Aboul-Fotouh, F. (2012). Refugees. In S. Ahmed & M. M. Amer (Eds.), *Counseling Muslims: Handbook of mental health issues and interventions* (pp. 281–305). New York, NY: Routledge.

Ahmed, S., Kia-Keating, M., & Tsai, K. (2011). A structural model of racial discrimination, acculturative stress, and cultural resources among Arab American adolescents. *American Journal of Community Psychology, 48*(3–4), 181–192.

Ajrouch, K. J. (2008). Social isolation and loneliness among Arab American elders: Cultural, social, and personal factors. *Research in Human Development, 5*(1), 44–59.

Al-Krenawi, A., & Graham, J. R. (2005). Marital therapy for Muslim Arab couples: Acculturation and re-acculturation. *The Family Journal, 13*(3), 300–310.

Allen, R. (2010). The bonding and bridging roles of religious institutions for refugees in a non-gateway context. *Ethnic and Racial Studies, 33*(6), 1049–1068.

Amer, M. M. (2005). Arab American mental health in the Post September 11 era: Acculturation, stress, and coping. *Dissertation Abstracts International: Section B: The Sciences and Engineering*, 1974.

Amer, M. M., & Hovey, J. D. (2007). Socio-demographic differences in acculturation and mental health for a sample of 2nd generation/early immigrant Arab Americans. *Journal of Immigrant and Minority Health, 9*, 335–347.

Arfken, C. L., Kubiak, S. P., & Farrag, M. (2009). Acculturation and polysubstance abuse in Arab-American treatment clients. *Transcultural Psychiatry, 46*(4), 608–622.

Awad, G. H. (2010). The impact of acculturation and religious identification on perceived discrimination for Arab/Middle Eastern Americans. *Cultural Diversity and Ethnic Minority Psychology, 16*(1), 59–67.

Bala, J., & Kramer, S. (2010). Intercultural dimensions in the treatment of traumatized refugee families. *Traumatology, 16*(4), 153–159.

Başoğlu, M., Livanou, M., Crnobarić, C., Frančišković, T., Suljić, E., Đurić, D., et al. (2005). Psychiatric and cognitive effects of war in former Yugoslavia: Association of lack of redress for trauma and posttraumatic stress reactions. *JAMA: The Journal of the American Medical Association, 294*, 580–590.

Bemak, F., Chung, C., & Pedersen, P. B. (2003). *Counseling refugees: A psychosocial approach to innovative multicultural interventions*. Westport, CT: Greenwood Press.

Berman, H. (2001). Children and war: Current understandings and future directions. *Public Health Nursing, 18*, 243–252.

Bracken, P., Giller, J. E., & Summerfield, D. (1997). Rethinking mental health work with survivors of wartime violence and refugees. *Journal of Refugee Studies, 10*, 431–442.

Bronfenbrenner, U. (1986). Ecology of the family as a context for human development. *Developmental Psychology, 22*, 723–742.

Burman, E., & Chantler, K. (2005). Domestic violence and minoritisation: Legal and policy barriers facing minoritized women leaving violent relationships. *International Journal of Law and Psychiatry, 28*, 59–74.

Cerhan, J. (1990). The Hmong in the United States: An overview for mental health professionals. *Journal of Counseling and Development, 69*, 88–92.

Courtois, C., Ford, J., Herman, J., & van der Kolk, B. (2009). *Treating complex traumatic stress disorders: An evidence-based guide*. New York, NY: Guilford Press.

Crumlish, N., & O'Rourke, K. (2010). A systematic review of treatments for post-traumatic stress disorder among refugees and asylum-seekers. *Journal of Nervous and Mental Disease, 198*, 237–251.

Dwairy, M., Achoui, M., Abouserie, R., & Farah, A. (2006). Parenting adolescent-family connectedness among Arabs: A second cross-regional research study. *Journal of Cross-Cultural Psychology, 37*(3), 248–261.

Ellis, B. H., MacDonald, H. Z., Lincoln, A. K., & Cabral, H. J. (2008). Mental health of Somali adolescent refugees: The role of trauma, stress, and perceived discrimination. *Journal of Consulting and Clinical Psychology, 76*(2), 184–193.

Ford, J. D., Courtois, C., van der Hart, O., Nijenhuis, E., & Steele, K. (2005). Treatment of complex post-traumatic self-dysregulation. *Journal of Traumatic Stress, 18*, 467–477.

Geltman, P. L., Grant-Knight, W., Ellis, H., & Landgraf, J. M. (2008). The "lost boys" of Sudan: Use of health services and functional health outcomes of unaccompanied refugee minors resettled in the U.S. *Journal of Immigrant and Minority Health, 10*(5), 389–396.

Goldston, D. B., Molock, S. D., Whitbeck, L. B., Murakami, J. L., Zayas, L. H., & Hall, G. C. N. (2008). Cultural considerations in adolescent suicide prevention and psychosocial treatment. *American Psychologist, 63*, 14–31.

Hakim-Larson, J., Kamoo, R., Nassar-McMillan, S. C., & Porcerelli, J. H. (2007). Counseling Arab and Chaldean American families. *Journal of Mental Health Counseling, 29*(4), 301–321.

Halcón, L. L., Robertson, C. L., Savik, K., Johnson, D. R., Spring, M. A., Butcher, J. N., et al. (2004). Trauma and coping in Somali and Oromo refugee youth. *Journal of Adolescent Health, 35*(1), 17–25.

Harvey, M. R. (1996). An ecological view of psychological trauma and trauma recovery. *Journal of Traumatic Stress, 9*(1), 3–23.

Henggeler, S. W., Schoenwald, S., Borduin, C., Rowland, M., & Cunningham, P. (1998). *Multisystemic treatment for antisocial behavior in children and adolescents*. New York, NY: Guilford.

Herman, J. (1997). *Trauma and recovery*. New York, NY: Basic Books.

Herstad, B. (2009). *The role of religious communities in addressing gender-based violence and HIV.* Washington, DC: Futures Group International, Health Policy Initiative, Task Order 1. Retrieved from http://www.healthpolicyinitiative.com/Publications/Documents/867_1_The_Role_of_Religious_Communities_in_Addressing_GBV_and_HIV_FINAL_9_24_09_acc.pdf

Hynes, M., & Cardozo, B. L. (2000). Sexual violence against refugee women. *Journal of Women's Health & Gender-Based Medicine, 9*, 819–823.

Ibish, H. (2003). *Report on hate crimes and discrimination against Arab Americans: The post September 11, 2001–October11, 2002*. Washington, DC: American-Arab Anti-Discrimination Committee.

Jackson, M. L., & Lee, C. C. (1997). Counseling Arab Americans. In M. L. Jackson & C. C. Lee (Eds.), *Multicultural issues in counseling: New approaches to diversity* (2nd ed., pp. 333–349). Alexandria, VA: American Counseling Association.

James, K. (2010). Domestic violence within refugee families: Intersecting patriarchal culture and the refugee experience. *Australian and New Zealand Journal of Family Therapy, 31*(3), 275–284.

Jamil, H., Farrag, M., Hakim-Larson, J., Kafaji, T., Abdulkhaleq, H., & Hammad, A. (2007). Mental health symptoms in Iraqi refugees: Posttraumatic stress disorder, anxiety, and depression. *Journal of Cultural Diversity, 14*, 19–25.

Kayyali, R. (2006). *The Arab Americans*. Westport, CT: Greenwood Press.
Keyes, E. F. (2000). Mental health status in refugees: An integrative review of current research. *Issues in Mental Health Nursing, 21*, 397–410.
Kira, I. A. (2001). Taxonomy of trauma and trauma assessment. *Traumatology, 2*, 1–14.
Kira, I. A. (2002). Torture assessment and treatment: The wraparound approach. *Traumatology, 8*(1), 23–51.
Kira, I. A. (2010). Etiology and treatments of post-cumulative traumatic stress disorders in different cultures. *Traumatology, 16*(4), 128–141.
Kira, I. A., Ahmed, A., Mahmoud, V., & Wassim, F. (2010). Group therapy model for refugee and torture survivors. *Torture, 20*(2), 108–113.
Kira, I. A., Ahmed, A., Wassim, F., McAdams-Mahmoud, V., Clorain, J., & Rai, D. (2012). Group therapy for refugees and torture survivors: Treatment models innovations. *International Journal of Group Psychotherapy, 62*(1), 63–83.
Kira, I. A., Hammad, A., Lewandowski, L., Templin, T., Ramswamy, V., Ozkan, B., et al. (2007). The physical and mental status of Iraqi refugees and its etiology. *Ethnicity & Disease, 17*, S3-79–S3-82.
Kira, I. A., Lewandowski, L., Somers, C., Yoon, J., & Chiodo, L. (2012). PTSD, trauma types, cumulative trauma, and IQ: The case of African American and Iraqi refugee adolescents. *Psychological Trauma: Theory, Research, Practice, and Policy, 4*(1), 128–139.
Kira, I. A., Lewandowski, L., Templin, T., Mohanesh, M., & Abdulkhalek, H. (2011, August). *The dynamics of internalized stigma of mental illness among Arab Americans, Muslims, and refugees patients: A traumatology perspective*. Paper presented in the American Psychological Association Annual Convention, Washington, DC.
Kira, I. A., Lewandowski, L., Templin, T., Ramaswamy, V., Ozkan, B., & Mohanesh, J. (2008). Measuring cumulative trauma dose, types and profiles using a development-based taxonomy of trauma. *Traumatology, 14*(2), 62–87.
Kira, I. A., Lewandowski, L. A., Templin, T. N., Ramaswamy, V., Ozkan, B., & Mohanesh, J. (2009). The effects of post-retribution inter-group forgiveness: The case of Iraqi refugees. *Peace and Conflict: Journal of Peace Psychology, 15*, 385–413.
Kira, I. A., Lewandowski, L., Templin, T., Ramaswamy, V., Ozkan, B., & Mohanesh, J. (2010). The effects of perceived discrimination and backlash on Iraqi refugees' physical and mental health. *Journal of Muslim Mental Health, 5*(1), 59–81.
Kira, I. A., Lewandowski, L., Templin, T., Ramswamy, V., Ozkan, B., Hammad, A., et al. (2006). The mental health effects of retributive justice: The case of Iraqi refugees. *Journal of Muslim Mental Health, 1*(2), 145–169.
Kira, I., Lewandowski, L., Yoon, J., Somers, C., & Chiodo, L. (2012). The linear and non-linear associations between multiple types of trauma and IQ discrepancy indexes in African American and Iraqi refugee adolescents. *Journal of Child & Adolescent Trauma, 5*, 47–62.
Kira, I. A., Smith, I., Lewandowski, L., & Templin, T. (2010). The effects of gender discrimination on refugee torture survivors: A cross-cultural traumatology perspective. *Journal of the American Psychiatric Nurses Association, 16*(5), 299–306.
Kira, I. A., Templin, T., Lewandowski, L., Clifford, D., Wiencek, P., Hammad, A., et al. (2006). The effects of torture: Two community studies. *Peace and Conflict: Journal of Peace Psychology, 12*(3), 205–228.
Kira, I. A., Templin, T., Lewandowski, L., Ramaswamy, V., Bulent, O., Abu-Mediane, S., et al. (2011). Cumulative Tertiary appraisal of traumatic events across cultures: Two studies. *Journal of Loss and Trauma: International Perspectives on Stress & Coping, 16*, 43–66.
Kira, I. A., Yoon, J., Lewandowski, L., Somers, C., & Chiodo, L. (2011, August). *The effects of bullying on IQ in two adolescent minority groups: A traumatology perspective*. Paper presented at the American Psychological Association Annual Convention, Washington, DC.
Kira, I., Ashby, J. S., Lewandowski, L., Alawneh, A. N., Mohanesh, J., & Odenat, L. (2013) Advances in continuous traumatic stress theory: Traumatogenic dynamics and consequences of intergroup conflict—The Palestinian adolescents case. *Psychology, 4*, 396–409.

Kira, I., Fawzi, M., & Fawzi, M. (2012). The dynamics of cumulative trauma and trauma types in adults patients with psychiatric disorders: Two cross-cultural studies. *Traumatology*, Advanced online publication.

Kruse, J., Joksimovic, L., Cavka, M., Wöller, W., & Schmitz, N. (2009). Effects of trauma-focused psychotherapy upon war refugees. *Journal of Traumatic Stress, 22*(6), 585–592.

Kulwicki, A., & Miller, J. (1998). Domestic violence in the Arab American population: Transforming environmental conditions through community education. *Issues in Mental Health Nursing, 20*(3), 199–215.

Lubin, H., Loris, M., Burt, J., & Johnson, D. R. (1998). Efficacy of psychoeducational group therapy in reducing symptoms of posttraumatic stress disorder among multiply traumatized women. *The American Journal of Psychiatry, 155*, 1172–1177.

Luthar, S. S., Cicchetti, D., & Becker, B. (2000). The construct of resilience: A critical evaluation and guidelines for future work. *Child Development, 71*(3), 543–562.

McColl, H., Higson-Smith, C., Gjerding, S., Omar, M., Rahman, B., Hamed, M., et al. (2010). Rehabilitation of torture survivors in five countries: Common themes and challenges. *International Journal of Mental Health Systems, 4*, 16. doi:10.1186/1752-4458-4-16.

McEvoy, P. M., Nathan, P., & Norton, P. J. (2009). Efficacy of transdiagnostic treatments: A review of published outcome studies and future research directions. *Journal of Cognitive Psychotherapy, 23*, 20–33.

Moradi, B., & Hassan, N. T. (2004). Arab American persons' reported experiences of discrimination and mental health: The mediating role of personal control. *Journal of Counseling Psychology, 51*, 418–428.

Mourad, M., & Carolan, M. A. (2010). An ecological approach to culturally sensitive intervention for Arab American women and their families. *The Family Journal, 18*(2), 178–183.

Murray, L. K., Cohen, J. A., Ellis, B. H., & Mannarino, A. (2008). Cognitive behavioral therapy for symptoms of trauma and traumatic grief in refugee youth. *Child and Adolescent Psychiatric Clinics of North America, 17*(3), 585–604.

Nassar-McMillan, S. C., & Hakim-Larson, J. (2003). Counseling considerations among Arab Americans. *Journal of Counseling and Development, 81*, 150–159.

Neuner, F., Schauer, M., Klaschik, C., Karunakara, U., & Elbert, T. (2004). A comparison of narrative exposure therapy, supportive counseling, and psychoeducation for treating posttraumatic stress disorder in an African refugee settlement. *Journal of Consulting and Clinical Psychology, 72*, 579–587.

Neville, H. A., & Heppner, M. J. (1999). Contextualizing rape: Reviewing sequelae and proposing a culturally inclusive ecological model of sexual assault recovery. *Applied and Preventive Psychology, 8*(1), 41–62.

Padela, A. I., & Heisler, M. (2010). The association of perceived abuse and discrimination after September 11, 2001, with psychological distress, level of happiness, and health status among Arab Americans. *American Journal of Public Health, 100*(2), 284–291.

Panagopoulos, C. (2006). Arab and Muslim Americans and Islam in the aftermath of 9/11. *Public Opinion Quarterly, 70*, 608–624.

Porter, M., & Haslam, N. (2005). Predisplacement and postdisplacement factors associated with mental health of refugees and internally displaced persons: A meta-analysis. *JAMA: The Journal of the American Medical Association, 294*(5), 602–612.

Rasmussen, A., Nguyen, L., Wilkinson, J., Vundla, S., Raghavan, S., Miller, K. E., et al. (2010). Rates and impact of trauma and current stressors among Darfuri refugees in Eastern Chad. *The American Journal of Orthopsychiatry, 80*(2), 227–236.

Richmond, J. M., Elliott, A. N., Pierce, T. W., Aspelmeier, J. E., & Alexander, A. A. (2009). Polyvictimization, childhood victimization, and psychological distress in college women. *Child Maltreatment, 142*, 127–147.

Saxe, G. N., Ellis, B. H., Fogler, J., Hanson, S., & Sorkin, B. (2005). Comprehensive care for traumatized children. *Psychiatric Annals, 35*, 424–430.

Saxe, G. N., Ellis, B. H., & Kaplow, J. B. (2007). *Collaborative treatment of traumatized children and teens: The trauma systems therapy approach*. New York, NY: Guilford Press.

Shaheen, J. G. (2003). Reel bad Arabs: How Hollywood vilifies a people. *The Annals of the American Academy of Political and Social Science, 588*, 171–193.

Soheilian, S. S., & Inman, A. G. (2009). Middle Eastern Americans: The effects of stigma on attitudes toward counseling. *Journal of Muslim Mental Health, 4*, 139–158.

Stockton, R. R. (1985). The Palestinians of Dearborn, Michigan. *Psychological Reports, 56*(1), 123–129.

Summerfield, D. (2004). Cross-cultural perspectives on the medicalization of human suffering. In G. M. Rosen (Ed.), *Posttraumatic stress disorder: Issues and controversies* (pp. 233–245). New York, NY: Wiley.

Szapocznik, J., & Coatsworth, J. D. (1999). An eco-developmental framework for organizing the influences on drug abuse: A developmental model of risk and protection. In M. D. Glantz & C. R. Hartel (Eds.), *Drug abuse: Origins & interventions* (pp. 331–366). Washington, DC: American Psychological Association.

U.S. Office of Refugee Resettlement [O.R.R.]. (2010). *Refugee arrival data: By country of origin and state of initial resettlement.* Retrieved March 10, 2011, from http://www.acf.hhs.gov/programs/orr/data/refugee_arrival_data.htm

Vogel, D., Heimerdinger-Edwards, S., Hammer, J., & Hubbard, A. (2011). "Boys don't cry": Examination of the links between endorsement of masculine norms, self-stigma, and help-seeking attitudes for men from diverse backgrounds. *Journal of Counseling Psychology, 58*(3), 368–382.

Wrobel, N., Farrag, M., & Hymes, R. (2009). Acculturative stress and depression in an elderly Arabic sample. *Journal of Cross-Cultural Gerontology, 24*(3), 273–290.

Chapter 10
Mental Health Risks in Arab Americans Across the Lifespan

Nancy Howells Wrobel and Ashley Paterson

The field of psychopathology has been heavily influenced by a developmental approach, which seeks to explore and comprehend the components impacting normal and abnormal development across the lifespan. A complex interaction of social, biological, and psychological processes is viewed as occurring over time in an individual to create either an adaptive or maladaptive outcome (Masten & Coatsworth, 1995). Of particular interest in this body of research is the study of those whose lives have included various degrees of hardship (Cicchetti & Toth, 2009). From such studies we are able to derive basic knowledge of resilience in the face of hardship, as well as determine what factors may contribute to a more maladaptive outcome. This knowledge in turn may aid intervention.

In addition to a more focused study of those facing hardship, there has been increased interest in, as well as a changing perspective on, addressing the study of psychopathology among minority group members. There appears to be multiple ways in which our study of psychopathology may benefit from examination across ethnic and cultural groups. Prior examination of these issues, with a focus on Latinos and other ethnic groups in the USA, have resulted in identification of a shift towards viewing adaptation in minority groups as reflecting "differences," rather than "deficits" (Garcia-Coll, Akerman, & Cicchetti, 2000; Garcia-Coll, Crnic, Lamberty, & Wasik, 1996). In simple terms, development that appears maladaptive in one culture may serve an adaptive function in another cultural context or environment. The hardships and stressors experienced by many minority groups readily lead to

N.H. Wrobel (✉)
Department of Behavioral Sciences, University of Michigan-Dearborn,
Dearborn, MI 48128, USA
e-mail: nwrobel@umd.umich.edu

A. Paterson
Department of Psychology, University of Windsor, 401 Sunset Avenue,
Windsor, ON N9B 3P4, Canada
e-mail: patersoa@uwindsor.ca

S.C. Nassar-McMillan et al. (eds.), *Biopsychosocial Perspectives on Arab Americans: Culture, Development, and Health*, DOI 10.1007/978-1-4614-8238-3_10,

examination of potential risks as well as alternative modes of adaptation to stress and trauma. Thus, there is a particular challenge for mental health professionals as they attempt to distinguish between adaptation that is "different" due to cultural context and that which is better described as maladaptation in minority groups.

In addition to examining the relation of hardship to mental health outcomes, the present chapter applies some of the notions of developmental psychopathology to a relatively understudied minority group, Arab Americans. Such an approach to mental illness risks and protective factors with this specific group appears particularly relevant. As one considers the complex historical and political context experienced by those whose families have emigrated from the Arab world over several decades, it seems important to consider that the impact of these events on mental health may vary greatly for individuals at different points in the lifespan. The timing of entry into the USA, and the relationship to historical and political events may also have an impact on the development and adjustment of Arab immigrants. In particular, identification with the designation of "Arab American" may vary a great deal depending upon when an individual immigrated to the USA, both historically and in terms of the age of the immigrant at the time (Wrobel, Farrag, & Hymes, 2009).

Historical Context

There have been a series of waves of immigration from the Arab countries, and each wave represents a pattern of historical and political circumstances (Abu-Baker, 2006; Erickson & Al-Timimi, 2001). Individuals arriving during these distinct waves of immigration had varying psychological experiences, both in terms of their identity and the degree of trauma experienced. Those arriving near the start of the twentieth century were motivated to seek the "American Dream" economically, and their tendency was to blend into the dominant American society. Subsequent groups of refugees came not so much out of "optimism" for a better lifestyle, but in response to stressful events in the Middle East. Thus, some had been displaced from their homeland due to the Israeli–Palestinian conflict of the 1940s, and others fled due to increasing tension and wars over the next 2 decades. Also of note here, in terms of the psychological experience, is that the Arab countries were no longer under European colonial rule (Erickson & Al-Timimi, 2001), and a greater sense of Arab identity was evident in these immigrants. Their settlement in densely populated Arab American communities, such as Dearborn, Michigan, allowed immigrants to maintain a cultural identity, including religious affiliations, and other customs, perhaps serving as protective mechanisms psychologically.

The most recent wave of immigration, beginning after the 1967 war, included immigrants who were motivated to escape political strife as well as to seek financial stability. Iraqi immigrants make up the largest proportion of this group. The social environment for this wave of immigrants can be characterized as involving increasing levels of anti-Arab sentiment. This, in turn, discouraged assimilation and encouraged the establishment of separate Arab and Muslim institutions. The complexity of the experience, and related mental health risk, for these immigrants is great, as many had already experienced significant trauma, including torture, prior to their emigration (Jamil et al., 2002).

Amer and Hovey (2007) also note that there are two sub-groups represented, one highly educated and the other at a much lower socioeconomic and educational level, with presumably greater risk for continued mental health difficulties. The circumstances have continued to be stressful as anti-Arab sentiment against those who have remained in the USA has been heightened by ongoing political events (Abu-Baker, 2006; Erickson & Al-Timimi, 2001; Naber, 2000). Reported perceptions of discrimination against Arab Americans (Moradi & Hasan, 2004; Zogby, 2001 cited in Moradi & Hasan, 2004) as well as documented discriminatory acts (Ibish, 2003) accelerated following 9/11.

Acculturation

Acculturation and Adaptation

Just as the political and social experiences of Arab Americans have varied over the decades, the degree of acculturation displayed, and degree of acculturative stress, varies between groups and individuals. Generally, acculturation involves the psychological adaptation that takes place when two or more cultural groups come into contact (Redfield, Linton, & Herskovitz, 1936, as cited in Trimble, 2003). Assimilation refers to an individual "relinquishing (their) cultural identity and moving into the dominant society" (Berry, 1990, p. 93), and the degree of assimilation varies for immigrants. Some may experience either total assimilation of one cultural group by a dominant host culture, or a multicultural circumstance, where separate cultures continue to exist (Rudmin, 2003). The relation between degree of assimilation and the chance of mental health risk or resilience is not entirely clear or universal. Berry's commonly cited model (1990) predicts that a moderate degree of assimilation allows individuals to maintain their identities as well as the support of their original ethnic group, while benefitting from the resources present in the dominant culture. Other views stress the flexibility of a bicultural form of adaptation (Gallagher-Thompson et al., 1997; Zamanian, Thackrey, Starrett, & Brown, 1992).

The relation between mental health and acculturation is complex, and it is clear that acculturation and the accompanying stress alone may not necessarily be the direct cause of mental health problems. In reality, acculturation may either enhance or detract from one's psychological well-being, depending upon a wide range of variables (Berry & Kim, 1988). In general, the duration of residency in the host country has been identified as a factor in psychological adjustment, with more recent immigrants displaying poorer adjustment (Kiefer et al., 1985), and greater resistance to cultural change (Ghaffarian, 1998). Faragallah, Schumm, and Webb (1997) describe the length of residence in the USA as a measure of exposure to the host culture, noting that with greater exposure immigrants have become more acculturated, either acquiring the host culture or rejecting it. Consequently, the risk of mental health problems was expected to be higher in more recent immigrants.

For Arab Americans, religious affiliation appears to be an important factor in adaptation, acculturation, and related mental health variables. Generally, many authors have concluded that Christian Arabs have more successfully adapted to American society. In addition to the greater likelihood of shared religious and cultural practices for Christian Arabs in the USA, they may be experiencing some relief from religious persecution they may have experienced while living in their homeland (Amer & Hovey, 2007). In their own examination of religious difference, Amer and Hovey found that among Arab Americans, Christians did report a greater degree of integration and assimilation, while Muslims had higher levels of ethnic identity, including both religious and cultural practices, such as maintaining their Arabic language, music, and traditional foods. Muslims also reported higher levels of intrinsic religiosity, and for them, this variable predicted lower levels of depression. While commonly accepted models of acculturation seemed relevant for the Christian groups, with separation and marginalization predicting depression, the pattern varied for Muslims. Although Muslims in the sample reportedly saw integration as desirable, integration did not predict a greater level of mental health adjustment (Amer & Hovey, 2007). Consistent with these findings, Awad (2010) reported that while Christian Arabs who were immersed in the dominant culture and thus higher in acculturation actually experienced less depression, Muslims who were more fully immersed in the dominant culture experienced a higher level of depression. For Muslims, to remain separated may protect them from stressors, such as discrimination, which may be more likely if they are integrated into the dominant group. In addition, Awad found that high ethnic identity predicted higher levels of discrimination, perhaps due to the higher visibility related to things like speaking in Arabic or wearing traditional clothing. This variation across religious groups at the time implies the most adaptive pattern of acculturation may depend upon an interaction of personal, cultural, and situational factors.

Acculturative Stress and Mental Health

Investigation of the relation between acculturation and mental health often addresses the negative aspects of acculturation separately, utilizing the concept of "acculturative stress" (Berry, Trimble, & Olmedo, 1986). Acculturative stress is defined as a type of stress in which "the stressors are identified as having their source in the process of acculturation" (Williams & Berry, 1991, p. 4). Immigrants may experience common practical stressors, such as finding employment, housing, and transportation, and in addition may face unique, acculturation related stressors, such as difficulties with language and varying customs. Knowledge of these stressors can be useful in both prediction of depression and anxiety disorders, as well as their prevention.

The majority of information on acculturative stress and mental health has focused on the larger immigrant groups in the USA, particularly Asian or Latino populations. For these groups, the results point to a relationship between acculturation related stressors and mental health symptoms and syndromes including depression, anxiety, and suicidal ideation (Gallagher-Thompson et al., 1997; Hovey, 2000; Hovey & King, 1996; Hovey & Magaña, 2000; Organista, Organista, & Kurasaki, 2003; Torres & Rollock, 2004), yet many factors mitigate the degree of stress experienced. Some of these factors relate to environmental stressors faced by the immigrant population, such as the relocation itself and loss of family support (Hovey & Magaña, 2002; Kiefer et al., 1985), while others involve personal characteristics or capacities of the individual, such as previously acquired skills or education.

For many immigrant groups, the level of education appears to facilitate adaptation to a new culture, (e.g., Kiefer et al., 1985), and appears to be a salient variable in the prediction of depression (Gallagher-Thompson et al., 1997) and resistance to cultural change (Ghaffarian, 1998). Thus, a focus on educational level may be useful in terms of protective factors. English language skills are also viewed as a particularly strong contributor to adaptation in the USA, (Ajrouch & Jamal, 2007; Bhattacharya & Schoppelrey, 2004; Mills & Henretta, 2001) and a lack of such skills may also be a factor contributing to mental health symptoms in various immigrant populations (Choi, 2001; Hovey & Magaña, 2002).

Poor English skills, as well as perceived stress related to these skills, have been predictive of depression in Arab Americans (Wrobel et al., 2009). Ajrouch (2007) has suggested that language acquisition is of particular concern for Arab Americans, as failure to learn English may contribute to greater exposure to hostility from many individuals in the dominant culture. There are also practical difficulties that create stress in those who are primarily fluent in Arabic. The fact that the alphabet itself is so distinct from the English alphabet makes relatively simple adaptations, like reading traffic signs or passing a citizenship test, more difficult than it may be for immigrants of Western origin. With regard to prevention of depression, it should also be noted that maintaining fluency in Arabic, while gaining sufficient skills in English, may facilitate bicultural adaptation, which has been associated with more positive adaptation in other groups (Berry, 1990). This may be increasingly important for immigrants who came during the more recent waves, who are more likely to value their Arab identity. Thus, for Arab Americans, pressure to attain English skills while maintaining their language of origin may exist.

Female gender may be viewed as a risk factor for mental health disorders, such as depression and PTSD, among Arab Americans. For females, post-migration stressors may increase risk for these disorders, even among women with significant pre-migration stressors, including persecution and torture (Norris, Aroian, & Nickerson, 2011). The influence of gender on the acculturation process and related post-immigration stressors is complex and varies in part due to variation in gender role ideologies across cultures. Females, however, have been reported by a number of researchers to have greater difficulty in adapting to the new culture (e.g., Hurh & Kim, 1990; Kiefer, 1985), because they either have fewer opportunities to acculturate when remaining in the home, or they experience increased demands of employment coupled with a traditional division of labor, which results in a heavy workload overall (Estiritu, 1999). Amer and Hovey (2007) note that Arab American women may be uniquely "at-risk" for mental health and physical problems as they are impacted by pressure to deal with Western cultural behaviors and influences on their children while at the same time experiencing their own social discomfort. Muslim women also appear to be readily targeted in terms of discriminatory acts (Hassouneh & Kulwicki, 2007) and may be somewhat more identifiable as a target than Muslim men due to distinctions in dress, such as the wearing of a hijab.

Immigration Status and Origin

In addressing the varying experiences of immigrants in the USA, it is important to note the immigration status and specifically whether the relocation itself was voluntary (Berry, 1990). As noted above, many of the early Arab American immigrants were personally motivated to come to the USA for economic or educational improvement. In recent waves of immigration, there is an increase in the number of immigrants of refugee status, who may perceive themselves as having less choice in the decision to leave their country of origin (Hovey, 2000; Hovey & Magaña, 2000). This includes a large influx of immigrants from Iraq who arrived following the Gulf War in Iraq as well as the invasion of Iraq by the USA following the 9/11 terrorist attacks. As a result of changes in immigration policy, over 32,000 Iraqi immigrants entered the USA in 2008–2009 alone (Schopmeyer, 2011). Immigrants with a less certain status and a history of mistreatment, such as these Iraqi refugees, may perceive themselves as threatened or treated unfairly by those in the mainstream group, and thus may feel less inclined to identify with that group (Ajrouch & Jamal, 2007).

Also of importance in terms of acculturative stress is the fact that recent Arab immigrants vary in country of origin. The country of origin has a major impact on assimilation, and even has an impact on their perception of racial identity. Immigrants from countries such as Lebanon and Syria, for example, are more likely to identify with a white, nonminority, and thus be more likely to assimilate (Ajrouch & Jamal, 2007). In contrast, Iraqi immigrants in one study reported higher levels of pressure to acculturate and learn the language of the host country relative to those from Lebanon or Palestine (Wrobel et al., 2009).

Arab Cultural Influences

Arab cultural values have important implications for the emergence of depression and anxiety disorders such as PTSD. These values must be considered within the context of the dominant culture in North America. Taken as such, they may provide opportunities for increased risk, or greater resilience in high-risk populations.

Social and Religious Influences

Collectivism

Individuals of Arab descent typically have a collectivistic cultural view that emphasizes cooperation and interdependence in which their identities are strongly linked to group goals and group identities (Triandis, 2001). Relationships are often prioritized over other functions, regardless of time and context (Abi-Hashem, 2008). Identifying with one's family and cultural community can be particularly gratifying and an important source of resilience as this environment can meet several psychological needs, including warmth, connectivity, belongingness, and meaning (Abi-Hashem, 2008). However, the circumstances and time of relocation may impact the availability of this support (Wrobel et al., 2009). For example, a person immigrating to the USA with a refugee status may have lost family members in their home country or may have relocated alone. The presence of family or community support may therefore strongly impact the course or presence of mental illness.

Religion

Religion is often integral to Arab life and provides a community through which needs for belonging, worship, celebration, and hope are met (Abi-Hashem, 2008). Especially in later life, religious affiliation can be an important source of resilience as it has been associated with less depression and higher well-being (Hoyer & Roodin, 2009; Levin, 2006). Having strong religious associations may provide someone with additional coping strategies when dealing with death or loneliness (Hoyer & Roodin, 2009). Across cultural groups, either a high degree of religious beliefs or no religious beliefs has been associated with greatest psychological well-being (Krause, 1995; Krause, Ingersoll-Dayton, Ellison, & Wulff, 1999). This relation, however, is complicated among Arab people because a high degree of religious association may also be a source of risk, given religion-based discrimination. In particular, Muslims are at greater risk to experience discrimination compared to Christians (Awad, 2010), especially Muslim females, as they are more likely to be a visible minority when they wear traditional clothing in the Western cultural context.

Among the key values in Arabic culture is the avoidance of public shame (e.g., Dwairy, 2009). This cultural stance has implications for several areas of functioning, including help-seeking behaviors. Asking for help from a mental health professional may be viewed as reflecting negatively upon the family (Al-Krenawi & Graham, 2000; Dwairy & Van Sickle, 1996), possibly, in part, because of the stigma associated with mental illness. Although knowledge of mental illness varies across countries and across families of varying levels of acculturation, some only include the more severe mental disorders such as schizophrenia in their understanding of psychology and the need for treatment (Hamdi, Amin, & Abou-Saleh, 1997; Soueif & Ahmed,

2001). Typically, assistance is sought from family members, from religious leaders in the community, or from physicians (Hakim-Larson & Nassar-McMillan, 2007), instead of from professionals in the mental health field.

Psychological Theory

Several early Arab philosophers provide a framework through which developmental psychopathology issues should be considered. First, Al-Farabi (AD 870–950) an Islamic philosopher and writer of *Citizens of a Noble City*, examined social psychological concepts that can be likened to the worldview of people of Arab descent and particularly Arab Muslims. Al-Farabi examined innate factors necessary for cohesion of large groups. These factors include similarities between physical characteristics, language, speech, and area of residence (Al-Farabi, 1948, as cited in Soueif & Ahmed, 2001). Arab Americans often meet these psychological needs by embracing a collectivistic orientation and joining with others of their country of origin. Researchers examining developmental psychopathological factors among Arab Americans have often combined data from several different Arab groups. This is controversial because, as mentioned previously, the Arab population in the USA is extremely diverse in terms of country of origin, race, and religion. However, cohesion among all Arabs exists because of the strong emphasis on language, as well as shared political perspectives or experiences. Al-Farabi also argues that in smaller groups, integration occurs by frequently being in contact, sharing meals and drinks, understanding a shared experience of conflict and world events, sharing in pleasure, and collectively confronting threats (Al-Farabi, 1948, as cited in Soueif & Ahmed, 2001). These values continue to be shared by many Arab Americans and the development and treatment of psychopathology should be considered in light of these factors.

In contrast, Western psychological theory is strongly rooted in individual processes that form personality and predict adaptive and maladaptive cognitions, emotions, and behaviors (Dwairy, 2002). For example, Dwairy (2002) argues that many of the psychological theories that lay the foundation of therapy in Western cultures are rooted in the process of individuation. That is a process that requires individuals to separate themselves from their family and others in an attempt to develop their own sense of self and identity. A behaviorist approach appears to be one of the few theoretical orientations that prioritizes external factors in explaining cognitions, emotions, and behaviors. However, individuals from traditional cultures must rely on family and close community members for support (Dwairy, 2002). This collective approach informs a very different conceptualization of personality and behavior. Arab scholars have historically drawn on collective values to inform personality and behaviors. For example, some argue that Al-Ghazzali (AD 1058–1111) was a pioneer of behaviorism (Farag, 2000). Using metaphors, he illustrated how nature and nurture affect personality. Also, Ibn-Sina (or Avicenna, AD 980–1037) examined the mutual relationship between the mind and body, and highlighted the importance of upbringing and childhood experiences in shaping personality development (Farag, 2000). Dwairy (2002) writes about the social factors that are integral to the development of personality and maladaptive functioning in his psychosocial dynamic personality theory. These different cultural emphases regarding the development of psychopathology will help guide diagnosis and treatment among Arab Americans.

Mental Health Risks and Disorders in Arab American Immigrants and Refugees

General Issues of Adulthood

In many ways, mental health symptoms and disorders among Arab Americans are similar to those identified in other developing or developed countries, with a high degree of anxiety and mood disorders, as well as disorders reflecting significant trauma, such as PTSD, paranoid and dissociative disorders (Abi-Hashem, 2008). A potentially high incidence of anxiety, depression, and PTSD can be attributed to the acculturative stress, prior trauma, as well as loss of family support and limited access to resources (Laffrey, Meleis, Lipson, Soomon, & Omidian, 1989). Arab American mental health profiles may also parallel other minority group patterns, as they may experience similar stressors related to discrimination. Jackson's model (Jackson, Williams, & Torres, 2003) suggests that chronic discrimination, which results in the anticipation of unpredictable threatening events, eventually leads to increased physiological responsiveness. This ultimately increases not only anxiety and depression, but also potentially increases anger, suspicion, and vigilance. Consistent with this model, for example, is the long-standing finding that ethnic minority group members, such as African Americans, tend to manifest sub-clinical levels of paranoia on measures of personality, such as the MMPI.

Quantifying the degree to which such disorders occur in Arab American samples is complicated by cultural factors, such as avoidance of shame, which may it turn contribute to stigma in reporting mental health concerns. The avoidance is not just of personal shame, but also of bringing shame to one's family or group, who would be expected to care for them if there is a need. The avoidance of shame and stigma, as well as strong cultural biases towards caring for and mentoring one's own may make it difficult to capture a clear sense of the number of individuals who might present with psychiatric symptoms, but do not seek mental health treatment and thus avoid diagnosis. Shame and a sense of stigma have been viewed as barriers to utilization of mental health services by other collectivist groups, such as Asian Americans (Leong & Lau, 2001).

In addition, the presentation of certain disorders may vary in Arab American samples. Depression, for example, is typically associated with increases in anxiety and somatic complaints but decreases in feelings of guilt, which is contrary to symptoms typically seen in North American populations (Erickson & Al-Timimi, 2001; Hamdi et al., 1997; Sayed, 2003). With the exception of expressions of anger in men, emotional expression is typically avoided (Al-Krenawi & Graham, 2000). Instead, symptoms may be presented as more socially acceptable bodily complaints (Nassar-McMillan & Hakim-Larson, 2003), and therefore it may not be evident that their symptomatology is consistent with depression or PTSD. Furthermore, Abi-Hashem (2008) stresses that the nature of religiosity among Arab Americans may contribute to a more spiritualized interpretation of their circumstances, with possible amplification of the "religious-existential components" of any difficulties. Interpreting symptomatology within the context of religion could therefore be highly informative.

A recent study of Iraqi immigrants provides an understanding of the varying levels of mental health disorders in Arab Americans who entered the USA over several decades (Jamil, Nassar-McMillan, & Lambert, 2007). This study is particularly important as it contrasts immigrants who arrived under differing circumstances, including refugees. Iraqi immigrants represent a large proportion of immigrants from the Middle East over the last 2 decades. The investigators sought a range of participants from the Arab American community through cultural and religious organizations as well as through the local media. The resulting group was evenly divided by gender and participants were classified in terms of arrival prior to 1980, between 1980 and 1990, and a post-Gulf War group who came after 1990. These groups are distinct. The earlier immigrants came for more economic reasons, and those immigrating during the Gulf War sought and experienced relief from conditions in their countries of origins. The post war immigrants experienced the highest levels of trauma, not only in Iraq, but subsequently in refugee camps and upon arrival to the USA.

In this study (Jamil, Nassar-McMillan, et al., 2007), the participants were interviewed extensively regarding their war-related experiences and were verbally administered a series of diagnostic questionnaires to assess symptoms of PTSD, depression, panic, and anxiety. The findings of this comparison clearly reflect the relations between the varying experiences of the groups, pre- and post-immigration, and resulting psychological symptoms and disorders. Consistently, the more recent immigrants, who experienced the most trauma, had the highest levels of mental health symptoms. Approximately 12 % met diagnostic criteria for PTSD, 24 % met criteria for an anxiety disorder, and 65 % met criteria for a depressive disorder, with 2/3 of those depressed individuals classified as having major depression. All groups had some self-reported cases of panic and the post-war immigrants experienced panic at a rate of 32 %. The authors caution that there is significant variation within the post-war group, suggesting that even within the most traumatized group, some individuals emerge with relatively sound mental health. Of interest here is the finding that the group who left the Middle East during the Gulf War only differed from those entering earlier in frequency of depression. This group may have adapted culturally over their years in the USA and thus appear fairly low in stress, but there may be some residual disappointment or loss of esteem as they may not have been able to attain the same professional status they may have held in their country of origin.

Further investigation specifically focusing on refugees was conducted on a sample of refugees who had presented at an Arab focused community mental health center in a community with a notably dense population of Arab Americans (Jamil, Farrag, et al., 2007). The sample included adult Iraqi immigrants, predominantly between 30 and 50 years of age, who were either seeking or receiving treatment at the center. Consistent with the finding in the community based sample (Jamil, Nassar-McMillan, et al., 2007), Iraqi refugees presenting for treatment had high levels of self-reported symptoms of anxiety, with over 80 % describing their recent symptom level as intense. Women were more likely to receive a diagnosis of depression, but both men and women self-reported symptoms of depression on the average, as occurring "quite a bit" or "extremely." It should be noted that these individuals are in an age group in which they would typically be heavily engaged in the tasks of early adulthood, such as fulfilling occupational, household, and child-rearing responsibilities. When questioned regarding whether their symptoms had an impact on eight major areas of their daily life, including work, household, family relationships, and leisure, 2/3 of the participants indicated that symptoms had affected all areas. The degree of reported psychological distress is not surprising, as over 90 % of all men and women had experienced wartime trauma, with most men and 1/3 of the women having been victims of imprisonment or torture.

Within the Arab American refugee community, the unique psychological impact of torture has been examined by Kira and his associates (2006). In their interpretation of findings from two community studies, these authors provide us with both a model of mental health risk, but also a view of resilience in the face of seemingly unspeakable trauma. Here and in other writings, Kira and his associates stress the notion of these experiences as involving cumulative trauma disorders, with either an acute response in which the most recent trauma triggers a more severe response to a series of events, or the development or exacerbation of more chronic symptoms. They predicted that survivors of torture would differ from other refugees in a number of ways, including: higher exposure to trauma, greater psychological and medical symptoms, and greater susceptibility to trauma related to recent backlash against Arab immigrants. They also predicted lower sociocultural adjustment and growth, less posttraumatic growth and optimism, and a decreased likelihood of forgiveness. Their findings met some of the first set of hypotheses, but were surprising with regard to others. Those who had experienced torture did, in fact report higher levels of trauma and higher levels of health related symptoms, and they were susceptible to greater exposure and reaction to backlash following the September 11 attacks, but cumulative trauma dose rather than torture itself predicted response to PTSD and cumulative trauma measures. *Cumulative trauma dose* in this case was defined as the number of types of trauma the person had experienced. Contrary to predictions, torture victims actually seemed to fair somewhat better than others in terms of posttraumatic growth and sociocultural adjustment. These authors note that such resilience may be a result of the torture actually strengthening a collective religious or political identity, and thus suggest that these elements be a focus of intervention for torture victims.

Racism, Discrimination, and Mental Health Symptoms

Discrimination has been linked to greater levels of psychological distress in Arab Americans (Moradi & Hasan, 2004), perhaps even among those who had successfully navigated the stressors of immigration. For Arab Americans, discrimination has been viewed as being related to the level of acculturation and adaptation processes, with some choosing to totally assimilate while denying their heritage, and others choosing to remain insulated within the Arab American cultural community (Abu-Baker, 2006). Conflicting thoughts about how to react to these events may in itself be a psychological stressor, with some feeling a great pressure towards acculturation, others feeling pressured not to acculturate, and some actually feeling both.

The potential impact of discrimination has been examined extensively in other minority populations, and self reported racism appears to have a major impact on negative mental health outcomes (Paradies, 2006). In the examination of racism and its relation to health and mental health, Paradies notes more recent exposure to racism seems generally to predict a more negative outcome. While racism is likely stressful, the impact of this stress on health and mental health over time may be modified by psychosocial factors, such as racial/ethnic identity, and the mode of coping (Noh & Kaspar, 2003). For example, religious or other cultural practices appear to attenuate the relationship between self-reported racism and depression in groups such as Native Americans (Whitbeck, McMorris, Hoyt, Stubben, & LaFromboise, 2002).

The events occurring on September 11, 2001 and the reactions of Americans to those events created a circumstance that had a notable impact on the Arab American community, and studies following these events yield some powerful information about the impact of discrimination. As noted, an increased incidence of discrimination following the 9/11 attacks has been documented (Ibish, 2003). Padela and Heisler (2010) examined psychological distress, health status, and happiness in relation to perceived abuse and discrimination in a sample of Arab Americans in the Dearborn, Michigan community about 2 years following the attacks. Of those surveyed, approximately one-fourth reported that either they or immediate household members had experienced abuse related to race or ethnicity during the post-September 11 time period, and the occurrence was slightly higher for Muslims than Christians. Reported abuse and discrimination predicted lower levels of happiness, decreased health status, and higher levels of psychological distress, as measured by a general screening instrument. While those who identified as Muslim had a greater exposure to discrimination, the impact of discrimination on mental and physical health was similar across religious groups.

In addition to acts of overt and covert discrimination, Arab American Muslims have been subject to an extremely high level of hate crimes, such as mosque burnings or bomb threats, creating an environment with a notable degree of stress that may exacerbate prior trauma and impact group identity. Rippy and Newman (2006) note that prior research with minority groups indicates that one's personal perception of whether a particular act is discriminatory is impacted by personal characteristics, such as strong group identification and being highly identifiable as part of an ethnic group, thus making them easily targeted. They specifically examined Muslims who varied in immigration history (immigrants, second generation, and Muslim converts) and ethnic origin (Arab, Southeast Asian, African American, or White American Muslims), in order to evaluate levels of perceived religious discrimination, and their relation to state and trait anxiety as well as paranoia. Of interest was the finding that the perception of increased discrimination against Arabs as a group was greater than perceptions of increased personal discrimination. Arab Muslims were unique in that they had a stronger bicultural identification than non-Arab Muslim groups, which may have contributed to ethnic differences in perceived societal discrimination. Although state and trait anxiety were not related to perceived discrimination in this study, exposure to perceived discrimination was predictive of increased suspicion, vigilance and mistrust among Muslim American males. They concluded that such mistrust may lead to social isolation, which in turn fosters further potential paranoia.

Within these studies, it is evident that chronic exposure to perceived hostile environments are present for Arab Americans, yet the response to these stressors and related mental health outcomes varies. Of interest here are those factors which may mediate response. Liebkind and Jasinskaja-Lahti (2000) found a clear link between discrimination and psychological distress in Arabs living in Finland, but noted that for some ethnic groups who were very likely to be targets of discrimination, the degree of that relationship was weaker. They attribute this finding to the possible tendency to develop external attributions for negative events, thus protecting self-esteem (Crocker & Major, 1989, cited in Liebkind & Jasinskaja-Lahti, 2000).

The role of personal control in mediating the impact of discrimination on mental health has been examined specifically in Arab Americans by Moradi and Hasan (2004). Their findings were consistent with the Finland study, in that there was a direct link between perceived discrimination and distress. Further analysis of the mediating variables in the Moradi and Hasan study, however, suggested that perceived discrimination was related to lower perception of perceived control over life events. Additionally, low perceived control was related to lower self esteem as well as to increased psychological distress. Perceived control, as fostered by sociopolitical involvement, has been examined in other minority groups as a protective factor which may enhance resilience (Zimmerman, Ramírez-Valles, & Maton, 1999).

Variations Across Ages and Stages: Risks Impacting Younger and Elderly Arab Americans

It is well established in developmental theory that the mastery of certain tasks has salience for individuals at various points in the life span. The skills gained are then utilized as they navigate life challenges (Burt & Masten, 2010). The particular stages and developmental tasks prominent for an individual at certain points in history may impact the degree and nature of exposure to potentially stressful events as well as the manner in which those stressful experiences impact further development. Completion of developmental tasks, such as identity formation, are of particular concern as Arab Americans navigate a complex bicultural environment. Even simple factors, like the age at which immigration occurs, may impact the potential for psychological distress and the development of symptoms or disorders.

Children and Adolescents: Parenting and Mental Health

There is little published research that specifically applies to the development of young Arab American children. As the major tasks of early development are based in attachment (Sroufe, 1979), we may presume that children are particularly impacted by the psychological status of their parents as well as parenting practices defined by the culture. These, in turn, may be impacted by stressors encountered by the parent. For example, refugees experiencing high levels of stress are reported to have difficulty navigating basic daily activities, and women in particular have high levels of depression (Jamil, Farrag, et al., 2007), both of which may impact their ability to serve optimally in their role as parents of young children.

There are defined cultural practices common among Arab Americans, often based on Arab traditions, which play a role in parenting For example, the collectivistic emphasis places family needs above those of the individual (Hakim-Larson & Nassar-McMillan, 2007). Psychological lore involving Baumrind's typology (1987) in the USA strongly favors an authoritative style of parenting in terms of mental health outcomes and well-being, and discourages either permissive or authoritarian parenting styles, yet this belief may not generalize to a more authoritarian/collective cultural context (Dwairy, Achoui, Abouserie, & Farah, 2006). Dwairy and associates examined the relation between parenting style and consistency on mental health outcomes and connectedness in over 2,800 Arab adolescents across eight societies. They concluded that while authoritative parenting is related to higher connectedness and better mental health, an authoritarian style did not have the same harmful impact on mental health that is observed in Western societies. An inconsistent mode of parenting emerged in factor analysis, and this pattern was actually the most detrimental to connectedness and mental health. It is suggested that mental health and school personnel should foster consistency rather than discouraging or stigmatizing authoritarian parenting styles within groups favoring a collectivistic cultural style. The notion that a stricter style may actually be preferred in fostering competence when the environment is perceived as dangerous (Masten & Coatsworth, 1995), may also support these practices among Arab American families who recognize potential threat due to discrimination.

The degree and nature of acculturation of the parents also may play a role in the child's mental health and development. The impact of bicultural upbringing on Arab American children appears to have some positive aspects in terms of development of self-concept for some. A comparison of college students in Egypt with students raised in traditional Arab American families in a community densely populated by Arabs in the USA (Soliman & McAndrew, 1998) had revealed that reported self-concept in the Arab Americans was higher than those raised in a more monocultural environment in Egypt. Alkhateeb (2010) extended a similar comparison to preadolescent children, ranging in age from 11 to 13. In this case, the Arab Americans were raised in an area which was less densely populated with other Arabs, and they received both full-time public school education and attended a private Arabic/Islam Sunday school; they were compared with Arab national students in Lebanon. Parents of the Arab American students were typical of "third wave" immigrants as most had immigrated after 1970, and tended to be well educated with a strong Arab identity. Results of this comparison suggest that across multiple areas, including physical appearance and ability, general school, and peer relations, the Arab American students reported higher self-concept. The author concludes that the children appear to gain competence across two cultures without a loss of identification with their Arab background.

Young Adults: The Formation of Identity

Formation of a cohesive identity is accepted as a fairly universal task of development in adolescence and early adulthood (Masten & Coatsworth, 1995), yet variations in identity formation appear to occur across cultural contexts (Portes, Dunham, & Castillo, 2000). Thus, development of cultural identity is of importance in the determination of well-being in this age group. Youth of Arab descent may find this process particularly difficult because of their minority status in North America. In addition to their general identity development, they must actualize an ethnic identity, a construct that captures an individual's feelings of ethnic belonging and pride that is conducive to their overall well-being (Phinney, 2003). Youth of Arab descent may have more difficulty integrating both their private and public worlds given the opposing worldviews (Abi-Hashem, 2006; Abu-Laban & Abu-Laban, 1999). Whereas Americans value independence, personal freedom, personal achievement based goals, and independent critical thought, people of Arab descent typically value communal achievements, parental involvement in decision-making, and respect for authority (Amer, 2002; Haboush, 2007). In fact, in a Muslim sample, Al-Issa (2000) found that Western ideals are sometimes viewed as selfish and irresponsible in collectivistic families. Abi-Hashem (2008) further argued that separation and individuation may lead to the risk of fragmentation, isolation, and loneliness.

For some, late adolescence is a significant transitional period as enrollment in college may provide much greater exposure to the dominant culture (Asvat & Malcarne, 2008). At this time, experiences related to acculturation and discrimination may contribute to discrepancies in aspects of identity, which in turn may contribute to symptoms of depression. Patterns identified in a general study of international students (Jung, Hecht, & Wadsworth, 2007) may generalize to young Arab American immigrants as well. Among these students, gaps were sometimes evident between three different levels of identity, including: their personal self-concept of identity; their relational identity, involving their perception of how others see them; and their enacted identity, involving how they communicate with others in the host culture. The impact of gaps in identity, along with the mediating roles of acculturation levels, social support, social undermining, and perceived discrimination were examined. Both discrimination and personal-enacted identity gaps had strong direct effects on level of depression. Additionally, they found that a higher level of acculturation predicted a decreased gap in identity, particularly the discrepancy between personal and relational identity. In contrast, perceived discrimination predicted greater gaps, with greatest impact on the personal/enacted gap. A personal-enacted identity gap also mediated the impact of acculturation and discrimination on depression. The role of both social support and social undermining in this process were also examined. Social undermining is viewed as perceived criticism or hindrance in attaining one's goals, while social support refers to the availability of support from those in the environment. Social undermining by family or acquaintances appeared to exacerbate the impact of discrimination on depression, but social support had no mediating effect.

Of interest in this study of international students (Jung et al., 2007) is that acculturation had no direct impact on depression. The authors suggest that a "sojourner" status may lessen these effects, as the individual may purposely limit contact to members of their home culture, with the idea that they are ultimately returning home. This pattern may be different for young immigrants or second generation Arab Americans, who do not have a "sojourner" status. Asvat and Malcarne (2008) shed some light on how this process may differ, particularly for Muslim students, whose culture of heritage differs significantly from the mainstream culture. They examined both the impact of personal acculturation levels on depression and the impact of discrepancies between the students' level of acculturation and their family level of acculturation. In this case, a strong personal identification with their heritage culture was associated with lower levels of lifetime depression, but had no impact on levels of depression reported in the last year. In contrast, strong identification with the mainstream culture actually contributed to depressive symptoms over the past year, possibly due to a greater exposure to or vulnerability to negative events as they entered college, but did not have an impact on lifetime depression. Generally, there appeared to be a discrepancy in the students' and their families' levels of acculturation, with the students having a more bicultural orientation overall. Students appeared most vulnerable to depression when their identification with the heritage culture was low and their family heritage cultural identification was high, possibly creating tension and a greater sense of acculturative stress.

Although biculturalism has often been favored in terms of predicting mental health outcomes, it is important to recognize that biculturalism is not a universal experience, and may be more accurately viewed as a continuum. For instance, Britto and Amer (2007) found that among Arab Muslim young adults, those who were either highly bicultural or high in Arab cultural identity reported a greater level of family support, and a lower degree of acculturative stress in the home than those who were moderately bicultural. Thus, it would appear that development of either a strong Arab cultural identification or a clear bicultural identity may be associated with positive mental health outcomes, and in turn, having a family which is supportive and lacking in acculturative stress may facilitate a strong formation of identity.

Henry, Stiles, Biran, and Hinkle (2008) also examined perceptions of parent acculturation behavior among 18–26 year olds who had either immigrated to the USA, or were born to parents of Arab origin residing in the USA. In their study of factors affecting well-being, they separated parental preservation of the culture of origin and openness and parental exposure to the new culture, and also explored parental control as a mediator between these variables and outcome. There was clearly an interaction between acculturation practices and control, as those whose parents were not open to cultural experiences fared better when parental control was low, and those whose parents favored openness tended not to be affected by the degree of control. In contrast, lower parental control led to a more favorable outcome when parents leaned toward the preservation of their culture of origin. In essence, preservation of the culture appeared more beneficial when there was some autonomy, allowing the emerging adult to engage in American cultural experiences, while still maintaining the support of the Arab cultural group.

Elderly Arab Americans

Published research addressing mental health issues among Arab American elderly populations is very limited. Salari (2002) describes elderly Arab Americans as particularly "invisible" in aging research. While Arab Americans have generally been understudied in general, due to them being classified merely as white, this is particularly true with the elderly because Arab immigrants have been a relatively young group, and thus have not had to deal with a significant number of elderly within their population until somewhat recently (The Zogby Study, 1997). The examination of elderly Arab Americans allows us an opportunity to study the effects of acculturation and related stress over time, particularly among those who have been present in the USA for varied, sometimes long periods of time. Acculturation among the elderly immigrants may be viewed as somewhat unique, as the elderly may have had limited contact with the dominant culture (Gong, Takeuchi, Agbayani-Siewert, & Tacata, 2003).

Prior studies involving other immigrant groups suggest that elderly immigrants are particularly impacted negatively by the experiences of adjusting to a new culture, and those described as "lower" in acculturation have been viewed as more prone to depression (Mills & Henretta, 2001; Zamanian et al., 1992). In theory, resistance to cultural changes may be more prominent in older groups (Ghaffarian, 1998), and existing psychological distress may be compounded by practical problems typically impacting aging ethnic populations, such as access to health care and appropriate housing (Harris, 1998). Additionally, elderly people who have recently immigrated may experience more isolation, limited independence, fear of failure to learn a new language, and demoralization than their younger counterparts (Carlin, 1990).

Ajrouch (2007) has examined the well-being of Arab American elders in the post 9/11 climate relative to available human and social capital. Those born outside the USA appeared to experience greater levels of negative mood, and lower levels of life satisfaction. This distinction between immigrants and non-immigrants seemed to be explained in large part by differences in language skills as well as level of education. When family relationships were explored, social relations with adult children or spouses did not have such a clear impact on the well-being of the immigrants; however it does appear that elderly Arab Americans utilize adult children as a source of support, particularly when they are experiencing a low mood. This is to be expected as the collectivistic approach common in Arab culture includes the practice of caring for the elderly in the family (Hakim-Larson & Nassar-McMillan, 2007). Ajrouch cautions, however, that solely relying on family members may not be optimal, particularly when needs are high.

More recent immigration into the USA as well as less permanent residency status (e.g., refugee or temporary status) has been found to predict greater degrees of acculturative stress and depression in elderly Arab Americans (Wrobel et al., 2009). Those from Iraq were higher in acculturative stress and depression relative to immigrants from Lebanon or Palestine. The measure of acculturative stress used allowed for separate evaluation of different aspects of acculturative stress, and revealed some patterns unique to this group. Compared with other minority immigrant groups, these Arab Americans reported very little pressure against acculturation, and little pressure regarding retaining competence in their native language. In addition, contrary to prior findings, the older the immigrants were, the less pressure they felt regarding English competency.

Although some members of the sample were able to avoid certain aspects of acculturative stress, elderly individuals did experience stress related to acculturation, and the multidimensional approach used here (Wrobel et al., 2009) allowed a clear view of the way in which specific aspects of acculturative stress played a role in contributing to a depressed mood. As predicted, demographic variables, such as lower skills in English, did appear to be related to higher levels of depression; however entering the acculturative stress variables into the equation revealed that the relation between poor English skills and depression was more complex. In essence it was not just the fact that one is lacking in English language fluency, but rather an interaction of poor English competency and the perception that this lack of skill is a stressor that was most predictive of depression. The fact that the individuals studied resided in an area with a dense population of Arabs may create an environment in which some elderly individuals who are not working outside the home are able to maintain their cultural practices and language of origin, and avoid requirements to be fluent in English. Those who reported more stressful experiences related to language skill, and in addition had poorer skills, logically had greater levels of emotional distress. Measurement of such perceived stress in the elderly can facilitate identification of those most at risk for mental health symptoms.

Methods of Assessment of Mental Health Disorders

Given that a large number of Arabs immigrated to North America because of conflicts and war in their home country (Ajrouch, 2000; Erickson & Al-Timimi, 2001), assessing for emotional disorders, such as PTSD and depression, is strongly encouraged, both for purposes of research and treatment. This process, however, may need to differ from typical assessments conducted with North American populations for several reasons. As described above, presentation of symptoms may vary, and thus the primary diagnosis may not be immediately apparent to professionals trained in Western cultural groups.

Assessment tools typically used with North American populations may bias results and must therefore be interpreted with caution. For example, in the assessment of suicide, it is encouraged to ascertain levels of suicidal ideation and guilt by direct means (Al-Krenawi & Graham, 2000; O'Connor, Warby, Raphael, & Vassallo, 2004). However, these thoughts are considered irreverent and may therefore be denied if questioned directly (Ali, Liu, & Humedian, 2004; Al-Krenami & Graham, 2000). A previous study of depression amongst Iraqis indicated that few individuals had thoughts of suicide or had attempted suicide (Bazzoui, 1970). However, approximately 25 % of those who were identified as depressed indicated a desire to escape into the wilderness and run away from home. Therefore, rather than questioning suicidal symptoms directly it may be more useful to use metaphors to ascertain suicidal ideations. The use of metaphors has been strongly encouraged as a core process in therapy (Dwairy, 2009).

Also, the interpretation of assessment tools must be done in light of their limitations. Norms of most assessment tools, regardless of whether or not they have been translated into Arabic, are often based on North American populations (Melikian, 1984; Soueif & Ahmed, 2001). Assessment tools also rely heavily on individuation processes rather than considering collectivist values and norms (Dwairy, 2002). Furthermore, English fluency may also affect the interpretation of projective tests (Haboush, 2007). Since Arabic is a more emotionally expressive language as compared to English, interpretations of the TAT and the Rorschach may depict a more disturbed person (Sayed, 2003). Alternatively, Dwairy (2002) suggests incorporating objects from the home to discuss family relations and dysfunction.

Critique

The goal of this chapter was to address mental health risks for a minority group whose members are likely to have experienced significant psychological stressors at various points in their lives. It is important to note that the body of research is in its infancy in many ways, and current research findings must be applied with some degree of caution. While thoughtful research is emerging, these individuals remain understudied to a large degree. When considering issues, including acculturation and acculturative stress, much of our understanding and application of these concepts is based on extrapolation from existing research on other minority groups, such as Latinos and Asians. Rudmin (2009) has cautioned against viewing acculturative stress globally, as groups may differ in their response to immigration in significant ways. While similarities may exist, there is some evidence that the impact of these experiences varies for Arab Americans, relative to the larger minority groups, due to unique aspects of their culture (Wrobel et al., 2009) as well as the current political climate which may harbor a particularly high degree of discrimination and tension. Even within the Arab community, there is variation in response to acculturation, with Christians tending to fare better than Muslim immigrants (Amer & Hovey, 2007). Both researchers and clinicians should also be aware that not all responses to acculturation are negative. Protective aspects of culture may actually foster more positive outcomes among Arabs relative to other groups, and thus we are encouraged to capitalize on these cultural means of healing and resilience (Abi-Hashem, 2008).

While research is emerging, data collection has been problematic for cultural and political reasons. The notions of shame and stigma described above prevent identification of those with mental illness, making it difficult to secure a clinical population to study. Those who do present for treatment or for a research study may either be more distressed, or perhaps have a greater level of sophistication about mental health issues. Additionally, those who are less influenced by the notion of shame may be more acculturated, and thus not at such a great risk as others. This makes a true representative sample difficult to acquire. In the post 9/11 climate disclosing personal data may be perceived as an even greater potential risk, and certainly those who have experienced oppressive regimes may also be hesitant to disclose information to those who appear to be in authority. It is notable that a large number of the studies reviewed involved populations from a region that is very densely populated with Arab Americans, such as Southeastern Michigan. Results of studies of such phenomena as discrimination and acculturative stress may be somewhat different for those living in a community where they may be able to remain somewhat insulated within their culture of origin, maintaining their language and customs. Studies using the internet to secure participants who are more widespread geographically are promising, but run the risk of being biased towards the more affluent or educated (Kraut et al., 2004). Studies of some Arab American groups, such as young Arab Americans, may be enhanced by research directions involving iPhone applications. Further studies of both elderly and young Arab Americans will foster our awareness of the changing needs of Arab Americans across the lifespan. Despite these limitations, the emerging base of information serves to foster a greater understanding of this ethnic minority group.

Implications for Research, Treatment, and Policy

Personal Growth of Practitioners

The increase in racism experienced by Arab Americans post 9/11 has been paralleled by an increase in prejudicial beliefs held by some members of the majority culture (Rose, 2002). Even individuals with strong multicultural values and people of Arab backgrounds must reflect on their beliefs and attitudes in relation to Arab communities living in the USA and abroad before embarking in a therapeutic relationship with a person of Arab descent because of the powerful influence of social factors that affect our unconscious (Greenwald, McGhee, & Schwartz, 1998). Without this self-examination, a mental health worker runs the risk of inadvertently expressing discriminatory views that will exacerbate symptoms rather than alleviate them, or they may engender a working relationship comparable to the sociopolitical relations between the USA and the Middle East (Roysircar, 2003). This self-reflection should include a self-examination of cultural and religious beliefs and how they are either in line or contrary to the worldview of clients (Hakim-Larson & Nassar-McMillan, 2007). It should also include a reflection on how the client may be interpreting the therapist's gender, race, ethnic background, religion, or culture. Even therapists of Arab descent must remain aware that conflict not only occurs between people of Arab descent and people of European descent, but the Arab world has a deep history of conflict between countries, regions within countries, religions, and Muslim sects (Haboush, 2007). This self-reflection will better prepare a psychologist to know if an open conversation regarding possible cultural barriers is necessary.

Awareness of Cultural Norms and Acculturation

A second necessary step for practitioners working with Arab population is a firm grasp on the culture-specific developmental factors that affect mental illness. It is important to understand, in relation to culture-specific values and beliefs, etiological factors that contribute to risk and resilience and to the manifestation of mental illness. Foremost, it is essential to ascertain levels of acculturation within the family. Although children may grow up in North America, which facilitates acculturation, parents may have spent the majority of their lives in their home country. Assessing level of acculturation across family members will provide a framework under which the level Arab and North American values can be interpreted. Similarly, Dwairy (2002) suggests assessing levels of individuation to determine the proportion of their personality that is formed from social norms, values, and expectations, and from private factors that are typically hidden from the social world. When experiencing mental health symptoms, Arabs may seek guidance from their physicians, family, or religious leaders, as these help-seeking strategies underlie core values upheld by Arabs, including the importance of family and community, the desire to save-face and avoid shaming the family, and the essence of religion as a way of life central to their identity. Understanding these and other values will help mental health workers recognize risk and resilience within the context of a client's developmental history that impact assessment and treatment.

Impact of Shame on Mental Health Related Behaviors

The notion of public shame and its avoidance has implications for several areas of functioning, including help-seeking behaviors, child behavior management, and disclosures of abuse. Communicating with family, physicians, and religious leaders are more acceptable as approaches to seeking help because they reduce the amount of shame a family will endure. Seeking help for children with developmental or learning disabilities may also draw negative attention to the family (Duvdevany & Abboud, 2003). Some parents may be unwilling to label their child with special needs and will, in turn, prevent them from integrating into the school setting (Haboush, 2007). This is complicated by the increased risk among some Arab families of having a child with a developmental disability or genetic disorder because of the encouraged practice of marrying cousins (Giger & Davidhizar, 2002; Haboush, 2007; Kulczycki & Lobo, 2002). Encouraging parents to seek the necessary help is in the best interest of the child in order to facilitate learning. Public policy should therefore encourage community outreach programming.

Behavioral approaches to treatment with children must be considered within the context of the shame-based culture. Specifically, parents often use shame instead of positive reinforcement to control child behaviors. As indicated above, an authoritarian parenting style has not been associated with greater distress among the children as it has among North American children; instead the consistency of parenting predicts outcomes (Dwairy et al., 2006). Furthermore, Baumrind (1987) has discussed the limitation of the application of her parenting styles with traditional cultures. That is, she and other scholars (e.g., Arnett, 2010), have indicated that many parents of traditional cultures adaptively raise their children with a high degree of demandingness and responsiveness. Parenting programs such as Triple P-Positive Parenting Program typically emphasize positive reinforcement as the preferred means to teach children appropriate behavior (Sanders, Markie-Dadds, & Turner, 2003). This specific approach has several aspects that appear to be adaptive across cultures, but also has a number of approaches that may be inconsistent with Arab culture values. For example, it encourages parental communication and collaborative teamwork. This approach may increase parental discord rather than reduce it by bringing to conscious reflection shameful repressed thoughts. Instead, using metaphorical approaches to understanding parental conflict will allow parents to process their difficulties without shame (Dwairy, 2009). In addition, Triple P does not consider the effectiveness of maintaining a strict home environment that is effective in collectivistic families. Therapists working with Arab families should therefore consider how shame and control could be adaptive within the Arab culture and integrate shame-based discipline methods. Without this, parents of Arab descent may not feel heard and understood, and in turn may not continue in treatment. Haboush (2007) suggested joining with the family first by encouraging the shame-based methods of behavioral control and then incorporating other methods such as positive reinforcement. Dwairy (2009) encourages therapists to conduct a culture analysis. This entails bringing to light conflicting cultural values that lead to maladaptive outcomes.

Disclosures of abuse must be treated with increased care since such disclosures may cause the family to disown the abused victim and in turn re-traumatize him or her (Abu-Baker & Dwairy, 2003). Abu-Baker and Dwairy (2003) suggest a culturally sensitive model that includes six stages: (1) verifying the presence of abuse, (2) mapping nuclear and extended family members as well as the hierarchical structure of the family to identify possible advocates for the youth, (3) meeting with various members of the community (e.g., teacher, social worker), trusted religious leaders identified by the family or youth, and the child advocate within the family to strengthen relationships between all those who have the child's interest at heart, (4) conducting a ceremony that includes condemnation of the behavior, an apology from the abuser, discussion of an appropriate punishment for the abuser, and the recognition of the courage of the extended family, (5) therapy that includes individual treatment for the abuser and the victim as well as family and couple's interventions, and (6) follow-up.

Notions of Authority

Throughout the lifespan it is important to consider that Arab populations express their respect for authority by avoiding disagreements. As such, obtaining appropriate informed consent for treatment and research may be difficult. Mental health professionals are viewed as figures of authority and may therefore not be questioned by clients. This is further complicated if working with children because the therapist is not only an authority by title, but an elder, who is respected. Therefore, it is important to obtain informed consent from adults and assent from children with care. This value also has implications for the therapeutic process. Because confrontation is avoided, clients may appear passive and avoid confrontation (Roysircar, 2003). Using a more active approach to therapy may be necessary (Abudabbeh & Aseel, 1999; Al-Krenawi & Graham, 2000).

Approaches to Therapy

Several approaches have been encouraged with Arab Americans to facilitate the therapeutic process. Foremost, fostering a strong working relationship with the client is paramount to therapeutic success (Abi-Hashem, 2008; Hakim-Larson & Nassar-McMillan, 2007). To facilitate this process, it is important to gain knowledge regarding the worldview of a typical person of Arab descent and ascertain the client's level of acculturation and individuation (Dwairy, 2002). Overall, scholars have discouraged psychodynamic and humanistic approaches to therapy as they are ambiguous and inconsistent with a collectivistic cultural perspective, and therefore may increase the anxiety experienced by the client (e.g., Dwairy, 2009). Instead, directive approaches, such as behavioral and cognitive interventions are more culturally sensitive and consistent with Arab values (Dwairy, 2009). Specifically, several therapeutic interventions are argued to be most effective with individuals of Arab descent: (1) use of metaphors, (2) content analysis, and (3) imparting a multi-systemic approach (Dwairy, 2009; Nassar-McMillan & Hakim-Larson, 2003).

People of Arab descent often use metaphors to describe emotions and experiences. Staying attuned to these metaphors during sessions and incorporating metaphors when discussing emotionally laden topics may be most effective. This method may be particularly useful because metaphors allow clients to process and confront unconscious and repressed thoughts that are causing distress without open discussion that may cause more discomfort (Al-Krenawi & Graham, 2000; Dwairy, 2009). Working with metaphors involves three stages. The client must first identify a metaphor that represents the problem, then describe how to change the metaphor, and finally apply this lessons to the actual problem (Dwairy, 2009; Kopp, 1995). Dwairy further suggests conducting a content analysis that could be useful to interpret and resolve conflicting values. That is, interpreting sources of conflict within the cultural values of the client and drawing on specific values that are consistent with the distressing thought may prove useful. In particular, this cultural analysis should consider the collectivistic orientation and religion. For example, a therapist could encourage a controlling husband in a Muslim family to remember the central role of A'isha, the Prophet's wife. In addition to the use of metaphors and conducting a cultural analysis of the presenting problem, imparting a multi-systemic approach to therapy, regardless of the client's age, will encourage clients to reach out to family and friends for support and will address systemic, family difficulties, rather than intrapsychic dysfunction (Nassar-McMillan & Hakim-Larson, 2003). By developing strong working relationships with the various members of this system, the therapist will be more effective at fostering support and resilience for the identified client.

Treatment Issues Across the Lifespan

Arab Americans will face similar and different challenges across the lifespan. For children, it is important to understand the differences between school systems and ways of behavioral management (e.g., Haboush, 2007). For adolescents, it is important to foster a strong identity that includes public and private life spheres (e.g., Abi-Hashem, 2006; Abu-Laban & Abu-Laban, 1999). For young adults and middle aged adults, who may face greater degrees of discrimination as they navigate the world of work, treatment implications include the need for therapists to be realistic with clients about the degree of control they have over discrimination, but at the same time to make them aware of opportunities for activism, or antidiscrimination policies which may provide them with a greater sense of mastery and control. For older adults, helping them navigate the stresses of acculturation by fostering support from family and by drawing on religious affiliations may be beneficial (Hoyer & Roodin, 2009).

Family support and support from the community, as a source of risk or resilience is an integral part of assessment and treatment for all age groups. Due to the cultural importance of family and religious life, these areas require special attention in a clinical interview as well as in intervention. If limited family and community support is available, seeking connections from others should still be encouraged. Arabs value hospitality and having neighbors and friends over to share a feast can have great therapeutic value (Abi-Hashem, 2008). Similarly assessing the importance of religion in the individual's and the individual's family's life will help guide functional therapeutic interventions. If religion is a core aspect of their social identity, then integrating prayer and religious affiliations into therapy can be useful tools to foster resilience. Also, speaking with a religious leader may not only be helpful to the client, but also to the therapist in the vein of gaining knowledge of practices (Dwairy, 2009).

Conclusions

Exploration of mental health risks and protective factors in Arab Americans clearly affords researchers and clinicians an opportunity to view the impact of hardship on mental health outcomes. In this chapter, we also recognized that adaptation may vary depending upon both historical and political events, current stressors, and the point in the lifespan development of the individual as these circumstances occur. Past research on acculturation suggests that the relationship between assimilation and resilience is not a direct or universal one (e.g., Berry & Kim, 1988). For Arab Americans, various personal, cultural, and situational factors mediate the outcome. For example, while separation and marginalization may predict depression in Christian Arabs, integration into the dominant culture may present a greater risk for Muslim Arab immigrants who may experience a more hostile response (Awad, 2010).

Across religious groups, acculturative stress does appear to predict mental health symptoms, including depression and anxiety. Poor language skills and low educational levels contribute to high mental health risk. Gender plays a complex role, yet females appear to be at greater risk due to conflicting cultural expectations (Amer & Hovey, 2007), and higher likelihood of being targeted for discrimination (Hassouneh & Kulwicki, 2007). Factors related to the immigration itself contribute to adjustment outcomes, with refugees, particularly those from Iraq, experiencing significant levels of distress currently. Exposure to war and other trauma prior to immigration has been related to higher levels of depression and PTSD for Iraqis and others (e.g., Jamil, Nassar-McMillan, et al., 2007).

While characteristics and practices unique to the culture may present mental health risk, other cultural elements present a degree of protection. Strong religious affiliation among Arabs is viewed as a source of resilience and decreased depression, particularly in later years, or when dealing with death or loneliness (Hoyer & Roodin, 2009). Similarly, identification with sociopolitical groups may enhance perception of control over discrimination and thus mediate related stress.

Of particular note is the collectivist nature of the culture, with family and community providing support across the lifespan. In contrast, a higher emphasis on avoiding public shame in such cultures results in notable levels of mental health stigma and a reluctance to engage in treatment when significant mental health disorders occur. Possible suppression and somatic presentation of emotion as well as religious interpretation of symptoms require a tailored approach to mental health symptoms in Arab Americans.

As highlighted above, approaches to mental health prevention and intervention may vary in focus depending upon the particular stage and developmental tasks which are prominent for the individual. Children's attachment and socialization are impacted by parental stress as well as cultural practices. Clinicians must be wary of the fact that optimal parenting styles may vary between collectivistic and more Westernized cultural groups (e.g., Dwairy et al., 2006). Formation of identity in adolescents, as well as tendencies for depression, was related to discrepancies between personal and family acculturation. Young adults appear to adapt best when parents allowed some engagement in American culture, while maintaining support of the Arabic cultural group (e.g., Henry et al., 2008). Acculturation risks for the elderly may be less severe as they are not required to venture into the dominant culture, yet perceived pressure regarding English language resulted in greater psychological stress, even among the elderly (Wrobel et al., 2009). Increasing language skills and education, as well as enhancing perceived control through political and cultural engagement may contribute to positive mental health outcomes across all age groups.

References

Abi-Hashem, N. (2006). The agony, silent grief, and deep frustration of many communities in the middle east: Challenges for coping and survival. In P. T. P. Wong & L. C. J. Wong (Eds.), *Handbook of multicultural perspectives on stress and coping* (pp. 457–486). Dallas, TX: Spring Publications. doi:10.1007/0-387-26238-5_20.

Abi-Hashem, N. (2008). Arab Americans: Understanding their challenges, needs, and struggles. In A. J. Marsella, J. L. Johnson, P. Watson, & J. Gryczynski (Eds.), *Ethnocultural perspectives on disaster and trauma: Foundations, issues, and applications* (pp. 115–173). New York: Springer Science+Business Media. doi:10.1007/978-0-387-73285-5_5.

Abu-Baker, K. (2006). Arab/Muslim families in the United States. In M. Dwairy (Ed.), *Counseling and psychotherapy with Arabs and Muslims* (pp. 29–43). New York: Teachers College.

Abu-Baker, K. A., & Dwairy, M. (2003). Cultural norms versus state law in treating incest: A suggested model for Arab families. *Child Abuse & Neglect, 27*, 109–123.

Abudabbeh, N., & Aseel, H. A. (1999). Transcultural counseling and Arab Americans. In J. McFadden (Ed.), *Transcultural counseling* (2nd ed., pp. 283–296). Alexandria, VA: American Counseling Association.

Abu-Laban, S. M., & Abu-Laban, B. (1999). Teens between: The public and private spheres of Arab-Canadian adolescents. In M. W. Suleiman (Ed.), *Arabs in America* (pp. 113–128). Philadelphia, PA: Temple University Press.

Ajrouch, K. J. (2000). Place, age, and culture: Community living and ethnic identity among Lebanese American adolescents. *Small Group Research, 31*(4), 447–469. doi:10.1177/104649640003100404.

Ajrouch, K. J. (2007). Resources and well-being among Arab-American elders. *Journal of Cross-Cultural Gerontology, 22*(2), 167–182. doi:10.1007/s10823-006-9033-z.

Ajrouch, K. J., & Jamal, A. (2007). Assimilating to a white identity: The case of Arab Americans. *International Migration Review, 41*(4), 860–879. doi:10.1111/j.1747-7379.2007.00103.x.

Ali, S. R., Liu, W. M., & Humedian, M. (2004). Islam 101: Understanding the religion and therapy implications. *Professional Psychology: Research and Practice, 35*(6), 635–642. doi:10.1037/0735-7028.35.6.635.

Al-Issa, I. (2000). The mental health of Muslim immigrants in Europe. In I. Al-Issa (Ed.), *Al-junun: Mental illness in the Islamic world* (pp. 253–274). Madison, CT: International Universities Press.

Alkhateeb, H. M. (2010). Self-concept in Lebanese and Arab American pre-adolescents. *Psychological Reports, 106*, 435–447. doi:10.2466/PR0.106.2.435-447.

Al-Krenawi, A., & Graham, J. R. (2000). Culturally sensitive social work practice with Arab clients in mental health settings. *Health & Social Work, 25*(1), 9–22.

Amer, M. (2002). *Evaluation of measures of acculturation and mental health for second generation and early immigrant Arab Americans*. Unpublished master's thesis, University of Toledo, Toledo, OH.

Amer, M. M., & Hovey, J. D. (2007). Socio-demographic differences in acculturation and mental health for a sample of second generation/early immigrant Arab Americans. *Journal of Immigrant and Minority Health, 9*, 335–347. doi:10.1007/s10903-007-9045-y.

Arnett, J. J. (2010). *Adolescence and emerging adulthood: A cultural approach* (4th ed.). Upper Saddle River, NJ: Prentice Hall.

Asvat, Y., & Malcarne, V. L. (2008). Acculturation and depressive symptoms in Muslim university students: Personal-family acculturation match. *International Journal of Psychology, 43*, 114–124. doi:10.1080/00207590601126668.

Awad, G. H. (2010). The impact of acculturation and religious identification on perceived discrimination for Arab/Middle Eastern Americans. *Cultural Diversity and Ethnic Minority Psychology, 16*, 59–67. doi:10.1037/a0016675.

Baumrind, D. (1987). A developmental perspective on adolescent risk taking in contemporary America. *New Directions for Child Development, 37*, 93–125. doi:10.1002/cd.23219873706.

Bazzoui, W. (1970). Affective disorders in Iraq. *The British Journal of Psychiatry, 117*(537), 195–203.

Berry, J. W. (1990). Acculturation and adaptation: A general framework. In W. H. Holtzman & T. H. Bornemann (Eds.), *Mental health of immigrants and refugees* (pp. 90–102). Austin, TX: Hogg Foundation of Mental Health.

Berry, J. W., & Kim, U. (1988). Acculturation and mental health. In P. Dassan, J. W. Berry, & N. Sartorius (Eds.), *Health and cross-cultural psychology: Towards application* (pp. 207–236). London: Sage.

Berry, J. W., Trimble, J. E., & Olmedo, E. L. (1986). Assessment of acculturation. In J. Lonner & J. W. Berry (Eds.), *Field methods in cross-cultural research* (pp. 291–324). Beverly Hills, CA: Sage.

Bhattacharya, G., & Schoppelrey, S. L. (2004). Preimmigration beliefs of life success, postimmigration experiences, and acculturative stress: South Asian immigrants in the United States. *Journal of Immigrant Health, 6*(2), 83–92. doi:10.1023/B:JOIH.0000019168.75062.36.

Britto, P. R., & Amer, M. M. (2007). An exploration of cultural identity patterns and the family context among Arab Muslim young adults in America. *Applied Developmental Science, 11*(3), 137–150.

Burt, K. B., & Masten, A. (2010). Development in the transition to adulthood; vulnerabilities and opportunities. In J. E. Grant & M. N. Potenza (Eds.), *Young adult mental health* (pp. 5–18). Oxford: Oxford University Press.

Carlin, J. E. (1990). Refugee and immigrant populations at special risk: Women, children, and the elderly. In W. H. Holtzman & T. H. Bornemann (Eds.), *Mental health of immigrants and refugees* (pp. 224–233). Austin, TX: Hogg Foundation of Mental Health.

Choi, N. G. (2001). Diversity within diversity: Research and social work practice issues with Asian American elders. *Journal of Human Behavior in the Social Environment, 3*(3–4), 301–319. doi:10.1300/J137v03n03_18.
Cicchetti, D., & Toth, S. L. (2009). The past achievements and future promises of developmental psychopathology: The coming of age of a discipline. *Journal of Child Psychology and Psychiatry, 50*(1–2), 16–25. doi:10.1111/j.1469-7610.2008.01979.x.
Coll, C. G., Akerman, A., & Cicchetti, D. (2000). Cultural influences on developmental processes and outcomes: Implications for the study of development and psychopathology. *Development and Psychopathology, 12*(3), 333–356. doi:10.1017/S0954579400003059.
Coll, C. G., Crnic, K., Lamberty, G., & Wasik, B. H. (1996). An integrative model for the study of developmental competencies in minority children. *Child Development, 67*(5), 1891–1914. doi:10.2307/1131600.
Duvdevany, I., & Abboud, S. (2003). Stress, social support and well-being of Arab mothers of children with intellectual disability who are served by welfare services in northern Israel. *Journal of Intellectual Disability Research, 47*(4–5), 264–272. doi:10.1046/j.1365-2788.2003.00488.x.
Dwairy, M. (2002). Foundations of psychosocial dynamic personality theory of collective people. *Clinical Psychology Review, 22*(3), 343–360. doi:10.1016/S0272-7358(01)00100-3.
Dwairy, M. (2009). Culture analysis and metaphor psychotherapy with Arab-Muslim clients. *Journal of Clinical Psychology, 65*(2), 199–209. doi:10.1002/jclp.20568.
Dwairy, M., Achoui, M., Abouserie, R., & Farah, A. (2006). Parenting styles, individuation, and mental health of Arab adolescents: A third cross-regional research study. *Journal of Cross-Cultural Psychology, 37*(3), 262–272. doi:10.1177/0022022106286924.
Dwairy, M., & Van Sickle, T. D. (1996). Western psychotherapy in traditional Arabic societies. *Clinical Psychology Review, 16*(3), 231–249. doi:10.1016/S0272-7358(96)00011-6.
Erickson, C. D., & Al-Timimi, N. (2001). Providing mental health services to Arab Americans: Recommendations and considerations. *Cultural Diversity and Ethnic Minority Psychology, 7*(4), 308–327. doi:10.1037/1099-9809.7.4.308.
Estiritu, Y. L. (1999). Gender and labor in Asian immigrant families. *American Behavioral Scientist, 42*(4), 628–647. doi:10.1177/00027649921954390.
Farag, S. (2000). Arab states: Egypt and the Arab states. In A. E. Kazdin (Ed.), *Encyclopedia of psychology* (Vol. 1, pp. 224–228). Washington, DC: American Psychological Association. doi:10.1037/10516-079.
Faragallah, M. H., Schumm, W. R., & Webb, F. J. (1997). Acculturation of Arab-American immigrants: An exploratory study. *Journal of Comparative Family Studies, 28*(3), 182–203.
Gallagher-Thompson, D., Tazeau, Y. N., Basilio, L., Hansen, H., Polich, T., Menendez, A., et al. (1997). The relationship of dimensions of acculturation to self-reported depression in older, Mexican-American women. *Journal of Clinical Geropsychology, 3*(2), 123–137.
Ghaffarian, S. (1998). The acculturation of Iranian immigrants in the United States and the implications for mental health. *The Journal of Social Psychology, 138*(5), 645–654. doi:10.1080/00224549809600419.
Giger, J. N., & Davidhizar, R. (2002). Culturally competent care: Emphasis on understanding the people of Afghanistan, Afghanistan Americans, and Islamic culture and religion. *International Nursing Review, 49*(2), 79–86. doi:10.1046/j.1466-7657.2002.00118.x.
Gong, F., Takeuchi, D. T., Agbayani-Siewert, P., & Tacata, L. (2003). Acculturation, psychological distress, and alcohol use: Investigating the effects of ethnic identity and religiosity. In K. M. Chun, P. B. Organista, & G. Marin (Eds.), *Acculturation: Advances in theory, measurement, and applied research* (pp. 189–206). Washington, DC: American Psychological Association. doi:10.1037/10472-012.
Greenwald, A. G., McGhee, D. E., & Schwartz, J. L. K. (1998). Measuring individual differences in implicit cognition: The implicit association test. *Journal of Personality and Social Psychology, 74*(6), 1464–1480. doi:10.1037/0022-3514.74.6.1464.
Haboush, K. L. (2007). Working with Arab American families: Culturally competent practice for school psychologists. *Psychology in the Schools, 44*(2), 183–198. doi:10.1002/pits.20215.

Hakim-Larson, J., & Nassar-McMillan, S. (2007). Middle eastern Americans. In G. McAuliffe (Ed.), *Culturally alert counselling: A comprehensive introduction* (pp. 293–322). Thousand Oaks, CA: Sage.

Hamdi, E., Amin, Y., & Abou-Saleh, M. (1997). Problems in validating endogenous depression in the Arab culture by contemporary diagnostic criteria. *Journal of Affective Disorders, 44*(2–3), 131–143. doi:10.1016/S0165-0327(97)00037-2.

Harris, H. L. (1998). Ethnic minority elders: Issues and interventions. *Educational Gerontology, 24*(4), 309–323. doi:10.1080/036012798024040.

Hassouneh, D. M., & Kulwicki, A. (2007). Mental health, discrimination, and trauma in Arab Muslim women living in the US: A pilot study. *Mental Health, Religion and Culture, 10*(3), 257–262. doi:10.1080/13694670600630556.

Henry, H. M., Stiles, W. B., Biran, M. W., & Hinkle, S. (2008). Perceived parental acculturation behaviors and control as predictors of subjective well-being in Arab American college students. *The Family Journal, 16*(1), 28–34. doi:10.1177/1066480707309126.

Hovey, J. D. (2000). Acculturative stress, depression, and suicidal ideation among Central American immigrants. *Suicide & Life-Threatening Behavior, 30*(2), 125–139.

Hovey, J. D., & King, C. A. (1996). Acculturative stress, depression, and suicidal ideation among immigrant and second-generation Latino adolescents. *Journal of the American Academy of Child and Adolescent Psychiatry, 35*(9), 1183–1192. doi:10.1097/00004583-199609000-00016.

Hovey, J. D., & Magaña, C. (2000). Acculturative stress, anxiety, and depression among Mexican farmworkers in the Midwest United States. *Journal of Immigrant Health, 2*(3), 119–131. doi:10.1023/A:1009556802759.

Hovey, J. D., & Magaña, C. G. (2002). Psychosocial predictors of anxiety among immigrant Mexican migrant farmworkers: Implications for prevention and treatment. *Cultural Diversity and Ethnic Minority Psychology, 8*(3), 274–289. doi:10.1037/1099-9809.8.3.274.

Hoyer, W. J., & Roodin, P. A. (2009). *Adult development and aging* (6th ed.). New York: McGraw Hill.

Hurh, W. M., & Kim, K. C. (1990). Correlates of Korean immigrants mental health. *The Journal of Nervous and Mental Disease, 178*(11), 703–711. doi:10.1097/00005053-199011000-00006.

Ibish, I. (2003). *Report on hate crimes and discrimination against Arab Americans*. Washington, DC: American-Arab Anti-Discrimination Committee.

Jackson, J. S., Williams, D. R., & Torres, M. (2003). Perceptions of discrimination and health: The social stress process. In A. Maney (Ed.), *Social stressors, personal and social resources, and their mental health consequences* (pp. 86–146). Rockville, MD: National Institute of Mental Health.

Jamil, H., Farrag, M., Hakim-Larson, J., Kafaji, T., Abdulkhaleq, H., & Hammad, A. (2007). Mental health symptoms in Iraqi refugees: Posttraumatic stress disorder, anxiety, and depression. *Journal of Cultural Diversity, 14*, 19–25.

Jamil, H., Hakim-Larson, J., Farrag, M., Kafaji, T., Duqum, I., & Jamil, L. H. (2002). A retrospective study of Arab American mental health clients: Trauma and the Iraqi refugees. *The American Journal of Orthopsychiatry, 72*, 355–361. doi:10.1037/0002-9432.72.3.355.

Jamil, H., Nassar-McMillan, S. C., & Lambert, R. G. (2007). Immigration and attendant psychological sequelae: A comparison of three waves of Iraqi immigrants. *The American Journal of Orthopsychiatry, 77*, 199–205. doi:10.1037/0002-9432.77.2.199.

Jung, E., Hecht, M. L., & Wadsworth, B. C. (2007). The role of identity in international students psychological well-being in the United States: A model of depression level, identity gaps, discrimination, and acculturation. *International Journal of Intercultural Relations, 31*(5), 605–624. doi:10.1016/j.ijintrel.2007.04.001.

Kiefer, C. W., Kim, S., Choi, K., Kim, L., Kim, B. L., Shon, S., & Kim, T. (1985). Adjustment problems of Korean American elderly. *The Gerontologist, 25*(5), 477–482.

Kira, I. A., Templin, T., Lewandowski, L., Clifford, D., Wiencek, P., Hammad, A., et al. (2006). The effects of torture: Two community studies. *Peace and Conflict: Journal of Peace Psychology, 12*(3), 205–228. doi:10.1207/s15327949pac1203_1.

Kopp, R. R. (1995). *Metaphor therapy: Using client-generated metaphors in psychotherapy.* Philadelphia, PA: Brunner/Mazel.

Krause, N. (1995). Religiosity and self-esteem among older adults. *The Journals of Gerontology: Series B: Psychological Sciences and Social Sciences, 50B*(5), 236–246.

Krause, N., Ingersoll-Dayton, B., Ellison, C. G., & Wulff, K. M. (1999). Aging, religious doubt, and psychological well-being. *The Gerontologist, 39*(5), 525–533.

Kraut, R., Olson, J., Banaji, M., Bruckman, A., Cohen, J., & Couper, M. (2004). Psychological research online: Report of board of scientific affairs advisory group on the conduct of research on the internet. *The American Psychologist, 59*(2), 105–117. doi:10.1037/0003-066X.59.2.105.

Kulczycki, A., & Lobo, A. P. (2002). Patterns, determinants, and implications of intermarriage among Arab Americans. *Journal of Marriage and the Family, 64*(1), 202–210. doi:10.1111/j.1741-3737.2002.00202.x.

Laffrey, S. C., Meleis, A. I., Lipson, J. G., Solomon, M., & Omidian, P. A. (1989). Assessing Arab-American health care needs. *Social Science & Medicine, 29*(7), 877–883.

Leong, F. T. L., & Lau, A. S. L. (2001). Barriers to providing effective mental health services to Asian Americans. *Mental Health Services Research, 3*(4), 201–214. doi:10.1023/A:1013177014788.

Levin, J. (2006). Religion. In R. Schulz, L. S. Noelker, K. Rockwood, & R. L. Sprott (Eds.), *The encyclopedia of aging* (4th ed., Vol. 1, pp. 1016–1022). New York: Springer.

Liebkind, K., & Jasinskaja-Lahti, I. (2000). The influence of experiences of discrimination on psychological stress: A comparison of seven immigrant groups. *Journal of Community & Applied Social Psychology, 10*(1), 1–16. doi:10.1002/(SICI)1099-1298(200001/02)10:1<1::AID-CASP521>3.0.CO;2-5.

Masten, A. S., & Coatsworth, D. (1995). Competence, resilience, and psychopathology. In D. Cicchetti & D. J. Cohen (Eds.), *Developmental psychology* (Risk, disorder, and adaptation, Vol. 2, pp. 715–752). New York: Wiley.

Melikian, L. H. (1984). The transfer of psychological knowledge to the third world countries and its impact on development: The case of five Arab gulf oil-producing states. *International Journal of Psychology, 19*(1–2), 65–77. doi:10.1080/00207598408247516.

Mills, T. L., & Henretta, J. C. (2001). Racial, ethnic, and sociodemographic differences in the level of psychosocial distress among older Americans. *Research on Aging, 23*(2), 131–152. doi:10.1177/0164027501232001.

Moradi, B., & Hasan, N. T. (2004). Arab American persons reported experiences of discrimination and mental health: The mediating role of personal control. *Journal of Counseling Psychology, 51*(4), 418–428. doi:10.1037/0022-0167.51.4.418.

Naber, N. (2000). Ambiguous insiders: An investigation of Arab American invisibility. *Ethnic and Racial Studies, 23*, 37–61.

Nassar-McMillan, S., & Hakim-Larson, J. (2003). Counseling considerations among Arab Americans. *Journal of Counseling and Development, 81*(2), 150–159. doi:10.1002/j.1556-6678.2003.tb00236.x.

Noh, S., & Kaspar, V. (2003). Perceived discrimination and depression: Moderating effects of coping, acculturation, and ethnic support. *American Journal of Public Health, 93*(2), 232–238. doi:10.2105/AJPH.93.2.232.

Norris, A. E., Aroian, K. J., & Nickerson, D. M. (2011). Premigration persecution, postmigration stressors and resources, and postmigration mental health: A study of severely traumatized U.S. Arab immigrant women. *Journal of the American Psychiatric Nurses Association, 17*(4), 283–293. doi:10.1177/1078390311408900.

O'Connor, N., Warby, M., Raphael, B., & Vassallo, T. (2004). Changeability, confidence, common sense and corroboration: Comprehensive suicide risk assessment. *Australasian Psychiatry, 12*(4), 352–360. doi:10.1111/j.1440-1665.2004.02126.x.

Organista, P. B., Organista, K. C., & Kurasaki, K. (2003). The relationship between acculturation and ethnic minority mental health. In K. M. Chun, P. B. Organista, & G. Marin (Eds.),

Acculturation: Advances in theory, measurement, and applied research (pp. 139–161). Washington, DC: American Psychological Association.

Padela, A. I., & Heisler, M. (2010). The association of perceived abuse and discrimination after September 11, 2001, with psychological distress, level of happiness, and health status among Arab Americans. *American Journal of Public Health, 100*(2), 284–291. doi:10.2105/AJPH.2009.164954.

Paradies, Y. (2006). A systematic review of empirical research on self-reported racism and health. *International Journal of Epidemiology, 35*, 888–901. doi:10:1093/ije/dy1056.

Phinney, J. S. (2003). Ethnic identity and acculturation. In K. M. Chun, P. Balls Organista, & G. Marín (Eds.), *Acculturation: Advances in theory, measurement, and applied research* (pp. 63–81). Washington, DC: American Psychological Association.

Portes, P. R., Dunham, R., & Castillo, K. D. (2000). Identity formation and status across cultures: Exploring the cultural validity of Eriksonian theory. In A. L. Comunian & U. P. Gielen (Eds.), *International perspectives on human development* (pp. 449–459). Lengerich, Germany: Pabst Science.

Rippy, A. E., & Newman, E. (2006). Perceived religious discrimination and its relationship to anxiety and paranoia among Muslim Americans. *Journal of Muslim Mental Health, 1*(1), 5–20. doi:10.1080/15564900600654351.

Rose, M. (2002). Teaching tolerance after terrorism. *Education Digest, 67*(6), 4–9.

Roysircar, G. (2003). Religious differences: Psychological and sociopolitical aspects of counseling. *International Journal for the Advancement of Counselling, 25*(4), 255–267. doi:10.1023/B:ADCO.0000005525.71147.e8.

Rudmin, F. W. (2003). Critical history of the acculturation psychology of assimilation, separation, integration, and marginalization. *Review of General Psychology, 7*(1), 3–37. doi:10.1037/1089-2680.7.1.3.

Rudmin, F. (2009). Constructs, measurements and models of acculturation and acculturative stress. *International Journal of Intercultural Relations, 33*, 106–123. doi:10.1016/j.ijintrel.2008.12.001.

Salari, S. M. (2002). Invisible in aging research: Arab Americans, Middle Eastern immigrants, and Muslims in the United States. *The Gerontologist, 42*(5), 580–588.

Sanders, M. R., Markie-Dadds, C., & Turner, K. M. T. (2003). Theoretical, scientific and clinical foundations of the Triple P-Positive Parenting Program: A population approach to the promotion of parenting competence. *Parenting Research and Practice Monograph, 1*, 1–24.

Sayed, M. A. (2003). Psychotherapy of Arab patients in the west: Uniqueness, empathy, and "otherness". *American Journal of Psychotherapy, 57*(4), 445–459.

Schopmeyer, K. (2011). Arab Detroit after 9/11: A changing demographic portrait. In N. Abraham, S. Howell, & A. Shryock (Eds.), *Arab Detroit 9/11: Life in the terror decade* (pp. 29–63). Detroit, MI: Wayne State University Press.

Soliman, D. R., & McAndrew, F. T. (1998). Self-concept in Arabs and Arab Americans. *Psi Chi Journal of Undergraduate Research, 3*(3), 124–126.

Soueif, M. I., & Ahmed, R. A. (2001). Psychology in the Arab world: Past, present, and future. *International Journal of Group Tensions, 30*, 211–240.

Sroufe, L. A. (1979). The coherence of individual development: Early care, attachment, and subsequent developmental issues. *The American Psychologist, 34*(10), 834–841. doi:10.1037/0003-066X.34.10.834.

The Zogby Study. (1997). *Detroit MSA ethnic census*. Dearborn, MI: ACCESS.

Torres, L., & Rollock, D. (2004). Acculturative distress among Hispanics: The role of acculturation, coping, and intercultural competence. *Journal of Multicultural Counseling and Development, 32*(3), 155–167. doi:10.1002/j.2161-1912.2004.tb00368.x.

Triandis, H. C. (2001). Individualism-collectivism and personality. *Journal of Personality, 69*(6), 907–924. doi:10.1111/1467-6494.696169.

Trimble, J. E. (2003). Introduction: Social change and acculturation. In K. M. Chun, P. B. Organista, & G. Marin (Eds.), *Acculturation: Advances in theory, measurement, and applied research* (pp. 3–13). Washington, DC: American Psychological Association.

Whitbeck, L. B., McMorris, B. J., Hoyt, D. R., Stubben, J. D., & LaFromboise, T. (2002). Perceived discrimination, traditional practices, and depressive symptoms among American Indians in the upper Midwest. *Journal of Health and Social Behavior, 43*, 400–418. doi:10.2307/3090234.

Williams, C. L., & Berry, J. W. (1991). The primary prevention of acculturative stress among refugees: Application of psychological theory and practice. *The American Psychologist, 46*, 632–641.

Wrobel, N. H., Farrag, M. F., & Hymes, R. W. (2009). Acculturative stress and depression in an elderly Arabic sample. *Journal of Cross-Cultural Gerontology, 24*(3), 273–290. doi:10.1007/s10823-009-9096-8.

Zamanian, K., Thackrey, M., Starrett, R. A., & Brown, L. G. (1992). Acculturation and depression in Mexican-American elderly. *Clinical Gerontologist: The Journal of Aging and Mental Health, 11*(3–4), 109–121. doi:10.1300/J018v11n03_08.

Zimmerman, M. A., Ramírez-Valles, J., & Maton, K. I. (1999). Resilience among urban African American male adolescents: A study of the protective effects of sociopolitical control on their mental health. *American Journal of Community Psychology, 27*(6), 733–751. doi:10.1023/A:1022205008237.

Chapter 11
Education and Employment Among Arab Americans: Pathways to Individual Identity and Community Resilience

Karen L. Haboush and Nicole Barakat

Introduction

Education and employment have traditionally represented pathways to both individual and family success in Arab culture (Al-Khatab, 2000). Both are deeply valued. Because Arab culture emphasizes the importance of family, activities that function to maintain this unit and its honor, such as education and employment, are highly regarded. Education has implications for employment; therefore, the two are interrelated.

The 2010 American Community Survey (ACS) provides estimates of US demographic information, although official counts are provided by the US Census (2010). Recent statistics indicate that Arab Americans report higher mean levels of both education and median income relative to the US population as a whole, in line with earlier US Census reports (Brittingham & de la Cruz, 2005; U.S. Census Bureau, 2010). At the same time, considerable variability exists among Arab Americans (Abu El-Haj, 2009; El-Araby Aly & Ragan, 2010) and more recent Arab immigrants, who are often displaced for political reasons, may have less formal education (Wingfield, 2006). Thus, reasons for immigration and degree of acculturation to Arab and Western values intertwine to influence trends for Arab Americans in both school and work settings. Additionally, the more recent sociopolitical context subsequent to September 11, 2001, has also played a role in shaping Arab American behaviors and lifestyles in relation to both school and employment, as both settings

K.L. Haboush (✉)
Graduate School of Applied and Professional Psychology, Rutgers University,
152 Frelinghuysen Road, Piscataway, NJ 08854, USA
e-mail: haboush@rci.rutgers.edu

N. Barakat
Rutgers University, 152 Frelinghuysen Road, Piscataway, NJ 08854, USA
e-mail: nicolembarakat@gmail.com

S.C. Nassar-McMillan et al. (eds.), *Biopsychosocial Perspectives on Arab Americans: Culture, Development, and Health*, DOI 10.1007/978-1-4614-8238-3_11,

have witnessed an increase in bias and harassment of Arab Americans (Abel, 2005; Abu El-Haj, 2009; Abu-Ras & Abu-Bader, 2009; Arab American Institute, 2002; Britto, 2008; Council on American-Islamic Relations [CAIR], 2008; Malos, 2010; Shammas, 2009; Sirin & Fine, 2007; Wingfield, 2006). Thus, contemporary experiences of Arab Americans in school and work reflect a convergence of deeply held cultural values along with adaptation to the current sociopolitical climate. Resilience enhances adaptation to adverse circumstances (Belfiore, Lee, Spicer, & Dexter, 2008).

Education not only equips Arab Americans with the necessary skills and knowledge to pursue specific occupations, but schooling also contributes to the critical psychological task of identity development, including cultural identity, in children (Sirin & Fine, 2007). Academic achievement enhances psychological resilience (Masten, 2007); educational success contributes to a positive self-image for Arab American youth since it is a deeply held cultural value (Al-Khatab, 2000) and cognitive competence also promotes resilience by setting the foundation for adult occupational success (Masten & Cicchetti, 2010). Many aspects of schooling, including the presence of supportive networks of professionals and peers, can promote academic and social competence (Allen, 1998; Belfiore et al., 2008). At the same time, neither schools nor jobs exist in isolation as enclosed systems, but rather, are social institutions that function within a myriad of other systems, all of which impact each other (Britto, 2008; Merrell, Ervin, & Gimpel, 2006; Muhtaseb, 2007; Wingfield, 2006). As socializing contexts, both schools and jobs mirror trends within the larger society. Thus, Arab Americans also require protective factors to promote positive adaptation to the increased harassment that has occurred in public schools and jobs following September 11, 2001.

Increased bias complicates the development of identity formation, with the result that some Arab Americans attempt to conceal their ethnic identity out of fear of retribution, while others have consciously opted to identify with Arab culture (i.e., enrolling in Arabic language classes and schools) along with directly confronting the accuracy of stereotypes about Arabs (Abu El-Haj, 2006, 2009). Some responses to increased harassment may actually reflect resilience on the part of Arab Americans, such as students engaging in critical discourse regarding US policies in the Middle East during a current events lesson. However, members of other ethnic groups may perceive these behaviors as confirming stereotypes of Arab Americans as terrorists, unpatriotic, and suspicious and mistakenly label these behaviors as reflecting Arab "cultural" norms (Abu El-Haj, 2006, 2009; Sirin & Fine, 2007). Thus, in a bidirectional manner, while academic and occupational achievement may enhance psychological resilience, the current sociopolitical climate in schools and work settings also calls for greater resilience on the part of Arab Americans in order to succeed. Resilience is a socially constructed process, not a static trait, which requires systemic factors that support its development (Beiten & Allen, 2005).

This chapter will focus on describing several factors that may be associated with Arab American resilience in both schools and work settings, building upon the contributions of both developmental and ecological systems theories. An overview of historical trends in immigration, as these have impacted education and employment patterns for Arab Americans, will be provided followed by a section on resilience as a theoretical construct and organizing framework for this chapter. Specific aspects of the experience of schooling and work for Arab Americans will be discussed in the context of this framework, especially in light of increased bias directed toward Arab Americans in both settings subsequent to September 11, 2001.

Historical Background

Overview of Education and Employment

Historically, both education and occupational success have been revered in the Arab world. Arab culture, with its strong reliance on the family unit, has traditionally viewed education as enhancing family survival by improving chances of economic success, increasing girls' desirability as marriage partners, and, for Arab Muslims, as an essential vehicle for transmitting knowledge ("*Ilm*") of the Koran ("*Qur'an*") (Ajrouch, 2000; Al-Khatab, 2000; Britto, 2008; Haboush, 2007). Education is associated with improving chances for upward mobility for both sexes (Al-Khatab, 2000; Crabtree, 2010). Given the value placed upon strong family ties, economic success enjoyed by families in the United States frequently allows them to provide financial support for extended family back home, thereby helping to ensure family stability (Ajrouch, 2000; El-Araby Aly & Ragan, 2010). Educational achievement lays the groundwork for occupational success and both success and achievement help to maintain family pride and honor, central values in Arab culture (Kovach & Hillman, 2002).

Data from the 2010 ACS suggests that Arab Americans report higher levels of education than the US population at large, despite some variability for Arab Americans depending on their country of origin (U.S. Census Bureau, 2010). Approximately 89 % have high school degrees or higher compared to 86 % of the total US population (U.S. Census Bureau, 2010). Roughly 27 % of Arab Americans have bachelor's degrees compared to 18 % of the larger US population. Eighteen percent of Arab Americans have postgraduate degrees compared to approximately 10 % of the US population (U.S. Census Bureau, 2010). Roughly 40 % of Arab Americans are under age 25 (U.S. Census Bureau, 2010). Approximately 6 % attend preschool, 36 % attend elementary school, 18 % attend high school, and 36 % attend college and graduate school (U.S. Census Bureau, 2010).

Education lays the groundwork for occupational success and each wave of Arab immigration to the United States has been characterized by specific employment patterns, largely dependent upon the opportunities in America at the time of immigration and the skill sets of immigrants. As with education, job success in Arab cultures is strongly connected to family success and brings honor to the family, in contrast to more individualistic Western cultures (Kovach & Hillman, 2002). From the outset of their immigration to the United States, Arab immigrants, as part of the acculturation process, have generally displayed a strong ability to adapt to American society and a drive toward accumulating wealth, often with the goal of creating a legacy to pass along to their children (Naaf, 1985). Arab Americans tend to work in professional occupations, have higher incomes than the average American, and are one of the wealthier ethnic groups (Brittingham & de la Cruz, 2005; U.S. Census Bureau, 2010). The most recent ACS found that the median income for Arab American households was $61,579 compared to a median income of $60,609 for all the US households. At the same time, many immigrants, particularly those who are newer and younger, are living at or near poverty levels: approximately 17 % of families and 18 % of adults between the employable ages of 18 and 64 years were living below poverty level (U.S. Census Bureau, 2010).

The development of these employment patterns has enabled Arab immigrants to assimilate themselves into the larger society and scholars have often emphasized the economic success of Arab Americans (Britto, 2008). However, it is important to recognize that acculturation is a complicated process for Arab immigrants with consequences for economic success (Berry & Sam, 1997) due to the psychological implications of what it means to identify with Western values, especially amidst a landscape of discrimination. Personal characteristics, including ethnicity, religion, and education, along with contextual factors such as discrimination and political climate are all mediators of acculturation (Yakushko, Backhaus, Watson, Ngaruiya, & Gonzalez, 2008). Generally speaking, a positive acculturation process increases cultural fluency and contributes to an immigrant's ability to attain educational and economic success (Yakushko et al., 2008).

Patterns of Immigration and Implications for Education and Employment

From the outset of their immigration to the United States, Arab Americans have displayed a drive toward accumulating wealth. Financial success has been viewed as enhancing family standing and cohesiveness; and males are especially expected to achieve (Ajrouch, 2000). For many of the first Arab immigrants, the means to accumulating wealth was through business entrepreneurship, sales, factory jobs in the mid-west automotive industry, and farming government-granted parcels in the Great Plains. Immigrants who came to the United States after World War II were largely well educated and recognized an opportunity to establish a more stable life for themselves and their families. In many cases, however, Arab immigrants found that the economic opportunities that presented themselves in this new land responded to their entrepreneurial and independent spirit but also required an adaptation to American social and cultural values.

Four Waves of Arab Immigration

Immigration from the 22 Arab states to the United States has occurred in several waves, with levels of education and trends in employment varying for each successive influx (Britto, 2008; Nassar-McMillan & Hakim-Larson, 2003). An overview of these trends is summarized in Table 11.1.

Table 11.1 Historical employment trends over four waves of Arab immigration

Immigration and employment factors	First wave	Second wave	Third wave	Fourth wave
Years	1878–1924[a]	Post-World War II to 1967[b]	1967–2003[a]	2000–2010
Approximate number of immigrants	Up to 9,000 per year in 1913 and 1914[a]	80,000 45,201[a]	757,626[a]	301,241[c]
Countries of origin/ nationality	Greater Syria (Syria, Lebanon, and Palestine)[a]	Palestine, Egypt, Syria, Iraq[b]	Palestinian, Lebanon, Egypt, Iraq, Syria[a]	Egypt, Iraq, Somalia, Morocco, Lebanon, Jordan, Sudan, Syria, and Yemen[c]
Religion	90 % Christian[a]	60 % Muslim[b]	Primarily Muslim[a]	Primarily Muslim[a]
Regions to which they immigrated	New York and the Northeast[a]	Large cities[b]	Dearborn, Michigan; Chicago[a]	New York, Los Angeles, Miami, Washington DC, and Chicago Metro Areas
Political context of countries of origin	Ottoman occupation of greater Syria[a]	Arab-Israeli War of 1948[b]; revolutions in Egypt, Syria, and Iraq[a]	Six Day War (1967), Lebanese Civil War (1975), Israel invasion of Lebanon (1982), Iran-Iraq War (1980) Gulf War (1990s)[a]	Iraq War (2003)[a], lack of economic opportunities in Egypt[a], political instability in Lebanon[a], Arab Spring of 2011
Labor class/level of education	Nonprofessional, primarily agrarian[a]	Highly educated and skilled professionals[b]	Professionals and nonprofessionals[a,d]	Professionals and nonprofessionals[c]
Industry	Peddlers, shopkeepers, suppliers, textile industry[a]	Engineers, doctors, highly skilled professionals[a]	Professionals, factory, farm, small business, restaurant, manual labor[a]; management, business, science, and arts; sales; service; production[d]	Management, business, science, and arts; sales; service; production[d]
US immigration policies	Relatively open immigration via Ellis Island[b]	1924 national origins quota system limited non-European immigration to skilled professionals[b]	Immigration Act of 1965 ended the quota system[b]	Homeland Security Act of 2002–2003

[a]Orfalea (2006)
[b]Naaf (1985)
[c]U.S. Census Bureau (2000). *Selected population profile in the United States. Arab*. American Community Survey
[d]U.S. Census Bureau (2010). *Selected population profile in the United States. Arab*. American Community Survey

The first wave of immigrants in the late 1800s was largely comprised of farmers who lacked formal schooling and primarily came to the United States seeking jobs. For many of the first Arab immigrants, the means to achieve wealth was through business entrepreneurship. For others, acquiring well-paying manufacturing jobs in the mid-west automotive industry or farming government grant parcels in the Great Plains was the road to self-sufficiency. Many left school in order to work in factories, such as the auto industry and linens, with the goal of accumulating enough wealth to return home. Sales, including peddling, was a popular route for employment and even open to women (Naaf, 1985).

Second-wave immigrants who came to the United States after World War II were largely well educated and recognized an opportunity to utilize their skills and establish more stable lives for themselves and their families. Many were highly educated English-speaking professionals who left professional well-paying jobs seeking greater stability in the United States (Ajrouch, 2000; Wingfield, 2006). In the 1970s as a result of various wars, (i.e., the Lebanese Civil War, Arab-Israeli Seven Day War), many immigrants left professional jobs seeking better opportunities in the United States (Al-Khatab, 2000). For some, this actually entailed a loss of well-paying positions in their country of origin.

Although the first immigrants were largely Christian, subsequent influxes included greater numbers of Muslim immigrants. Some evidence suggests that Christian Arab Americans may more easily assimilate to life in the United States than Muslim Arab Americans, perhaps owing to diminished visibility and, therefore, diminished likelihood of experiencing discrimination (Britto, 2008; Wingfield, 2006).

More recently, many third- and fourth-wave immigrants have come to the United States in response to political unrest and war (Britto, 2008). For example, approximately 60 % of Iraqis living in the United States entered as refugees after 1990, coinciding with the Persian Gulf War invasion and more recent US invasion (Arab American Institute, 2002; Jamil et al., 2002; U.S. Census Bureau, 2010). Arab political refugees may arrive in the United States with disrupted educational histories and features of trauma which impede their functioning, including a higher incidence of anxiety and depression (Abu-Ras & Abu-Bader, 2009; Jamil et al., 2002; Nassar-McMillan & Hakim-Larson, 2003; Wingfield, 2006). Limited English proficiency as a by-product of disrupted schooling further hinders chances for educational and employment success.

Extensive exposure to war and political unrest has often been pointed to as suggesting that Arabs have a long, collective history of surviving hardships and developing coping skills and resilience (Beiten & Allen, 2005). Resilience refers to the capacity to survive and even succeed and adapt in adverse situations (Belfiore et al., 2008). The increased discrimination and bias Arab Americans have experienced in schools and jobs following September 11, 2001, may be considered an example of adverse conditions. Thus, resilience is the organizing theoretical framework for this chapter. Specific features of both schools and jobs that may be associated with Arab American resilience will be discussed in the following section.

Theoretical Constructs: Schools and Work as a Context for Identity Development

Identity development is a lifelong process with personal identity being comprised of numerous facets. Throughout the lifespan, various developmental tasks coalesce in the formation of personal identity and self-concept, including ethnic, academic, and occupational identity (Ajrouch, 2000; Al-Khatab, 2000; Britto, 2008; Merrell et al., 2006). Identity development is a fluid process whereby identity is constructed as an outgrowth of social experiences and interactions within the surrounding environment (Ajrouch, 2000; Britto, 2008). Identity construction is, therefore, a "socially negotiated process" which becomes complicated when interactions with others convey negative messages about one's group membership, including ethnicity (Al-Khatab, 2000; Britto, 2008).

According to ecological models such as Albert Bandura's reciprocal determinism (Al-Khatab, 2000; Merrell et al., 2006), development does not occur in isolation, but rather involves an interaction between the individual and his or her environment: individuals function in and are impacted by numerous systems while simultaneously impacting these same systems. Membership in an ethnic minority group impacts the behavior of group members as well as that of others in the surrounding environment, including teachers, fellow students, employers, and colleagues, in a reciprocal manner (Al-Khatab, 2000). In schools, for example, children's academic achievement may be as much a function of their innate ability as it is their perception of their ability to succeed. In turn, these beliefs are influenced by the manner in which others respond to the student. For example, teachers with lowered expectations for ethnic minority students may not expect high levels of academic achievement and may, in turn, reinforce lower levels (Al-Khatab, 2000; Merrell et al., 2006). In such contexts, academic achievement, often considered a source of resilience for Arab Americans, may decline (Abu El-Haj, 2006, 2009; Al-Khatab, 2000).

Along with Bandura's model of reciprocal determinism, Urie Bronfenbrenner's ecological systems theory, one of the best known ecological models, posits that children exist within multiple systems, each of which influences the child's development (Britto, 2008; Merrell et al., 2011). For youth, the immediate system (i.e., microsystem) includes home and classroom, both of which are surrounded by increasingly larger systems such as the entire school system and surrounding community and, ultimately, the larger cultural context, which reflects broad cultural values and laws. The employment context for adults is also surrounded by multiple systems, culminating in the larger sociopolitical context which, at present, includes increased levels of discrimination directed toward Arab Americans. All individuals function within multiple social contexts throughout their lifespan (Britto, 2008; Merrell et al., 2006).

The interaction between the individual and specific settings such as schools and work environment influences many psychological tasks. In schools, an Arab American child's academic achievement may be influenced by perceptions of their abilities which arise in response to interactions with others within school. Kovach and Hillman (2002) found that Arab American students were highly motivated to succeed academically and that the school environment played a key role in their motivation, thereby enhancing academic resilience. However, both ethnic and academic identity development become more difficult when the environment does not promote a positive identity and individuals who are exposed to negative messages about their own group become susceptible to accepting them (Al-Khatab, 2000; Britto, 2008; Britto & Amer, 2007; Sirin & Fine, 2007). Resilience can promote adaptation to adverse conditions in school and work, but simultaneously, is also required to navigate these systems (Belfiore et al., 2008).

Areas of competence which serve to protect children and adults from adverse experiences are considered "protective factors" (Belfiore et al., 2008). In keeping with an ecological model, the following sections address the interplay between cultural factors which Arab American children and adults bring to school and work settings along with features of those systems that may impact resilience. Following a developmental trajectory, education will be discussed first as academic competence may enhance subsequent occupational success.

School Climate and Resilience: An Overview

Climate refers to a school's atmosphere for learning, including the degree to which a school feels like a safe learning environment (Lehr, 2004). It encompasses the feelings people have about a school and has implications for both academic achievement and identity formation (Lehr, 2004). Schools are socializing contexts in which a child's identity is constructed through social interactions, including experiences of bullying and discrimination. Importantly, many features of schools can serve as protective factors, including the presence of supportive friendly networks of peers and adults, despite the increased harassment of Arab American students following September 11, 2001 (Abu El-Haj, 2006; Belfiore et al., 2008; Britto, 2008; Britto & Amer, 2007; Shammas, 2009; Sirin & Fine, 2007; Wingfield, 2006).

Among Arab American students, resilience may be mediated by various factors which reflect the interplay between developmental stages and Arab cultural values. In her study of Muslim adolescents, Sheikh (2009) found that peer support was rated as more helpful than support from parents, religious leaders, and school mental health professionals. However, for younger children, parental support may be more important and may intersect other mediating variables, such as trauma and refugee status. In their research on Iraqi child refugees between 12 and 16 years of age, Lewandowski, Chiodo, Peterson, and Kira (2007) found that parental support was a strong protective factor. Thus, developmental stage, degree of acculturation, immigration status, and presence of trauma are examples of some of the many variables that may mediate student's resilience alongside Arab cultural values that shape the experience of schooling.

Trauma and Schooling

Arab American students whose families are recent refugees may present with histories of trauma (Abu-Ras & Abu-Bader, 2009) accompanied by features of post-traumatic stress disorder (PTSD). The effects of trauma on learning and school performance have been well documented: both the hyperarousal and numbing associated with PTSD can significantly impact academic performance as well as disrupt social interactions with peers (Saigh, Yasik, Oberfield, Halamandaris, & Bremner, 2006). Trauma affects the structure of the brain thereby interfering with the affective and behavioral regulation processes that make students available for learning and facilitates appropriate perceptions of peer interactions. As a result, memory, concentration, attention, fluid reasoning, and verbal reasoning are impaired (Haboush, Selman, & Sievering, 2008).

Peer relationships may also be disrupted by traumatized children's tendency to protect themselves by scanning their environment for future harm, thereby contributing to their sometimes misreading social cues (Haboush et al., 2008). However, increased discrimination in schools may also exacerbate this tendency. Care should be taken to distinguish between hypervigilance as a result of trauma and reactions to actual experiences of harassment directed toward Arab American students.

Although research supports the impact of trauma on learning and school relationships, its effects may be mediated by numerous factors, especially the presence of supportive adults such as parents and teachers (Belfiore et al., 2008; Lewandowski et al., 2007). Adaptation to American schools may be associated with multiple factors. Features of Arab schools and cultural values pertaining to education in Arab countries often differ from practices within the United States, and these differences may impact the educational experience and adjustment to school in the United States. In particular, recent Arab immigrants may carry expectations about education rooted in experiences from their country of origin that differ from the prevailing practices often encountered in the US public schools.

Education in Arab Countries

Both education and respect for authority figures are deeply valued in many Arab countries. This extends to teachers who are generally held in high regard and afforded a good deal of authority (Haboush, 2007; Haj-Yahia, 2001). Arab students are often expected to assume a less active role because instructional practices emphasize rote memorization and students are expected to absorb teacher's instruction rather than actively challenge it through critical discourse (Britto, 2008; Crabtree, 2010). These practices may be more consistent with widely held cultural values involving respect for authority, an external locus of control related to beliefs about the central role of religion in determining fate, and the political climate in some Arab countries which does not encourage open, critical questioning of ideas.

Al-Khatab (2000) and Britto (2008) have also noted that for Arab Muslims, education strongly encourages acceptance of and adherence to the Koran as it is written. In line with these values, Arab American parents may also be less accustomed to the role of advocate for their children regarding their schooling (Haboush, 2007).

Gender

Arab culture values education for both males and females as it is seen as enhancing the economic standing of the family (Ajrouch, 2000). For boys, advancement may come through better job opportunities while for girls, education has traditionally enhanced desirability as a marriage partner along with the ability to be gainfully employed (Ajrouch, 2000). Variability does exist in terms of the extent to which education for females is commensurate with that of males. Ajrouch (2000) found that for some Arab American females, leaving home to attend college was the only viable way to separate from their family.

Observant Arab Muslims may prefer that boys and girls be educated separately (Hoot, Szecsi, & Moosa, 2003). For religious Arab American Muslims, education is also valued as a female's knowledge of the Koran is important in regard to marriage and child rearing. Transmission of knowledge regarding religion is an important aspect of a mother's role.

Speaking Arabic and Second Language Acquisition

Another issue related to immigration patterns is the possibility that students may be fluent in languages other than, or in addition to, English. The most recent estimates from the ACS reported that 56 % of Arab Americans above the age of 5 spoke another language at home (U.S. Census Bureau, 2010). Students may speak Arabic, which has a number of dialects (Al-Khatab, 2000), as well as other languages such as French, Chaldean, and Hebrew.

Speaking Arabic may in itself be a source of pride (Al-Khatab, 2000) and potential source of resilience among both Christian and Muslim Arab Americans, both of whom have preserved the Arabic language in their worship and liturgies (Abudabbeh, 1996). Many Arab American Muslims feel especially proud that the Koran (*Qur'an*) is written in Arabic. Seymour-Jorn (2004) found that many Arab Muslim college students, including those born in the United States and not raised to speak Arabic, want to learn Arabic in order to read and understand the Koran in its original form. For others, speaking Arabic was a source of pride connecting students with their extended family in the Arab world and strengthening ethnic identity. Some public schools offer Arabic as a foreign language option whereas Islamic schools routinely teach it so that students can read the Koran (Al-Romi, 2000; Seymour-Jorn, 2004).

Education of Children with Disabilities

Education of children with disabilities is a field that is receiving increasing recognition in Arab countries. Historically, Arab children with disabilities remained at home due to concerns about maintaining family honor and avoiding shame. This contrasts with federal law in the United States which guarantees the right to a public education to children with disabilities (Haboush, 2007; Merrell et al., 2006). The centrality of religion in Arab countries has meant that disabilities have generally been viewed as having religious or spiritual causes (i.e., the evil eye) and warranting faith-based interventions, similar to traditional views about mental health issues and treatment (Gaad, 2001). Opdal, Wormnaes, and Habayeb (2001) give the example of how the term "mental retardation," when translated into Arabic, may be interpreted as referring to mental illness.

Nevertheless, inclusion of children with disabilities is an increasingly recognized concept in the literature on Arab education (Opdal et al., 2001). Children with physical disabilities (i.e., orthopedic impairment, blindness) may more readily be included than those with emotional and behavioral disabilities as the latter may be associated with views of mental illness and mental health treatment which have historically been sources of shame (Gaad, 2001; Nassar-McMillan & Hakim-Larson, 2003).

Education: Proposed Sources of Resilience

In examining resilience among Arab American couples following September 11, Beiten and Allen (2005) describe resilience as a socially constructed process, not a fixed trait. As noted in section "Four Waves of Arab Immigration," resilience refers to protective factors which enhance coping, and schools may play an essential role in fostering its development. By building a sense of cultural identity and self-esteem, resilience is enhanced so that students are able to assume greater responsibility and work harder than those who do not see themselves in as positive a light (Al-Hazza & Bucher, 2008; Allen, 1998). Interaction with other students, teacher expectations, and educational materials can all serve to promote resilience provided they present a positive cultural identity (Al-Hazza & Bucher, 2008; Britto, 2008; Wingfield, 2006).

Roughly 76 % of Arab Americans between the ages of 18 and 24, which includes college- and postgraduate-aged students, have reported experiencing anti-Arab discrimination (Abu El-Haj, 2006; Arab American Institute, 2002; Britto, 2008; Britto & Amer, 2007; Shammas, 2009; Wingfield, 2006). Reports of students being called "traitor" and "Little bin Laden" (Wingfield, 2006), threats to beat Arab American students (Wingfield, 2006), and accusations of students carrying bombs (Abu El-Haj, 2006) are examples of various forms of reported harassment. Not surprisingly, given the influence that the school environment has on students' learning, Britto (2008) found that Arab American students frequently describe feeling isolated and misunderstood by their peers.

Culturally Relevant Instruction

Educational materials and teachers have also been found to perpetuate inaccurate information (i.e., "All Arabs are Muslims"), as well as stereotypic and biased messages about Arab Americans (Al-Hazza & Bucher, 2008; Britto, 2008; David & Ayouby, 2005; Schwartz, 1999), and/or fail to include any discussion about Arab culture and historical contributions (Wingfield, 2006). Sources from the popular media, i.e., cartoons like "Aladdin" and movies such as "Delta Force One" and "The Seige," further perpetuate negative stereotypes about Arabs (Al-Khatab, 2000; Suleiman, 2001).

Teachers

Because social support is a key factor in enhancing resilience in children (Allen, 1998), teachers are integral to this process. Schools serve as socializing contexts by providing opportunities to either reinforce or challenge stereotypical beliefs about different groups, including Arabs (Al-Hazza & Bucher, 2008). Students' self-perception is affected by the way others perceive them and teacher expectations of students strongly influence the way they interact with their students (Al-Khatab, 2000; Wingfield, 2006). As with other forms of bullying, immediate intervention on the part of teachers to stop harassment of Arab American students has been recommended (Abu El-Haj, 2009), yet reports of teachers failing to intervene and/or making discriminatory comments are common (Wingfield, 2006). In her interviews with Arab American students, Abu El-Haj (2009) heard accounts of teachers telling students to either remove their *hijab* (headscarf) or face disciplinary action, telling a student "You look like a disgrace in that thing (headscarf)," and telling an Iraqi boy to "Go back where you came from." Many teachers acknowledge having limited teacher training in both Arab culture and history along with misinformation regarding Islam, which may contribute to their difficulty intervening (Hoot et al., 2003). Insufficient training may also contribute to teachers' selection of inaccurate educational materials (Britto, 2008; David & Ayouby, 2005), stereotypical and biased messages about Arab Americans (Al-Hazza & Bucher, 2008; Schwartz, 1999), and failure to incorporate discussion about Arab culture and historical contributions into their curriculum (Wingfield, 2006). Schwartz (1999) found that textbooks on the Middle East and Islam were frequently inaccurate.

Fortunately, numerous resources do exist to aid teachers in selecting culturally relevant and accurate instructional materials. Al-Hazza and Bucher (2008) provide a comprehensive list of children's literature dealing with Arab Americans and recommended instructional techniques. Hoot et al. (2003) list resources for teaching about Islam in the United States. Some educational materials directly from the Arab world may also provide useful primary sources of information, (see, e.g., Saudi Aramco World magazine, http://saudiaramcoworld.com) Weiss (2011).

Supporting Critical Discourse and Culturally Relevant Instruction

Infusion of discussion of Arab culture, historical events, and contributions (i.e., the calendar, the alphabet, contributions to medicine, and the arts) is a frequently recommended strategy for creating a classroom climate which is supportive of Arab American students (Al-Hazza & Bucher, 2008; David & Ayouby, 2005; Wingfield, 2006). However, researchers have noted that although inclusion of culturally relevant instructional materials is essential to combat negative stereotypes, many of these same materials either contain inaccurate information or present Arabs as a homogeneous group (Al-Hazza & Bucher, 2008; David & Ayouby, 2005; Schwartz, 1999). Further, David and Ayouby (2005) note that even positive portrayals of Arab culture can have negative outcomes in terms of fostering an image of a group as static and distinct and reinforcing a sense of Arab Americans as "foreign" and "the other." Considerable variability exists among Arab Americans in terms of values, behavior, and beliefs, including religion (Abu El-Haj, 2006). In this vein, just as resilience may be viewed as a socially constructed process, culture may also be thought of as a process through which meaning is created: Arab culture is not static but rather, diverse and changing (Abu El-Haj, 2006, 2009).

Abu El-Haj (2009) suggests that in order to combat inaccurate perceptions of Arabs and Arab Americans, teachers must incorporate instructional strategies that allow for critical examination of current events in the Middle East and US–Arab relations. Allowing for critical discussion of these topics helps to set a tone whereby the classroom is seen as more inclusive of the viewpoint of Arab American youth. In her research, Abu Haj found that when such a climate was lacking, there was a greater tendency for Arab American student's expression of their opinions to be viewed as "unpatriotic" or construed as supportive of anti-American terrorism, thereby contributing to further discrimination. For example, an Arab American student might express disagreement about the US decision to enter Iraq if they have family members who were injured or displaced. Such discussions are in line with the concept of using "teachable moments" when class discussions about the Middle East occur. Abu El-Haj documents the manner in which the lack of classroom climate that supports critical discourse can give rise to perceptions of Arab American students as "unpatriotic" and further promote bias against Arab American students. Although students' capacity to express their beliefs may be viewed as a source of resilience, the current sociopolitical climate may render the impression that such behavior is unpatriotic and Arab American students have been suspended and expelled for comments that have been construed as threats (Abu El-Haj, 2009).

Islamic Schools

As with other Arab American groups, education is deeply valued by devout Arab Muslim students who study the Koran (Britto, 2008; Hoot et al., 2003; Sabry &

Bruna, 2007). Although the largest percentage of Arab Americans are Christian (Nassar-McMillan & Hakim-Larson, 2003; Wingfield, 2006), Arab Muslim students may be especially vulnerable to increased harassment in public schools because certain practices enhance their visibility. Female students who wear the "*hijab*," children who cannot eat pork and other products not considered "*halal*," fasting on certain holidays, prayer during the school day, and limited participation in physical and sex education may all render Arab Muslim youth increasingly visible (Al-Romi, 2000; Hoot et al., 2003; Sabry & Bruna, 2007; Sirin & Fine, 2007). Numerous reports, for example, describe the harassment of female Muslim students who wear the *hijab* including being hit in the lip with a belt, having the *hijab* torn off by teachers, being suspended for wearing it to school, and being cursed at (Britto, 2008; Seymour-Jorn, 2004; Wingfield, 2006).

In response to misinformation and bias about Arab Muslims, there has been an increase in the number of Islamic schools in the United States (Al-Romi, 2000). These schools serve the purpose of protecting Muslim students from discrimination as well as enhancing transmission of accurate knowledge about Islam (Al-Romi, 2000). Islamic schools allow religious practices pertaining to diet, holiday observances, prayer during the school day, modest dress, and limited interaction between males and females to be observed. The greater sense of community provided by Islamic schools may be a source of resilience for students who identify with their faith (Al-Romi, 2000; Hoot et al., 2003). Interestingly, interviews with female students who opt to wear the *hijab* sometimes suggest that the very act of wearing it is a source of pride and resilience (Muhtaseb, 2007; Sheikh, 2009; Sirin & Fine, 2007). Though disliking the harassment they experience, many girls report a sense of purpose through educating others about Islam and a concomitant sense of satisfaction and pride (Sirin & Fine, 2007).

Employment

As with education, job success in Arab cultures is strongly connected to family success and brings honor to the family, especially for males (Kovach & Hillman, 2002). The strong family and community ties of Arab Americans have contributed enormously to their success in the United States. Arab Americans' communal orientation is well illustrated by the first wave of immigrants' creation of support networks for peddlers. First-wave Arab Americans were met at Ellis Island by representatives from the Arab community who would usher them to Washington Street in Manhattan where suppliers would provide them with the trappings of a peddler, often given completely on credit (Orfalea, 2006). Although peddling was largely solitary work, at the end of the week, peddlers would meet at common destination points, where they would eat, lodge, and trade stories. By the turn of the century, entire networks of peddling settlements had been established across the country (Naaf, 1985).

In terms of an immigrant's experience of occupational success and career development, resilience has been defined by Yakushko et al. (2008, p. 370) as "a dedication to persevere despite difficulties, insight as an ability to have clear understanding of oneself and the world of work, and identity as a developed sense of career goals." Resilience works together with acculturation to contribute to an immigrant or immigrant group's career success. Immigrants who arrive as refugees versus those who move voluntarily seeking career advancement and quality of life improvements may have very different experiences establishing career paths in their new country. Refugees typically come to a host country having experienced psychological and physical duress. This type of immigration stress, combined with individual personality factors, may contribute to difficulties with acculturation and therefore impact the immigrant's work prospects. However, a strong immigrant community can be a source of resilience and may mitigate some of the challenges facing refugees (Yakushko et al., 2008).

The first-wave Arab Americans' ingrained sense of community provided a supportive network that eased their transition into to their unfamiliar new home. The community constituted a source of resilience and provided for new immigrants, taking them under its wing from the moment they stepped off the boat and helping them through the initial transition to life in America. From finding work to learning English, the first-wave Arab Americans relied upon the strength of their communities to help them establish their presence in their new country.

This first generation of Arab American immigrants was characterized by its relative ease of assimilation into American society. Working as peddlers presented opportunities to observe American customs and learn English. They quickly adapted to the American lifestyle and their children were absorbed into the mainstream. Some cultural customs continued to be practiced in the privacy of their homes, such as preparing traditional foods and speaking Arabic. Christian religion was an advantage for this first wave of Arab immigrants, when considering ease of assimilation into mainstream America. Success was equated with adopting American attitudes in the public sphere in order to allow them to take advantage of the opportunities available to them in America at that time, and this was largely achieved.

Arab Muslims made up less than 10 % of the first wave of Arab immigrants and began arriving in the United States around 1900 (Orfalea, 2006). Some Muslims worked in the textile factories of the East, such as in Quincy, Massachusetts, or became peddlers like the Christian Arabs. Many began to congregate in industrial cities such as Pittsburgh and New Castle, Pennsylvania, where they worked in steel factories; Michigan City, Indiana, where they settled using the Homestead Act, whereby the government gave away acres of land to those hearty individuals willing to farm it. The first mosques in the United States were therefore established in locations such as Detroit, Michigan City; Ross, North Dakota; and Cedar Rapids, Iowa.

Second- and third-wave immigrants who fled unstable political conditions in their homelands expanded the professional classes, as the United States sought highly trained individuals. Loosened immigration policies were largely responsible for the third wave of Arab immigrants arriving in the United States from 1967 to 2003, many of whom were Palestinians and professionals (Orfalea, 2006).

Due to these immigration patterns, for the past several decades, Arab Americans have trended toward being wealthier and more educated than the US population at large. At the same time, nonprofessional immigrants and refugees have established themselves in factories, farms, and small businesses and restaurants. Examples include the community of Christian Iraqi Chaldeans in Detroit which has taken to small business ownership; Yemenis, who are largely young males working in the Detroit auto and cargo industries who send most of their earnings home; and Palestinians, 15 % of whom have settled in Chicago, where many work for low wages and live in poor conditions (Orfalea, 2006).

With political events that have taken place in the Middle East since the 1990s, the trend toward financial success may be changing. More recently, many Arabs have immigrated in response to political unrest and war (Britto, 2008). For example, approximately 60 % of Iraqis living in the United States entered as refugees after 1990, coinciding with the Persian Gulf War invasion and more recent US invasion (Brittingham & de la Cruz, 2005; Jamil et al., 2002; United States Department of Homeland Security, 2011). With the Arab Spring of 2011, immigration from the Middle East seems likely to continue, although it is uncertain how these recent events will affect political and immigration trends.

The Fourth Wave: Arab Americans Today

Data from the 2000 Census and most recent ACS (2010) provide a sketch of the economic contributions of Arab Americans to the overall US economy. In 2010, the median household income of Arab Americans was higher than that of the total population (U.S. Census Bureau, 2010). This was largely due to the greater percentage of Arab Americans making above $100,000 compared to the total population. Although still higher than the US population as a whole, the median income of Arab Americans has trended down since 2000, to become more aligned with the overall American population. This may be due to an increased percentage of the population living in poverty, as the poverty rate of Arab Americans climbed from 2000 to 2010, to exceed the total population's poverty rate by over 4 % (U.S. Census Bureau, 2010).

Employment and unemployment rates of Arab Americans have tended to mirror the total population and rose from around 3 % in 2000 to 7 % in 2010. Although many historians and sociologists have emphasized the economic success and wealth of Arab Americans, it is important to recognize that many Arab Americans, particularly newer immigrants and the young, may be living at or near poverty level. Refugee status may also be a contributing factor. Tables 11.2 and 11.3 summarize data from the 2000 and 2010 Department of Homeland Security American Community Survey findings.

The statistics from the 2010 US Census Bureau American Community Survey (ACS) reveal that Arab Americans trend toward the mainstream in their job industry and choice of occupation. For example, with 22 % of Arab Americans working in education, social services, and health care, Arab Americans are right in line with

Table 11.2 Employment rates of the total US population compared to Arab Americans in the years 2000 and 2010

	2000[a]		2010[b]	
Employment factors	Arab Americans	Total population	Arab Americans	Total population
Population 16 years and older	866,961	217,168,077	1,222,539	243,832,923
Employed (%)	61	59.7	55.7	57.0
Unemployed (%)	3.3	3.7	7.1	6.9
Not in labor force (%)	35	36.1	36.9	35.6

[a]U.S. Census Bureau (2000). *Selected population profile in the United States. Arab.* American Community Survey

[b]U.S. Census Bureau (2010). *Selected population profile in the United States. Arab.* American Community Survey

Table 11.3 Income and poverty rates of the total US population, compared to Arab Americans in the years 2000 and 2010

	2000[a]		2010[b]	
Household incomes and poverty rates	Arab Americans	Total population	Arab Americans	Total population
Median household income	\$47,459	\$41,994	\$51,273	\$50,046
Below \$25,000 (%)	26	28.6	–	–
\$25,000–49,999	26 %	29.3	–	–
\$50,000–99,999 (%)	30	29.7	–	–
≥\$100,000 (%)	18	12.3	–	–
Poverty rate (all families)	10.9	9.2	16.9 %	11.3 %
Poverty rate (all people)	13.9	12.4	19.6 %	15.3 %

[a]U.S. Census Bureau (2000). *Selected population profile in the United States. Arab.* American Community Survey

[b]U.S. Census Bureau (2010). *Selected population profile in the United States: Arab.* American Community Survey

national figures which place 23 % of total Americans in these industries. Likewise, 11 % of Arab Americans are in professional and management positions, compared to 10.6 % of all Americans. There are some notable exceptions to these trends, however, which highlight the uniqueness of the Arab American population. By occupational category, more Arab Americans work in management, business, science, and the arts than the overall population (45 % versus 36 %). These figures may reflect the historic trend for Arab Americans to work in business and sales industries. In addition, fewer Arab Americans work in service occupations than the overall population (13 % versus 18 %). These figures may reflect the trend for Arab Americans to be more highly educated than the mainstream. One industry category that particularly distinguishes Arab Americans from overall Americans is retail trade: 18 % of Arab Americans work in this sector, which ranks it second only after education and health care, while in the overall population, only 11.7 % work in retail trade. Occupation and industry data from the ACS 2010 are summarized in Figs. 11.1 and 11.2.

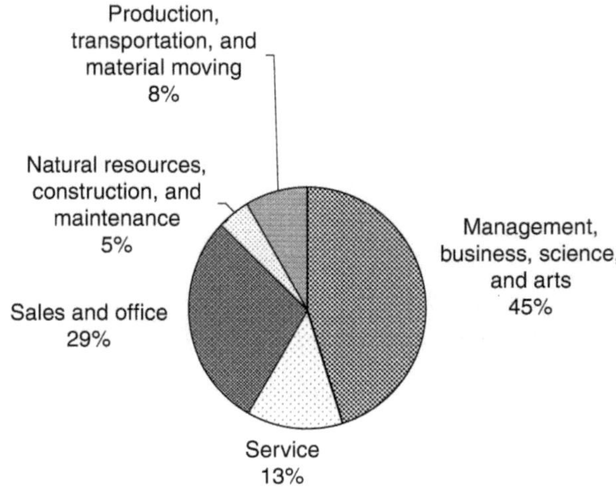

Fig. 11.1 Occupation types of Arab Americans, 2010. Data were taken from the U.S. Census Bureau (2010). *Selected population profile in the United States*. Arab American Community Survey

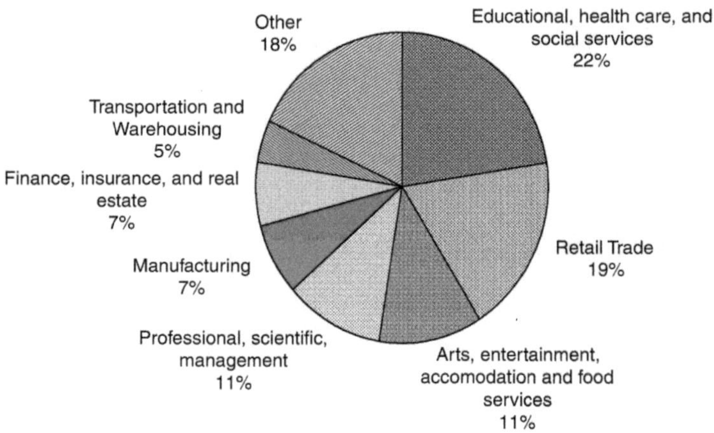

Fig. 11.2 Industry of Arab Americans, 2010. Data were taken from the U.S. Census Bureau (2010). *Selected population profile in the United States*. Arab American Community Survey

Employment Discrimination and Issues Affecting Arab Americans Today

Arab Americans have been often dubbed "the invisible minority" due to their successful assimilation into mainstream America. This assimilation has been aided by many factors, including Arab Americans' economic success, majority Christian religion, and white appearance. Despite their overall success as an immigrant group, historical and contextual factors (e.g., terrorist attacks of September 11, the military presence of the United States in the Middle East, the Western world's suspicious stance toward Islam, and stereotypic representations of Arabs in the media) have led to an overall climate of mistrust toward people of Arab descent and the solidification of a culturally held notion of the Arab as an enemy to America. In addition, more recent Arab immigrants are more likely to hold views that differ from the American mainstream in response to Middle East politics. They are more likely to be politically active and expressive of their viewpoints and therefore less likely to quietly assimilate into the mainstream.

Following the terrorist attacks of September 11, incidences of hate crimes against Arab Americans, Muslims, or those perceived to be Muslims increased dramatically across the United States (Arab American Institute, 2002; Council on American-Islamic Relations 2006; South Asian American Leaders of Tomorrow, 2001). Consistent with the increase in hate crimes, there was also a rise in employment-related discrimination. In November 2001, the Equal Employment Opportunities Commission (EEOC), the Justice Department, and the Labor Department jointly initiated an anti-discrimination statement in order to protect individuals who are or are perceived to be Muslim from harassment and discrimination and to increase public sensitivity to this topic.

The Council on American-Islamic Relations (CAIR), an advocacy organization whose mission is to enhance understanding between American Muslims and the American mainstream, keeps records of discrimination and harassment incidences against Muslims. The most recent figures available from their 2008 Civil Rights report state that over 10 % (281 total) of incidents of civil rights discrimination against Muslims are workplace related. When ranked by place of occurrence, 17 % (452 total) of cases of discrimination against Muslims occurred in the workplace, followed by a government agency, and a Muslim organization or mosque. CAIR further reports that of the 2,600 complaints they received in 2007, 63 % of the events were triggered because of the person's religion, ethnicity, or because they had a Muslim-sounding name. In the 2008 annual report, CAIR states that their current figures point to a downward trend in discrimination against Muslims and a hopefulness that the post-September 11 backlash is coming to an end (CAIR, 2008). The Arab American community has responded to harassment and employment discrimination by reaching out to victims and launching public awareness campaigns. CAIR collects and reports instances of anti-Muslim discrimination. Both CAIR and the Arab American Institute have responded to increased discrimination with campaigns to educate the public about Muslims and Arab Americans and dispel common misconceptions and misinformation. The response of such organizations to discrimination reveals their communities' strong desires to be legitimized in the eyes of mainstream America and to be accepted as a part of American society.

Some research findings have revealed that discrimination has had a direct effect on Arab men's economic success. Davila and Mora (2005) examined the direct impact of post-September 11 xenophobic attitudes on Arab men's earnings. Davila and Mora document that the monetary earnings of Arab men declined from the year 2000 to 2002 and, further, that this decline is not explainable by factors other than differences related to ethnicity. Davila and Mora examined a large data sample collected by the Census Bureau's American Community Survey. When compared to the US-born non-Hispanic white men with comparable education and experience, Middle-Eastern Arab men experienced a decline in wages during the year following September 11. The strongest effects occurred in regions that had the highest concentrations of Arab Americans, indicating that due to their increased visibility, they were more likely to become targets of discrimination.

Although Arab Americans may have been overlooked as "the invisible minority" in the past, political events of recent years, such as September 11, have heightened Americans' awareness of this group. In addition, since the second wave of immigration, Arab Americans are more likely to be Muslim, have Arabic-sounding names, and be more politically visible than in the past. Arab Americans are no longer the "invisible minority." To the contrary, they experience increased scrutiny in America today. These complex political factors have resulted in Arab Americans' difficulty successfully integrating into the workforce and increased experiences of employment discrimination.

Women's Roles and Issues in the Workplace

Arab American women's relationship to the public workplace is a complex and multifaceted one. While Arab American women are a highly educated group, having the highest levels of education of immigrant groups after Filipinas (Read & Cohen, 2007), they are less likely to be employed when compared to equally well-educated women in the United States. Although level of education can be used to predict employment rates among white, black, and Hispanic women in the United States, high education does not predict employment for Arab American women (Read & Cohen, 2007). Instead, cultural values prioritizing women's roles as mothers impact their decisions to work or not work.

In their 2008 study, Read and Oselin found that among Arab American women, the role of mother was most highly valued and emphasized. Study participants espoused that the most important role a woman has is to raise children, with an emphasis on instilling cultural and religious values. Although women are encouraged to attain college and professional education, many of them stop working once they have children, in order to fulfill what is seen as their primary role, that of mothering. Read and Oselin conclude that in contrast to other ethnic groups in the United States, Arab American women's education serves to support and maintain traditional gender roles. A mother's education is viewed as a communal asset that will better enable her to contribute to the well-being of the children and socioeconomic success of the whole family.

Employment and the **Hijab** *(the Veil)*

For Muslim women who wear the veil, finding employment can be difficult. In the West, the veil has become a powerful and politically charged symbol. It may represent women's subjugation to some, while for others it has come to symbolize empowerment and equality (Zine, 2006). Due to the high visibility of the veil and its multiply charged cultural meanings, women who wear it may be more likely to experience biased reactions from others. This is especially the case for women seeking employment.

According to Burgoon's expectancy violation theory (1986), which states that individuals evaluate others based on stereotypes they have formed, those who violate cultural stereotypes will be judged more harshly. Ahlam Muhtaseb (2007) used this theory to illustrate some of her own experiences as a college professor who wears the *hijab*. Muhtaseb reported that her students often respond to her perceived "foreignness," including her accent and *hijab*, with suspicion and end of the semester reviews that focused more on her personal characteristics than her teaching. She poignantly described the efforts she made to overcome her students' negative reactions to her by working extra hard to earn their trust and demonstrate her qualifications.

For women who wear the veil, finding employment in the United States is likely to be challenging. The veil may induce a strongly biased reaction in employers and cause them to question the candidate's appropriateness for the position. Once employed, women may face culturally biased reactions from their supervisors, coworkers, or clients. According to expectancy violation theory, a veiled woman's qualifications and performance may be more harshly judged than members of the in-group; in order to compensate for this, she will likely work extra hard to make others feel comfortable with her and to prove her abilities. Despite the prejudice and misunderstanding they typically experience, women who wear the veil often view it as a source of strength, constructing it not as a symbol of their subjugation, but as a rejection of the Western discourse that sexualizes women and commodifies beauty (Zine, 2006). Their deviation from the dominant discourse can lead women to experiences of bias and discrimination and to ultimately feel isolated from society, including employers and coworkers in the workplace (Zine, 2006).

Women who wear the *hijab* in the public arena and workplace may experience themselves as different, exotic, or even rejected by employers and coworkers. For women who do wear the veil, their belief in the veil as a positive religious symbol that supports and protects femininity, and the support they garner from their community are important sources of acceptance and strength. Due to its particular poignancy as a cultural symbol, women who wear the veil are likely to experience particularly strong dissonance, as their beliefs clash with Western perceptions of the veil. While the veil may be a source of resilience for these women as it represents their community and cultural ties, it is just as likely to present challenges to acculturation due to its high visibility and the politico-cultural associations the West has imbued it with.

American values emphasizing individualism may conflict with Arab American women's cultural traditions and cause acculturation stress for recent immigrants as well as successive generations. The female children of Arab immigrants may experience an even greater degree of distress as they grapple with the gap between the culture they are raised in and peer expectations and the traditions taught at home and familial expectations. For example, first-generation females may struggle with decisions regarding whether or not they should work while raising a family.

Methodology: Approaches, Critique, and Future Directions

The vast majority of research on Arab American education and employment has been qualitative in nature. Although the sources consulted for this chapter do not constitute an exhaustive literature search, they are believed to be largely representative of the available resources, given the overall dearth of empirical studies on Arab Americans. Empirical investigations of Arab Americans have partially been limited by their smaller representation in the US population as a whole, along with challenges to building trust in order to gain access to samples. The use of qualitative measures includes focus groups, individual and/or group interviews, and surveys, including Internet-based measures. Archival data are also used. Objective sources of data, when utilized, have involved the use of rating forms including self-report measures.

Neither schools nor jobs readily lend themselves to empirical investigations; as such, qualitative studies are a better fit with the context. Gaining access to adequate sample sizes of Arab Americans for empirical investigations is difficult. Although schools can provide physical access to children, there are often restrictions on researcher's access to students. Necessarily, this limits the representativeness of available samples. Some geographic regions of the country may have larger numbers of Arab American students than others and not all students attend public schools.

Among qualitative studies with students, focus groups have been more widely utilized. Such groups often allow the researcher more time to build trusting relationships which may elicit more discussion (see, e.g., Abu El-Haj, 2009; Ajrouch, 2000; Sheikh, 2009). The benefit of building more trusting relationships over time may be an important strength of this approach, especially in light of the current sociopolitical context. However, concerns about the potential for eliciting shame in the presence of the researcher and other group members may elicit less discussion as the relationship between the evaluator and students changes over time. Concerns about potential shame may be especially strong regarding some more taboo areas such as data, sex, and religiosity. In their work with Iraqi immigrants with trauma histories, Nassar-McMillan and Hakim-Larson (2003) noted that the high degree of mistrust on the part of these individuals limited their willingness to talk in a group and may therefore suggest that Arab Americans with trauma histories may also be more reluctant to participate in group context. Other advantages of using focus groups may include the use of Arabic-speaking researchers and frequent checking on understanding which cannot be done on the Internet or paper and pencil surveys and rating forms.

Outside of schools, qualitative research on education has been conducted in religious institutions such as mosques and community centers. Abu El-Haj (2009) interviewed youth in a community center. Sheikh (2009) interviewed members of two mosques in her study of Muslim adolescent girls; even so, gaining access to this population required the assistance of the religious clerics, called *Imams*. Research involving religiously observant children in religious settings may only be generalizable to children of the same faith and similar degrees of religious observance. Concerns about social appropriateness may be a limitation. Adult samples, such as parents, have also been recruited from mosques for focus groups pertaining to education (see, e.g., Sirin & Fine, 2007).

Interviews with adults are found in research on both education (i.e., teachers, parents) and employment (see, e.g., Hoot et al., 2003; Sabry & Bruna, 2007). Types of interviews, nature of questions, and degree of structure may vary. Sabry and Bruna (2007) conducted open interviews of teachers regarding their knowledge of Islam. Semi-structured life-history interviews may also be found in the literature (see Ajrouch, 2000). Seymour-Jorn (2004) combined surveys and interviews with college students.

Future research could elicit more statistical data on the effects of bias on student's mood and behavior through the use of behavior rating scales. For example, the Achenbach System of Empirically Based Assessment (ASEBA) has subscales which examine both internalizing mood symptoms as well as externalizing behaviors in children (Merrell et al., 2006). The ASEBA is widely used in schools, has corresponding scales for parents, teachers, and youth, and has been translated into Arabic.

Future research regarding the experience of education and employment for Arab Americans is desirable along with a focus on understanding those factors that promote resilience. In addition to continuing to examine incidents of bias against Arab American youth, research on the effectiveness of initiatives to enhance teacher awareness of bullying of Arab American youth is recommended. Although schools are increasingly addressing bullying through systemic interventions (Lehr, 2004; Merrell et al., 2006), qualitative reports of teacher's failure to intervene on behalf of Arab American students may suggest that teacher training needs to specifically address bias against these youth. As part of these initiatives, surveys of teacher's knowledge of Arab culture and awareness of bias directed at Arab American students might be conducted. Statistical data regarding outcomes for teacher training (i.e., reduced incidence of bias) subsequent to specific training on Arab American youth could help to clarify whether teacher's failure to intervene is due to their own biases against these students or a lack of sensitivity in recognizing such occurrences. Additionally, because the literature has underscored the role of the media, including instructional materials in perpetuating negative images of Arab Americans, student perceptions could be surveyed following more school-wide initiatives to increase knowledge of Arab culture among the student body. School-wide programs that highlight Arab culture, use of Arab music, art, and literature in lessons, and holiday celebrations are just possible examples of approaches for increasing awareness of Arab culture.

Finally, as anti-bullying initiatives are often implemented by school psychologists and other school mental health professionals, collecting survey data on their understanding of Arab culture and discrimination against students is also recommended.

Current research on Arab Americans in the workplace, including statistical data, is limited. Census data from the US Census Bureau American Community Survey 2000 and 2010 were utilized to formulate a contemporary understanding of employment and economic factors of Arab Americans. Current research trends regarding Arab Americans' issues in the workplace include studies of the impact of September 11 on increased prejudice against and stereotypes of Arab Americans and how these affect employment rates and opportunities. Survey and self-report data taken on Muslim Americans by the CAIR reflected increased incidences of discrimination post September 11. Census data were analyzed by Davila and Mora in order to determine that Arab American men's incomes declined in the years following September 11. Several sources shed light upon Arab American women's' issues with regard to employment, including culturally valued ideals for women and the perception of the *hijab* by employers and potential employers. Read and collaborators contribute qualitative data regarding work issues specific to Arab American women, gleaned from interviews and ethnographic sources.

The September 11 tragedy prompted a reactionary examination of stereotypes, racism, and violence faced by Arab Americans in various contexts in the United States, as well as a proactive response by some institutions such as the EEOC, which recognized the problem of discrimination against Arab Americans at work, and made official statements in the months following September 11 imploring fair treatment of Arab Americans. However, these examinations tapered off in the early 2000s, and little research has been conducted since then. The lack of attention to this issue perhaps reflects the small size of the Arab American population compared to more sizable minority groups in America. It is unknown to what extent concerns regarding immigration status may limit the willingness of Arab Americans to report discrimination in the workplace. Both work and schools may be viewed as extensions of the government which may limit the willingness of Arab Americans to report instances of bias.

Future directions for employment research should continue to examine issues of acculturative stress that may negatively impact immigrants' career success in the United States. Topics specific to Arab Americans include the effects of September 11 on discrimination in the workplace, including the manner in which discrimination may disproportionally impact individuals whose cultural traditions are most visible (i.e., women who wear the *hijab*, individuals with Arabic-sounding names). Studies on the impact of trauma on the acculturative process of war refugees and their subsequent ability to find employment may shed some light on how best to support such individuals. Finally, research on the career choices of recent immigrants and their offspring may shed some light on current trends regarding which industries are favored by Arab Americans.

Conclusion

Arab immigrants have historically experienced a high degree of economic and educational success in the United States. Many factors have contributed to their resilience and successful acculturation, including the presence of a strong community orientation and deeply held cultural values endorsing education and career achievement. However, sociopolitical factors following September 11, 2001, have created a climate of heightened suspicion and discrimination toward Arab Americans in both schools and employment settings. Both the maintenance of traditional values, such as family cohesiveness, education, economic success, and religion as well as resilience in adapting to the current sociopolitical climate, will support Arab Americans' ability to experience success and fulfillment in the United States.

References

Abel, J. (2005). Americans under attack: The need for federal hate crime legislation in light of post-September 11 attacks on Arab Americans and Muslims. *Asian Law Journal, 12*, 41–65.

Abu El-Haj, T. R. (2006). Race, politics, and Arab American youth: Shifting frameworks for conceptualizing educational equity. *Educational Policy, 20*, 13–30.

Abu El-Haj, T. R. (2009). Becoming citizens in an era of globalization and transnational migration: Re-imagining citizenship as critical practice. *Theory into Practice, 48*, 274–282.

Abudabbeh, N. (1996). Arab families. In M. McGoldrick, J. Giordano, & J. Pearce (Eds.), *Ethnicity and family therapy* (pp. 333–347). New York: Guilford.

Abu-Ras, W., & Abu-Bader, S. H. (2009). Risk factors for depression and posttraumatic stress disorder (PTSD): The case of Arab and Muslim Americans Post 9/11. *Journal of Immigrant & Refugee Studies, 7*, 393–418.

Ajrouch, K. J. (2000). Place, age, and culture: Community living and ethnic identity among Lebanese American adolescents. *Small Group Research, 31*, 447–469.

Al-Hazza, T. C., & Bucher, K. T. (2008). Building Arab Americans' cultural identity and acceptance with children's literature. *The Reading Teacher, 62*, 210–219.

Al-Khatab, A. (2000). In search of equity for Arab-American students in public schools of the United States. *Education, 120*, 254–266.

Allen, J. R. (1998). Of resilience, vulnerability, and a woman who never lived. *Child and Adolescent Psychiatric Clinics of North America, 7*, 53–71.

Al-Romi, N. H. (2000). Muslims as a minority in the United States. *International Journal of Educational Research, 33*, 631–638.

Arab American Institute. (2002). *Healing the nation: The Arab American experience after September 11*. Retrieved from http://aai.3cdn.net/64de7330dc475fe470_h1m6b0yk4.pdf

Beiten, B. K., & Allen, K. R. (2005). Resilience in Arab American couples after September 11, 2001: A systems perspective. *Journal of Marital and Family Therapy, 31*, 251–267.

Belfiore, P. J., Lee, D. L., Spicer, E., & Dexter, D. (2008). Resilience in the classroom: The role of behavioral momentum. In D. H. Molina (Ed.), *School psychology: 21st century issues and challenges* (pp. 213–233). New York: Nova Science.

Berry, J. W., & Sam, D. L. (1997). Acculturation and adaptation. In J. W. Berry, M. H. Segall, & C. Kagitcibasi (Eds.), *Handbook of cross-cultural psychology* (pp. 291–326). Boston: Allyn & Bacon.

Brittingham, A., & de la Cruz, G. P. (2005). *We the people of Arab ancestry in the United States: Census 2000 special reports*. United States Census Bureau. Retrieved from http://www.census.gov/prod/2005pubs/censr-21.pdf

Britto, P. R. (2008). Who am I? Ethnic identity formation of Arab Muslim children in contemporary U.S. society. *Journal of the American Academy of Child and Adolescent Psychiatry, 47*, 853–857.

Britto, P. R., & Amer, M. (2007). An exploration of cultural identity patterns and the family context among Arab Muslim young adults in America. *Applied Developmental Science, 11*, 137–150.

Council on American-Islamic Relations. (2006). *Western Muslim minorities: Integration and disenfranchisement*. Retrieved from http://sun.cair.com/Portals/0/pdf/policy_bulletin_Integration_in_the_West.pdf

Council on American-Islamic Relations. (2008). *The status of Muslim civil rights in the United States: Without fear of discrimination*. Retrieved from www.cair.com/Portals/0/pdf/civilrights2008.pdf

Crabtree, S. A. (2010). Engaging students from the United Arab Emirates in culturally responsive education. *Innovations in Education and Teaching International, 47*, 85–94.

David, G. C., & Ayouby, K. K. (2005). Studying the exotic other in the classroom: The portrayal of Arab Americans in educational source materials. *Multicultural Perspectives, 7*, 13–20.

Davila, A., & Mora, M. (2005). Changes in the earnings of Arab men in the US between 2000 and 2002. *Journal of Population Economics, 18*(4), 587–601.

El-Araby Aly, A., & Ragan, J. F., Jr. (2010). Arab immigrants in the United States: How and why do returns to education vary by country of origin? *Journal of Population Economics, 23*, 519–538.

Gaad, E. E. N. (2001). Educating children with Down's syndrome in the United Arab Emirates. *British Journal of Special Education, 28*, 195–203.

Haboush, K. L. (2007). Working with Arab-American families: Culturally competent practice for school psychologists. *Psychology in the Schools, 44*, 183–198.

Haboush, K. L., Selman, J. S., & Sievering, K. (2008). Traumatized youth: New roles for school psychologists. In D. H. Molina (Ed.), *School psychology: 21st century issues and challenges* (pp. 117–155). New York: Nova Science.

Haj-Yahia, M. M. (2001). Culturally sensitive supervision of Arab social work students in Western universities. *Social Work, 42*, 166–173.

Hoot, J. L., Szecsi, T., & Moosa, S. (2003). What teachers of young children should know about Islam. *Early Childhood Education Journal, 31*, 85–90.

Jamil, H., Hakim-Larson, J., Farrag, M., Kafaji, T., Duqum, I., & Jamil, L. H. (2002). A retrospective study of Arab American mental health clients: Trauma and the Iraqi refugees. *The American Journal of Orthopsychiatry, 72*, 355–361.

Kovach, B. S., & Hillman, S. B. (2002). *African and Arab American achievement motivation: Effects of minority membership*. Paper presented at the 110th American Psychological Association Convention, Chicago, IL.

Lehr, C. A. (2004). *Positive school climate: Information for educators*. Retrieved from http://www.nasponline.org/communications/spawareness/schclimate__ho.pdf.

Lewandowski, L. A., Chiodo, L., Peterson, B., & Kira, I. (2007). *The effects of cumulative trauma on emotional and physical health, and risky behavior of adolescents: PTSD symptomatology and parental emotional support as mediators*. Paper presented at the 18th International Nursing Research Congress Focusing on Evidence-Based Practice, Vienna, Austria.

Malos, S. (2010). Post-9/11 backlash in the workplace: Employer liability for discrimination against Arab- and Muslim-Americans based on religion or national origin. *Employee Responsibilities and Rights Journal, 22*, 297–310.

Masten, A. S. (2007). Resilience in developing systems: Progress and promise as the fourth wave rises. *Development and Psychopathology, 19*, 921–930.

Masten, A. S., & Cicchetti, D. (2010). Developmental cascades. *Development and Psychopathology, 22*, 491–495.

Merrell, K. W., Ervin, R. A., & Gimpel, G. A. (2006). *School psychology for the 21st century: Foundations and practices*. New York: Guilford Press.

Merrell, K. W., Ervin, R. A., & Peacock, G. G. (2011). *School psychology for the 21st century (Second edition): Foundations and practices*. New York: Guilford Press.

Muhtaseb, A. (2007). From behind the veil: Students' resistance from different directions. *New Directions for Teaching and Learning, 110*, 25–33.
Naaf, A. (1985). *Becoming American: The early Arab immigrant experience*. Carbondale/Edwardsville, IL: Southern Illinois University Press.
Nassar-McMillan, S. C., & Hakim-Larson, J. (2003). Counseling considerations among Arab Americans. *Journal of Counseling and Development, 81*, 150–169.
Opdal, L. R., Wormnaes, S., & Habayeb, A. (2001). Teachers' opinions about inclusion: A pilot study in a Palestinian context. *International Journal of Disability, Development and Education, 48*, 143–162.
Orfalea, G. (2006). *The Arab Americans: A history*. Northampton, MA: Olive Branch Press.
Read, J. G., & Cohen, P. N. (2007). One size fits all? Explaining U.S.-born immigrant women's employment across 12 ethnic groups. *Social Forces, 85*, 1713–1734.
Read, J. G., & Oselin, S. (2008). Gender and the education-employment paradox in ethnic and religious contexts: The case of Arab Americans. *American Sociological Review, 73*, 296–313.
Sabry, N. S., & Bruna, R. K. (2007). Learning from the experience of Muslim students in American schools: Towards a proactive model of school-community cooperation. *Multicultural Perspectives, 9*, 44–50.
Saigh, P. A., Yasik, A. E., Oberfield, R. A., Halamandaris, P. V., & Bremner, J. (2006). The intellectual performance of traumatized children and adolescents with or without posttraumatic stress disorder. *Journal of Abnormal Psychology, 115*, 332–340.
Schwartz, W. (1999). Arab American students in public schools. *ERIC Digest, 142*, 1–7.
Seymour-Jorn, C. (2004). Arabic language learning among Arab immigrants in Milwaukee, Wisconsin: A study of attitudes and motivation. *Journal of Muslim Affairs, 24*, 109–122.
Shammas, D. S. (2009). Post-9/11 Arab and Muslim community college students: Ethno-religious enclaves and perceived discrimination. *Community College Journal of Research and Practice, 33*, 283–308.
Sheikh, M. F. (2009). *An exploratory study of the challenges of living in America as a Muslim adolescent attending public school*. Unpublished doctoral dissertation, Rutgers University, New Brunswick, NJ.
Sirin, S. R., & Fine, M. (2007). Hyphenated selves: Muslim American youth negotiating identities on the fault lines of global conflict. *Applied Developmental Science, 11*, 151–163.
South Asian American Leaders of Tomorrow. (2001). *American backlash: Terrorists bring home war in more ways than one*. Retrieved from www.saalt.org/attachments/1/American Backlash report.pdf
Suleiman, M. F. (2001). *Image making of Arab Americans: Implications for teachers in diverse settings*. Paper presented at the Annual Meeting of the California Association for Bilingual Education, Los Angeles, CA.
U.S. Census Bureau. (2000). *Selected population profile in the United States: Arab*. American Community Survey. Retrieved from http://factfinder2.census.gov/faces/tableservices/jsf/pages/productview.xhtml?pid=DE C_00_SF4_DP2&prodType=table
U.S. Census Bureau. (2010). *Selected population profile in the United States: Arab*. American Community Survey. Retrieved from http://factfinder2.census.gov/faces/tableservices/jsf/pages/productview.xhtml?pid=ACS_10_1YR_S0201&prodType=table
United States Department of Homeland Security. (2011). *Yearbook of immigration statistics: 2010*. Washington, DC: U.S. Department of Homeland Security, Office of Immigration Statistics. Retrieved from http://www.dhs.gov/xlibrary/assets/statistics/yearbook/2010/ois_yb_2010.pdf
Weiss, J. (2011). Classroom guide. *Saudi Aramco World, 62*, 44–45.
Wingfield, M. (2006). Arab Americans: Into the multicultural mainstream. *Equity & Excellence in Education, 39*, 253–266.
Yakushko, O., Backhaus, A., Watson, M., Ngaruiya, K., & Gonzalez, J. (2008). Career development concerns of recent immigrants and refugees. *Journal of Career Development, 34*, 362–396.
Zine, J. (2006). Unveiled sentiments: Gendered Islamophobia and experiences of veiling among Muslim girls in a Canadian Islamic school. *Equity and Excellence in Education, 39*, 239–252.

Chapter 12
Promoting Environmental Health in the Arab American Community

Hikmet J. Jamil

Promoting Environmental Health in the Arab American Community

Promoting environmental health in the Arab American community is based on understanding the background history of Arab Americans and the meaning of environmental health from a worldwide perspective. This chapter includes information about the background of Arab American immigrants as child development is affected by complex environmental factors as described by Urie Bronfenbrenner in his ecological theory (e.g., Bronfenbrenner, 1990, 1994). The theory describes five major environmental factors which have an impact on the child's development. These factors are: the microsystem (such as the family or classroom); the mesosystem (which is two microsystems in interaction); the exosystem (external environments which indirectly influence development, e.g., parental workplace); the macrosystem (the larger sociocultural context); and the chronosystem (the evolution of the external systems over time). Although this chapter will address environmental health in the Arab countries in general, the country of Iraq will be focused upon as a specific example of how information from Arab countries can enrich our knowledge of environmental health issues among Arab Americans in the USA.

This chapter also addresses the environmental health of individuals living within the Arab American community. Health is defined as a "state of complete physical, mental and social well-being and not merely the absence of disease or infirmity" (WHO, 1948, p. 100). Environmental health is defined as "the physical, chemical, and biological factors external to a person, and all of the related factors impacting behaviors. It encompasses the assessment and control of those environmental factors that can potentially affect one's health. It is targeted towards preventing disease and

H.J. Jamil (✉)
Wayne State University, 6530 Post Oak Drive,
West Bloomfield, MI 48322, USA
e-mail: hjamil@med.wayne.edu

S.C. Nassar-McMillan et al. (eds.), *Biopsychosocial Perspectives on Arab Americans: Culture, Development, and Health*, DOI 10.1007/978-1-4614-8238-3_12,

creating health-supportive environments" (WHO, 2012). This definition excludes behavior related to the social and cultural environment, and genetics, but it does include the work environment (WHO, 2012). The term "community" is defined as "social groups of any size whose members reside in a specific locality, share government, and often have common cultural and historical heritage. So any geographic area whose size should be determined by members includes economic, environmental, and social/cultural features of that area" (Hart, 1998). In summary, the goal of environmental health in the Arab American community means that Arab Americans need to understand how to overcome environmental hazards that could affect their health and consequently their productivity.

History of Arab American Communities

Arab Americans started to immigrate to the USA in the 1880s, and according to the Arab American Institute, there are at least 3.5 million Arab Americans (Arab American Institute, 2010). While Arab Americans live in all states, two thirds are concentrated in ten states. Of these, one third of the total lived in California, New York, and Michigan until the economic problems emerged in 2008. Since 2008, immigrants including Iraqi refugees, started to move to whatever State gave them the best chance to get work. Environmental health issues affected each succeeding wave of Arab American immigrants as discussed further below.

The first wave was between 1870s and 1924 when people emigrated from greater Syria (Syria, Lebanon, and Palestine), because they were the ones most affected by the wars in that region at that time. The reasons for immigration were both political, marked by the fall of the Ottoman Empire, as well as economic (Arab American Institute, 2011; Malvasi, 2006). Only 5–10 % of all Arab immigrants at that time were Muslims, and an even smaller fraction were Druze, an ethnic group who lived mainly in Lebanon, Syria and Israel (Naff, 1985). The settlement of this first wave of immigrants carries several problems as they came from countries which were lacking in public health and environmental health policies. Such deficiency could have been reflected in their settlement behavior once they arrived in the USA. This might have been the case especially if they were already suffering from health problems, or if they had to adjust to a new industrial work environment which they had never before been exposed to. Prior to immigration, large numbers from this first wave were farmers in their country of origin. After immigration, many had to work in industry which may have exposed them to various environmental hazards.

The second wave period, which occurred during the Great Depression, was much slower due to restrictive quotas on immigration to the USA from the 1920s to the 1940s. The 1948 Arab–Israeli War resulted in the displacement of over 750,000 Palestinians, out of a population of 1.3 million (Orfalea, 2006). From then until 1966, only 80,000 Arabs, primarily Palestinian and Egyptian, officially immigrated to the USA (Orfalea, 2006). While 90 % of first wave Arab immigrants were Christian, only 40 % professed Christianity in the second wave (Orfalea, 2006). Moreover, this group tended to be better educated and had a better financial status than the first wave immigrants (Arab American Institute, 2010). Those who emigrated in the second wave were susceptible to occupational and environmental hazards because of their lack of knowledge about the dangers which could affect their health in their new place of settlement (Haddad & Lummis, 1987).

The third wave period began when the USA passed new immigration reforms allowing a new wave of Arab Americans immigrants. Between 1967 and 2003 over 750,000 Arab immigrants came to the USA, due to Arab–Israeli conflicts, widespread "intra-Arab warfare", and a general increase in regional tensions (Orfalea, 2006). Islamism in the Middle East also resulted in a reduction of the native Christian populations (Kayyali, 2006). A large proportion of the immigrants were Palestinians and Iraqis (Orfalea, 2006). Many Iraqi immigrants during this time were Christians known as Chaldeans. For instance, between1960 and 2003 in Southeastern Michigan, the Iraqi Christian community grew from 3,000 to 80,000, out of a total population of around 150,000 Iraqi Christians in the USA (Orfalea, 2006).

In summary, in the third wave, more Arabs came from the war-torn and politically unstable countries in the Middle East to the USA (Abraham & Abraham, 1983). Some of them held student or work visas. Again, those who emigrated were suffering from several issues, including a lack of knowledge about public health and environmental health policy. The Arab countries were unable to implement such health policies for several reasons, such as a lack of trained professionals in public and environmental health.

Many Arab immigrants in the USA settled in enclaves to be near their relatives or friends. Such settlements led to the establishment of several communities based on ethnicity or religion. This tended to isolate these immigrants from the general American community. Such community establishments allowed individuals to behave as if they were still living in their country of origin. Lack of understanding of the public health and environmental policies of the USA resulted in this new group of Arab immigrants being exposed to several health problems and environmental hazards which may have affected their health and productivity.

In the years that followed the September 11, 2001 terrorist attacks, it was expected that America would see a decline in immigration from Arab regions. However, demographic information actually shows that immigration has not been affected by the attacks, and Arab Americans continue to make up a steady 4 % of immigrants (Brittingham & de la Cruz, 2005). While there are around 3.5 million Arab Americans estimated to live in the USA, Arab Americans are one of the fastest-growing immigrant groups, mainly due to the wars and political unrest in the Middle East. Almost 490,000 of the 3.5 million live in Michigan alone, and of those more than one-third (36 %) identify Lebanon as their country of origin (Abraham & Shryock, 2000; Arab American Institute, 2005; Rice et al., 2006).

A Personal History of Environmental Health Research with Arab Americans

I served as a primary health care physician in Iraq during the period 1964–1972. Then, I traveled to the UK and spent 6 years specializing in occupational and environmental health. After returning to Iraq in 1978, I noticed that the occupational and environmental health and safety knowledge among community people was limited or absent not only in Iraq, but in other Arab countries. This need for information led me to attempt to disseminate this knowledge to the Arab communities in Iraq and other Arab countries through different means over a period of about 20 years before I immigrated to the USA. Assessment surveys examining the needs of the people in Iraq and other Arab countries were undertaken during this time (Jamil, 1982, 1995; Jamil & Ismail, 1994), and personal communications and interactions took place with specialists who work in the environmental health departments in different Arab countries. Results of the surveys and my communication with other professionals consistently showed that the local communities generally lacked awareness of environmental health issues even though most, if not all of the Arab countries had signed all of the regulations issued by World Health Organization (WHO)/International Labor Office (ILO) regarding occupational and environmental health. However, the subject of environmental health and safety was not included in the syllabi of any level of primary or secondary education institutions in the Arab countries, with the exception of a few titles related to public health. This information explains why the Arab American community in the 1990s and into the 2000s needed special programs on public and environmental health; they had never before been exposed to such knowledge. Also, there were no post-graduate studies of environmental health and safety in most Arab countries; only Egypt and Tunisia had established a Diploma (1 year course) for physicians and non-physicians that allowed them to work in the industries and governmental offices as inspector officers. However, in Egypt, Cairo University, College of Medicine and Ein Shams University, College of Medicine went a bit further and established postgraduate studies (MSc and PhD). These programs attracted people from different Arab countries to study in this area (A. Masoud, personal communication, February 1984). The survey assessment (Jamil, 1982) also showed a few environmental health and safety specialists in some Arab countries who had their degrees from Europe or the USA. However, most if not all of those who held postgraduate degrees were holding administrative positions at governmental offices to run issues related to occupational, environmental health and safety with no or very limited awareness about health and environmental hazards within the community.

Occupational, Environmental Health and Safety Activities in Arab Countries 1978–1997

Based upon the "needs assessment survey" (Jamil, 1982), and on personal communication with department chairs and directors in Jordan, Syria, Iraq, and Egypt, an occupational, environmental health and safety syllabus was added to the curriculum of different undergraduate and postgraduate studies for physician and non-physician students. Contacts included the chair of the department of community medicine, Jordan University; the director of the Institute of Occupational Safety and Health, Jordan-Amman; the chair of the department of community medicine, Damascus

University; the director of the Institute of Occupational Safety and Health, Syria-Damascus; the director of the division of occupational and environmental medicine, Ain Shames University; and the director of the Institute of Safety, Iraq-Baghdad, who was trained in Egypt-Cairo at WHO/ILO Institute. The nonprofit scientific organization, The Iraqi Society of Occupational Health and Safety (ISOHS), was established in 1991 and took responsibility for publishing a monthly newspaper (ISOHS, 1992) and holding short courses in occupational, environmental health and safety. Media presentations and numerous publications of scientific studies based on existing occupational, environmental health, and safety problems were submitted and disseminated to relevant professionals and officials. Relevant recommendations were made to the policy makers. Also, eight conferences and several workshops and seminars about different occupational, environmental health and safety related topics were held during a 10-year period, and more than 79 oral presentations were given at different national (e.g., Egypt, Libya, Yemen, Jordan, UAE, Kuwait, Sudan, Syria, Tunis) and international (e.g., India, Finland, Ireland, USSR, Singapore, Japan) scientific meetings (seminars, workshops, conferences).

Changing the behavior of people in the Arab countries toward a healthier lifestyle and living environment is not easy. Many Arab governments have still not implemented an educational curriculum which would lead children to adopt the knowledge that would help them live in a healthy environment. Theories such as Bronfenbrenner's (1994) hold promise because they emphasize the importance of the broader social environment on the child. For example, the governments of Arab countries could provide support for nonprofit organizations or any educational institute that demonstrates interest in disseminating knowledge about occupational, environmental health, and safety issues through an internet webpage, Face book, YouTube, television, radio and cellular phone applications. This approach would make the information more accessible to the youth and even younger children. Thus, the new generation will grow up with a better understanding of why it is important to live in a healthy environment. The initial steps described in the above activities were undertaken to increase the awareness of people about possible personal health hazards which could arise from not following environmental health policies.

Author Activities in the USA (1997–2011)

Since moving to Michigan in 1997, the State with the most densely populated Arab American community, I have continued pursuing the dream of increasing awareness within this community about healthy environments, especially among the younger generation who will have an impact in the future on the policy makers on issues related to environmental health. However, the success of this goal depended on securing collaboration with others who were concerned and who shared the final goal of leading the Arab American people to be healthier and more productive. To achieve a healthy environment for Arab American communities in the USA, living conditions were studied in as much depth as possible, including demography, socioeconomic status, life style, and health behaviors. This was achieved through involvement in community based studies and community activities. This included joining with the Arab Community Center for Economic and Social Services (ACCESS), the Arab American and Chaldean Council (ACC), Chaldean American Association for Health Professionals (CAAHP), National Arab American Medical Association (NAAMA), a church parish, mosques, and the Wayne State University Department of Family Medicine and Public Health Sciences. Additional research collaborators since 1998 include the American Chaldean Federation (ACF), Lutheran Social Services of Michigan (LSSM), Kurdish Human Right Watch (KHRW), the US Committee for Refugees and Immigrants (USCRI), Centro Multicultural La Familia (CMLF), and Catholic Services of Macomb (CSM). In addition to more than 48 scholarly research publications among Arab Americans who are residents in Michigan, other activities included participating in several environmental health related community events, writing articles for local magazines (e.g., Jamil, 2003) and speaking for several radio broadcast programs (e.g., Channel MZK 667) to increase the awareness of people on topics related to environmental health problems in the Arab American community.

Methodological Approaches to Environmental Health and Education

Environmental health education in general is part of the larger educational reform process that is taking place in many parts of the world, including the Arab countries. There are many gaps in basic educational data available to the public and the information given is often outdated. In view of the general crisis of education in the Arab world (Jamil, Mukliis, & Al-Habboubi, 1981), it is not surprising to know that most Arab immigrants lived either their early lives or part of their lives in Arab countries where the level of environmental health education and awareness was fairly low in comparison to levels in other areas of the world such as the USA. Also, there was no implementation of health and safety or environmental health policies by the governments of many Arab countries. This resulted in a lack of knowledge among the general Arab population including many Arab immigrants to the USA. However, efforts are continuing to be made to address this problem. The objectives of environmental health education at this level are to establish a relationship between the individual and his or her natural and social environment, to help children and youth to gain skills, direction, and values pertaining to environmental health problems and responsibilities, and to align behavior in a positive and interactive way towards environmental health (Jamil et al., 1981). The effort to promote the environmental health of the Arab people will be based on the knowledge of health behavior and health education theory (Glanz, Rimer, & Viswanath, 2008), and on several community based studies on environmental health and safety, which I conducted in Iraq and in Jordan. These studies showed that workers and the people in the community were suffering from various health problems because they did not know how to protect themselves from hazards at work or present in their surrounding environment (Abdel-Khaleq & Jamil, 1996; Jamil, Al-Tawil, & Radhi, 1989; Jamil, Al-Timimi, Al-Ghabban, & Qasim, 1987). These studies also indicated that there was a lack of occupational and environmental health and safety policies both at work and in the community.

Although the results of these studies cannot be generalized to all Arab countries, we know that Iraqis and Jordanians share several environmental health and safety issues in common with other Arab countries. For example, a WHO report indicates that the prevalence of tobacco smoking is high in most Arab countries as compared to Europe or the USA (WHO, 2010); also, they share a sedentary life style, eating unhealthy diets, worksite and motor vehicle injuries, family and gun violence, non-adherence to prescribed medicine, and drug abuse. Additionally they share language, religions, background history, culture, and ethnicity. Therefore, we can speculate that these results may be representative in most if not all Arab countries. These studies concluded with recommendations toward a healthy environment. For example, road traffic accidents have been identified as a public health problem in Arab countries, and in many, it is counted as the leading cause of death among the general population (Jamil et al., 1981; Jamil & Arabiat, 1999), which suggests that the basics of road safety are still below the WHO standard road precautions (Al-Ani & Jamil, 1991; Jamil 1986a, 1986b; Jamil, Amen, & Farhoud, 1986). In addition, the numbers of work-related injuries among factory workers are also very high, according to the mean rate of work related injury published by WHO which indicates that the workers and/or the employers do not follow or enforce the safety regulations. In general, there appear to be difficulties in the implementation of the regulations and laws of occupational and environmental health and safety in the work place; there may also be difficulties in the qualifications of the personnel who are considered specialists in environmental health or occupational safety and hygiene (Jamil, 1984, 1985a, 1985b, 1986a, 1986b; Jamil & Ali, 1989; Jamil & Hussen, 1989). A high number of accidents were reported in elementary schools which indicate that safety regulations for children are not enforced (Jamil, Abdulla, Al-Noorachi, & Saeed, 1983).

Also, the work environment of most factories were determined to be unhealthy regarding high exposure to health hazardous materials based on blood level or urine level of the agent that the workers were handling in their respective occupations. In most cases, the amount of the identifying agent was well above threshold levels, which indicated that no environmental control regulations were implemented in those factories, and that the workers themselves were not aware of the hazards, and therefore could take no precautions. Studies examining the blood levels of several toxic agents in the blood of workers showed for example that lead is one of the major air contaminant in all Arab countries, because of the prevalent use of leaded gasoline in most Arab countries. This means that vulnerable groups are at a high risk of lead poisoning (Al-Ajzan, Jamil, & Tman, 1990; Al-Timimi, Jamil, & Abu-Tommam, 1988; Jamil, Al-Timimi, Al-Ajzan, & Al-Ghabban, 1991; Jamil,

Al-Timimi, Al-Ghabban, & Al-Niami, 1987; Jamil, Al-Timimi, Al-Ghabban, & Qasim, 1987).

Similar or different hazards were found among workers who deal with other elements such as chromium (Abdel-Khaleq & Jamil, 1996; Al-Shamma, Ismall, & Jamil, 1985; Al-Tawil, Al-Shamma, Ismal, Fakhre, & Jamil, 1988); nickel (Jamil, Al-Tawil, & Radhi, 1989); mercury (Al-Shammary & Jamil, 1992); and fluoride (Petrus & Jamil, 1993). Other studies in the community showed that contact dermatitis was more prevalent in Arab countries as compared to European countries (Hussien & Jamil, 1992; Jamil & Aziz, 1985; Jamil & Haboubi, 1992; Jamil, Haboubi, & Alrawi, 1989; Jamil & Jamil, 1994). Other indications of an unhealthy environment in Arab countries are the high numbers of smokers. WHO reports indicate that 77 % of adult men and 35 % of adult women in Arab countries used tobacco, which is much higher than that in Europe and the USA (WHO, 2010). These results were confirmed by several studies conducted not only in Iraq (Jamil, Haboubi, & Al-Tikriti, 1989; Jamil, Mukhlis, & Al-Tikriti, 1991; Jamil, Mukhlis, & Jamil, 1992), but also from WHO data.

An additional three field surveys on health and environmental health were conducted in different villages by faculty staff from different colleges at the University of Baghdad during the summers of 1993–1995. The results of these studies indicated that only 40 % of people drink clean water, 17–43 % were illiterate, and 55–70 % of the study samples reported themselves as healthy. Most of the children (97 %) were under fed and 12–21 % of the women were anemic (Hussain, Jamil, & Al-Sharbtti, 1996; Jamil, 1995; Jamil & Ismail, 1994). The general environment of these villages included housing, roads, electricity, and sewage systems that were found to be primitive. Most of the people worked on farms without any knowledge of the hazards of pesticides or the equipment they were using. Also, there was not a single safety measure that could be found in the villages. All of these observations indicated that the people who live in rural areas in Iraq are far from having any knowledge of environmental problems, and how it may have impacted their health or well-being. After 1991 and again in 2005, large numbers of people from these villages immigrated to the USA for various reasons and most of them settled in Michigan.

Our studies also involved identifying common health problems to understand public knowledge of diseases in general and chronic diseases in particular, so as to establish awareness programs. Studies were conducted among workers at different factories. The topic of these studies was based on factory physician suggestions while other studies were conducted among people in the community to identify some common illnesses. The studies conducted in Iraq (one in Jordan) addressed general illnesses among factory workers; varicose veins; back-pain hypertension; diabetes (Hussien & Jamil, 1993a, 1993b); occupational diseases (El-Khawaldeh & Jamil, 1994; Jamil & Jamil, 1994); brucellosis; and mortality in Iraq (Hermis, Mohammed, & Jamil, 1993; Mohammed, Hermis, & Jamil, 1993). These studies reflect the lack of environmental health education among the Iraqi and Jordanian people. However, WHO studies conducted in some of the other Arab countries support what was found in Iraq especially when we examine the prevalence of tobacco smoking in all Arab countries, the use of lead gas in the cars, or the prevalence of automobile injuries compare to Europe and USA (WHO, 2002, 2011).

We may conclude that people from the Arab world are not aware of the possible impact of environmental pollutants that many of them were exposed to. This lack of environmental health education is only part of the general suffering and neglect that people of these countries have faced. Among this list are substandard income, lack of religious freedom, exposure to violence and trauma, issues related to their daily life such as fear of having male children conscripted and sent to war at age 18 (Ai, Peterson & Ubelhor, 2002; Genesee County Health Department, 2003). All of these factors help to explain both the legal and illegal behavior of Arab immigrants as they seek to resettle in countries where they feel that the quality of living will be much better, especially for their children. Arab immigrants entering the USA, already carry with them a host of problems that greatly affect their environmental health. A lot of effort from health professionals, community leaders, societies or associations, including the nonprofit organizations is spent to achieve the dream of Arab Americans living in a healthy environment. In spite of all of these studies being conducted during the last 20 years, the present situation does not seem to be improved. If anything, it seems to have gotten worse in Iraq, Palestine, Egypt, Yemen, Libya, and Syria, based on my direct contact with academic institutions concerned with occupational, environmental health and safety in the Arab countries. After immigrating to the USA, I have made frequent visits to several Arab countries including Iraq, Egypt, Syria, Lebanon, Jordan, Kuwait, Qatar, United Arab Emirates, and Dubai to observe and learn more about the status of the environmental health problems of these countries.

I have come to the conclusion, based on studies done in Iraq and Jordan and the reports based on studies published by WHO, that people in these countries will continue to suffer the consequences of an unhealthy ecology, because most of the laws and regulations related to a healthy environment especially at the workplace are not seriously enforced. This is primarily due to a lack of dedicated specialists in the field of environmental health or occupational safety and hygiene. To make matters worse, the workers receive very little education in the topics of environmental health and occupational, health and safety during their education at school or during job training. Also, to my knowledge, very little effort has been made to include safety precautions and to identify risks in job descriptions. There are still no safety brochures or manuals provided, even to workers in high risk positions, as is the case in Europe or the USA, so that they understand what precautions they should take at work in order to avoid any work hazards.

Environmental Health of Arab Americans in the State of Michigan

Based on the previous section, we know that there are many environmental health risks that have faced the non-US born Arab Americans in their countries of origin. This prompted me to conduct an assessment survey of needs in different areas of environmental health hazards in order to understand the present situation that Arab Americans in Michigan are facing compared to other major ethnic groups and the American population at large. The primary purpose here is to provide policy makers with recommendations and suggestions about what is needed to increase the awareness of Arab Americans to environmental health hazards they might face, in order to achieve healthier behaviors. Working with non-profit community organizations and Wayne State University, as well as being involved in community based research, community activities, community services, mosques and parish councils has increased our understanding of what Arab Americans need to improve their environmental health culture. A number of community based studies were conducted with Arab Americans and other ethnic groups, but in this chapter special attention is given to topics related to environmental hazards (e.g., air pollution with metal elements, and smoking), chronic disease (e.g., asthma, heart diseases, diabetes, depression, and obesity), and the Hepatitis C virus as major public health problems among people in Arab countries (WHO, 2010). The results of these studies highlight the differences in the environment of Arab Americans compared to that of other ethnicities.

Environmental, Occupational Health and Safety

The term "special populations at risk" has been defined as workers "more likely to experience increased risks of diseases and injuries in the workplace as a result of biologic, social, and/or economic characteristics such as age, race, genetic susceptibility, disability, language barrier, literacy, culture, and low income" (CDC, 2005, 2009). One study demonstrated that the incidence of traumatic injuries, particularly those which are work-related, were higher among Arab Americans in Wayne County, compared to the number of injuries of other ethnic groups working in other areas of Michigan (Johnson, 1995). We examined the general knowledge of occupational health and safety of 300 Arab Americans people who attended a non-profit community organization for different reasons. Scores were lower in men who only spoke Arabic, were born in Arab countries, and had never worked in the USA before. Arab American job seekers have been found to be at a low level of occupational health and safety knowledge (Jamil, Simpson, Upfal, Blessman, & Hammad, 2003).

Air Pollution with Trace Heavy Elements

The Arab American community continues to grow over the years in the Southeastern part of the Detroit metropolitan area of Michigan, a birthplace of the automotive industry which has led to other related industries in the area (Savoie & Nriagu, 1999). Large quantities of pollutants have been released into the local ecosystem for nearly 100 years. Most Arab Americans in Southeastern Michigan live and work in close proximity to the Ford Rouge Plant, and have thus been exposed to high levels of air pollutants, including traces of different types of heavy metals and lung irritant dusts (Environment Protective Agency (EPA), 1996; Savoie & Nriagu, 1999). Literature reveals that clips of toenails are often used as a biomarker of exposures, as many of these dangerous elements bind well to keratin, the fibrous proteins present in the nails (Hopps, 1976). In a study (Slotnck, Nriagu, Johnson, Jamil, & Hammad, 2005) of trace elements (Al, V, Cr, Mn, Co, Ni, Cu, As, Se, Mo, Cd, Ba, Tl, and Pb) in toenails of 263 Arab Americans in the Detroit, there was a noticeably elevated level of Ni, in addition to significant differences in the mean concentration of Al, V, Cr, Mn, Cd, Pb, and Se. The results provide insight into exposures and factors such as socioeconomic status, diet, and factors related to culturally conditioned risk behavior, which all could influence exposures in this population. Differences in nickel were found based on the country of origin with those from Iraq having significantly higher levels than those from Lebanon. City of residence also made a difference in lead levels with those in the more industrialized Hamtramck having higher lead levels than those in Oak Park, Michigan.

Lead

Lead (Pb) was used for years in many popular and cheap products such as house-paint and toys (e.g., Scelfo & Flegal, 2000). Although most of these products are not using lead any more, at least in the USA, childhood lead exposure still persists (Brody, Pirkle, & Kramer, 1994; Detroit Department of Health and Wellness Promotion, 2005). Children under 5 years old are especially susceptible to the effects of lead exposure (CDC, 2005; Cohen Hubal et al., 2000). In Michigan in 2004, the estimated prevalence of lead poisoning was around 6 % of all children aged 6 years or younger who were tested for blood lead (Detroit Department of Health and Wellness Promotion, 2005). Immigrants and refugees are often of low socioeconomic status, and usually reside in low income areas such as Detroit or Hamtramck in Michigan, where old leaded paintchips may still be present in and around homes. A study was conducted on clients who attend Women Infant Child (WIC) clinic to examine multiple sources of environmental lead exposure, as it is still one of the most important hazardous elements to children in low income communities, as it affects the mental development of young children (Nriagu, Senthamarai-Kannan, Jamil, Fakhori, & Korponic, 2011). The study explored the hypothesis that level of acculturation is a risk factor for childhood lead poisoning in the Detroit area of Michigan. Blood lead levels (BLLs) were determined in 429 Arab American and African American children, aged 6 months to 15 years, who were receiving well-child examinations. Mean BLL was 3.8 ± 2.3 lg/dL (range: 1–18 lg/dL) and 3.3 % of the children tested had blood lead values above the 10 lg/dL level of concern. Neither the age of the dwelling units nor ethnicity of the child was significantly associated with the BLL. Acculturation-related factors that were associated with blood lead levels included paternal education, language spoken at home, home ownership, smoking in the home, and exposure of child to home health remedies. The blood lead level was higher among Arab American children from families who spoke Arabic language only versus children whose families spoke Arabic and English at home. This study provides information showing that immigrant children may be at heightened risk of being poisoned by lead which can be useful in identifying groups at risk of atypical exposures. With a geographic information system, we identified two possible high risk areas marked by poor housing conditions, low income residents and predominantly ethnic minorities (Nriagu et al., 2011). The study also showed that housing problems (e.g., houses built before 1970, most probably painted with paints containing lead) and child behavioral characteristics (e.g., children with pica syndrome) were related to potential risk factors favoring lead poisoning. If the adult community of Arab Americans was made more aware of prevention strategies, the risk of lead poisoning to children could be reduced.

Smoking

Unfortunately, many Arab Americans brought their smoking habits with them when they came to the USA, as smoking is an acceptable social and cultural behavior in Arab countries (Shafey, 2007), and smoking inside the home is considered to be within the range of common behaviors (Al-Omari & Scheibmeir, 2009). Offering a cigarette or hookah to someone is considered hospitable in Arab countries (Kulwicki & Rice, 2003; Lewis, 1995; Yadav & Thakur, 2000). Tobacco is still a major public health risk in many developing countries, with some studies reporting a high prevalence: Iraq (40 %), Palestine (48 %), Kuwait (52 %), Saudi Arabia (53 %), Lebanon (58 %), Jordan (65 %), and Tunisia (76 %) (Jamil, Haboubi, & Al-Tikriti, 1989; WHO, 2005). Several studies of tobacco smoking were conducted among Arab Americans of different age groups including youth in Michigan (Aswad, 2001; Kulwicki & Dervartanian, 1995; Rice & Kulwicki, 1992; Weglicki, Templin, Rice, Jamil, & Hammad, 2008). These studies showed that the number of hookah smokers among Arab Americans ranged between 17 % and 38 % versus non-Arab Americans (21 %). The prevalence of cigarette smoking ranged between 29 and 34 %, which is much higher than that of non-Arab Americans, and those who smoke both cigarettes and hookah was about 18.8 %. Other studies (Rice, 2006; Rice et al., 2006) show that there are a variety of personal, psychological, sociocultural, and environmental predictors in tobacco use for Arab Americans adolescents. Among these predictors are: friends or siblings who smoke, mother born in USA, being male, receiving offers of tobacco, and three or more people who smoke at home. Tobacco use by friends and family members was the strongest predictor of cigarette and hookah smoking.

Chronic Diseases

To better understand the general health of those residing in Arab American communities, it is necessary to consider the chronic diseases in the population. Arab Americans have worse health outcomes than do non-Hispanic Whites (Aswad, 2001; Dallo & James, 2000; de la Cruz & Brittingham, 2003; Jaber, Brown, & Hammad, 2003; Kridli, Herman, Brown, Fakhouri, & Jaber, 2005). However, the Arab American population is not a homogeneous group and is made up of individuals from various countries and regions (Brittingham & de la Cruz, 2005). Immigrants and refugees in general and Arab Americans in particular often have limited access to the health care system, so large numbers do not have health insurance because of low economic status (Refugee Council, 2011). All of these factors reflect the lack of health care, whether it is not a priority or not being able to afford private insurance, even although they know that they are suffering from different chronic diseases.

In a cross-sectional convenience sample study of community participants from Michigan, the overall age and sex adjusted prevalence of having one or more self-reported chronic conditions was 44 % (Jamil et al., 2009). The estimated number of chronic diseases was lower for Iraqi Christian (Chaldean) Americans as compared to those who identified themselves as Arab, White, or Black. Results also showed the frequency and proportion of individuals with zero, one, two, or three or more chronic conditions. Arab Americans were less likely to have one chronic condition as compared to Blacks or Whites. However, Arab Americans were more likely to have three or more chronic conditions compared to Blacks or Whites.

Asthma

Asthma is on the top of the list of chronic diseases in relation to environmental pollution (Meliker et al., 2001). In addition, asthma has been related to lifestyle factors and decreased ventilation in residencies (Magnusser, Jorres, & Nowak, 1993; Von Mutius et al., 1994). A study of Arab Americans living in metro Detroit showed that environmental risk factors and surrogates for socioeconomic status were found to be predictors of asthma prevalence among Arab American (Johnson, Nriagu, Hammad, Savoie, & Jamil, 2005). These variables may reflect environmental exposures in communities involved in this study. The results also show the main asthma triggers (perfumes, cleaning supplies, dust, pets, air pollution, pollens, trees, fresh cut grass, mold, smoke, cockroaches, and certain foods) detected in the Arab American community. Asthma prevalence was highest among the moderately acculturated immigrants in comparison to new immigrants, and those who were well acculturated. This suggests that risk factors associated with new immigrant status have been replaced by Western risk factors as this population becomes more acculturated

(Beasley, Crane, Lai, & Pearce, 2000). Factors such as cultural beliefs, income, and low socioeconomic status may influence health care access and its utilization; also, problems associated with translocation and acculturation may exacerbate asthma symptoms among immigrants (Chaudhuri, 2004; Eggleston, 2000; Holguin et al., 2005; Nriagu et al., 1999; Rottem, Szyper-Kravitz, & Shoenfeld, 2005; Sandel & Wright, 2006).

Environmental health problems among Arab Americans were recognized for the first time when the Arab American Environmental Health Project was initiated, and its results clearly displayed the impact of environmental pollution on asthma, obesity, and hypertension (Johnson, Nriagu, Hammad, Savoie, & Jamil, 2008). It is important to note that this does not mean other ethnic groups are not affected by the same factors (Braman, 2006; LeNoir, 1999; Rana, Nieuwdorp, Jukema, & Kastelein, 2007). There is some evidence that shows that immigrant status may be related to asthma (Holguin et al., 2005; Rottem et al., 2005), as well as metabolic and cardiovascular health problems (Gilbert & Khokhar, 2008; Wylie-Rosett, Mossavar-Rahmani, & Gans, 2002). In the results of the health assessment survey, asthma prevalence was lower in Arab Americans than in non-Middle Eastern Whites. Such differences could be due to genetic or environmental risk factor which could exacerbate asthma (Jamil et al., 2011) especially since we know that asthma prevalence differs between countries, as well as between populations within the same country (Arif, Delclos, & Serra, 2006; Moorman et al., 2007).

Diabetes

Diabetes mellitus is one of the public health problems that disproportionately affect minorities (Junga, 2006; Norman, 2006). The prevalence of self-reported diabetes among Arab Americans in Michigan ranges from 7.0 to 23.0 % (Jaber et al., 2003; Jaber, Slaughter, & Grunberger, 1995), in comparison to 9.3 % in the US population (Cowie, Rust, & Byrd-Hold, 2006). In one study comparing the prevalence of diabetes among different ethnic groups, the sex- and age-adjusted prevalence of diabetes was found to be lower for Chaldeans as compared to Arabs, Whites, and Blacks residing in Southeast Michigan (Jamil et al., 2008). However, after adjusting for all demographic background covariates, this association between ethnicity and diabetes was not statistically significant. This suggests that there are no differences in the prevalence of self-reported diabetes when comparing Chaldeans, Arabs and Blacks to Whites in Michigan. These results were inconsistent with that of another study conducted by Cook and Rafferty (2005) in which Blacks showed higher rates of diabetes than Whites in Michigan. The differences in the prevalence of diabetes between the Cook and Rafferty (2005) study and the Jamil, Fakhouri et al. (2008) study may be due to differences in the samples and the sampling designs. In addition, the study by Cook and Rafferty (2005) compared Blacks to Whites, while the Jamil, Fakhouri et al. (2008) study included Chaldeans and Arabs. The "White" group in the Cook and Rafferty (2005) may have included some Chaldeans and Arabs, while in the Jamil, Fakhouri et al. (2008) study,

Chaldeans and Arabs were specifically identified. Also, the Cook and Rafferty (2005) study is a population-based telephone survey, while the Jamil, Fakhouri et al. (2008) study was a self-administered convenience sample.

Heart Disease

Heart disease also disproportionately affects minority women (Lethbridge-Cejku & Vickerie, 2006). The prevalence of self-reported heart disease among Arab Americans in two studies was 3.7 % (Hassoun, 1995) and 7.6 % (Aswad, 2001). The overall prevalence of heart disease was 5.1 %. Estimates of prevalence were higher for Arab Americans (7.1 %), lower for Christian (Chaldean) Iraqi Americans (6.6 %), and lowest among African Americans (1.8 %) (Jamil, Fakhouri et al., 2008). However, there was shown to be no difference between these groups in relation to heart disease after adjusting for factors like socioeconomic status, healthcare characteristics, chronic conditions, and health behaviors. It is possible that occupational and environmental hazards can have an impact on heart disease (Steenland, Johnson & Nowlin, 1997).

Depression

Somatic or psychological symptoms of depression and the ability of health professionals to detect it in ethnic minorities vary worldwide (Bhugra & Mastrogianni, 2004). Histories of trauma and stress exposure have been linked to depression in both African Americans (Alim, Graves, & Mellman, 2006) and Arab Americans, and may account for some of the variance in depression that is typically observed within and across primary care settings in urban communities (Jamil et al., 2002). Depression is the second leading cause of disability in the USA (Apfeldorf & Alexopoulos, 2003) and it is predicted to become the second leading cause of disability after heart disease worldwide by the year 2020 (Alim et al., 2006). In the Arab world, depression has been historically stigmatized (Dwairy, 2002; Jumaian, Alhmoud, & Al-Shunnaq, 2004). Persons suffering from depression relied on those in their immediate social network for help (El-Islam, 1984). Only after the failure of these efforts would the families seek outside professional assistance (Al-Issa, 2000). However, resistance may persist even today because of the associated stigma of potentially heritable mental illness (El-Sendiony, 1981). Recent reports of depression in clinical samples of Arab Americans have varied from 22.4 to 49 % (Jamil et al., 2002, 2005; Jamil, Nassar-McMillan, & Lambert, 2006). The most common factors associated with depression are chronic illnesses (Sherina, 2002) such as type 2 diabetes (Dorsey, Rodriguez, & Brathwaite, 2002), heart failure, age, sex, and race (Gottlieb, Khatta, & Friedmann, 2004). Patients with poorly controlled hypertension are more than six times as likely to suffer from depression as non-hypertensive patients (American Society of Hypertension, 2003). In a health assessment survey study (Jamil, Fakhouri et al., 2008) which was conducted at the Arab

American and Chaldean Council, Division of Public Health in 2005, 2,878 persons were chosen to study the prevalence of depression among Arab, Chaldean, and African American population. The overall prevalence of self-rated depression among study groups was 18.2 %. By ethnicity, Arab Americans had the highest prevalence of depression (23.2 %), compared to African Americans (15.0 %). By country of origin, Iraqis had the highest prevalence (36.8 %) followed by Palestinians (18.8 %), Lebanese (16.2 %), Christian (Chaldean) Iraqis (13.3 %), the Yemenis (12.3 %), and Jordanians (Jamil et al., 2006). In a representative US sample from 1988 to 1994, the lifetime prevalence of major depression was 9.5 % (Riolo, Nguyen, & Greden, 2005). Other studies (Jamil et al., 2002) among Arab Americans with mental health disorders showed that 49 % had depression as a primary disorder, and given that depression is often under-reported, our Arab American prevalence of 23.3 % may be credible (Jamil, Grzybowski et al., 2008). Another study of 116 Iraqi refugees attending a community clinic reported a 22.4 % prevalence of depression (Jamil et al., 2005).

There is a well-known association between depression and occupational injury. In one study (Peele & Tollerud, 2005), they found that depression may serve as a precursor to occupational injury for women. In another study (Lerner et al., 2011), productivity was most influenced by depression severity. However, depressive symptoms are associated with unemployment, absenteeism, low productivity, loss of family income, and increased costs and utilization of health care (Adler et al., 2006; Tsutsumi, Kayaba, Theorell, & Siegrist, 2001; Whooley et al., 2002).

Obesity

The body mass index of Arab Americans in Southeast Michigan was reported to be 30.4 ± 6.8 kg/m^2 (Jaber et al., 1995). This finding is consistent with 2006 Michigan data (28.8 %) and is slightly higher than the 2006 national data (25.1 %) (CDC, 2008). The prevalence of obesity did not differ by race/ethnicity group although the risk factors did vary. Among Arab Americans, the factors most closely associated with obesity were smoking, number of children less than18 years old in the house, available automotive transportation, and self-reported depression. Similar results have been found in a Southeastern Michigan-based Arab American study (Hatahet, Khosla, & Fungwe, 2002), which also assessed risk factors for heart disease, as well as in a Lebanese study (Ibai, Hwalla, & Adra, 2003; Sibai, Hwalla, Adra, & Rahal, 2003).

Critique and Chapter Summary

In summary, the outcome of this chapter indicates that a large percentage of Arab Americans, including Chaldean Americans, in the USA are still living under unhealthy environmental conditions. This could be explained by the following: Arab

Americans were born in countries that did not enforce laws and regulations related to environmental health and safety issues. Furthermore, according to the government and academic community medicine faculty members in the Arab world, individuals were not exposed in their native countries during the mandatory primary years of school to programs related to environmental health and safety apart from some elementary lessons in public health (T. Yousuf/Professor of Community Medicine at Al-Kindy medical college, University of Baghdad/personal communication, 2011; F. Lami/Associate Professor of Community Medicine at Baghdad Medical College, University of Baghdad/personal communication, December 11, 2011). They were not exposed to educational material related to occupational, environmental health and safety in high school and college in their native countries (A. Boran/Associate Professor of Occupational & Environmental Health at College of Medicine Irbid-Jordan/personal communication, May 29, 2010). In addition, most if not all, Arab Americans were not exposed to training courses related to occupational and/or environmental health and safety before starting jobs when they lived in their native countries. This might explain the high rates of work-related injuries in those countries in comparison to developed countries (WHO, 2009). Because of the lack of emphasis on environmental health issues, there is also a dearth of specialists in the fields of occupational and/or environmental health and safety in the Arab countries (A. Boran, personal communication, May 29, 2010; N. Yahea, personal communication, December 10, 2011).

Among Arab Americans who were not American-born, large numbers were forced to leave or flee their native countries for political reasons, oppressive dictatorships, civil and factional wars, armed conflicts with other countries, and economic hardships (Jamil et al., 2010). When arriving to the USA, they may not have merged readily with the wider community, but instead tended to isolate themselves from the general population for a variety of reasons. These reasons included a lack of language skills, lack of means of transportation, feelings of discrimination, facing difficulties in finding jobs, and holding diverse cultural and traditional values and norms (Arnetz, Rofa, Ventimiglia, Arnetz, & Jamil, 2013). This means that many Arab Americans continue to live with the same or similar environmental health risk factors that were prevalent in their native countries such as the habit of smoking (especially the hookah), eating more or less similar types of food, lack of exercise and avoiding mixing with the general population as large numbers of them refused to learn the English language. However, some Arab American immigrants and those who arrived on work or study visas have not accepted the American way of life as they feel that it clashes with their religious and moral beliefs (Aswad, 2001). Living in an unhealthy environment leads to a larger prevalence of many of the chronic diseases. In addition, asthma and smoking of tobacco and the hookah were found to be higher than the general population (Jamil et al., 2009, 2010, 2011).

In order to overcome these problems and achieve a healthier environment for Arab Americans in the USA in general and specifically in those cities and states where they form relatively big congregations (e.g., Dearborn, Michigan; California; New York; Chicago, Illinois), a number of recommendations have been made through studies conducted among Arab Americans, especially in Michigan.

Arab American community leaders in the field of environmental health can play a major role in achieving a healthy environment among Arab Americans. Scientifically approved need assessment studies (pilot studies) that target the Arab Americans community can provide the basis for financial support for programs initiated at the State and Federal levels. The pilot studies should be followed by community-based research involving Arab Americans. The research should target the community health problems in order to help Arab Americans live a better life and to assimilate with the general community of the USA, while preserving their cultural dignity and their personal beliefs and love for their native homeland. Arab American leaders from academia, scientific societies and associations, religious leaders, teachers, and others who are interested in environmental health, public health, and preventive medicine, should allocate some of their time (either as volunteers or as paid advisors) to work together on strategies and community based research studies to promote the achievement of healthy occupational and daily living environments for Arab Americans. All nonprofit organizations who serve Arab Americans should be invited to participate in these activities. Involvement of other Arab Americans community organizations or associations (e.g., social clubs, youth clubs, athletic clubs, art and educational clubs) is crucial because they are the core of the community gatherings and through them several activities could be implemented to achieve the goal of healthier environments. The collaboration of the decision makers who are responsible for approving programs related to healthy environment needs to be fostered. This includes Arab American leaders (as mentioned above) and the nonprofit organizations and other community organizations (e.g., clubs, and social, religious, community art, and athletic events). Through such team efforts, it will be possible to achieve healthier environments and better awareness of environmental safety practices not only for the Arab American community, but for the community at large.

References

Abdel-Khaleq, A. S. A. M. J., & Jamil, H. (1996). A study of biological monitoring among electroplating Jordanian workers exposed to chromium and some occupational health hazards. *Journal of Community Medicine Iraq, 9*, 9–12.

Abraham, S. Y., & Abraham, N. (Eds.). (1983). *Arabs in the New world: Studies on Arab-American communities*. Detroit: Wayne State University Press.

Abraham, N., & Shryock, A. (Eds.). (2000). *Arab Detroit: From margin to main-stream*. Detroit: Wayne State University Press.

Adler, D. A., McLaughlin, T. J., Rogers, W. H., Chang, H., Lapitsky, L., & Lerner, D. (2006). Job performance deficits due to depression. *The American Journal of Psychiatry, 163*, 1569–1576.

Ai, A., Peterson, C., & Ubelhor, D. (2002). War-related trauma and symptoms of posttraumatic stress disorder among adult Kosovar refugees. *Journal of Traumatic Stress, 15*, 157–160.

Al-Ajzan, J. K., Jamil, H., & Tman, W. (1990). Lead in teeth of a sample population of Baghdad. *Journal of Community Medicine, 3*, 3–8.

Al-Ani, J. K. J., & Jamil, H. (1991). Epidemiological study of injured people in road traffic accidents in Baghdad City. *Journal of Community Medicine., 4*, 63–70.

Alim, T. N., Graves, E., & Mellman, T. A. (2006). Trauma exposure, posttraumatic stress disorder and depression in an African-American primary care population. *Journal of the National Medical Association, 98*, 1630–1636.

Al-Issa, I. (Ed.) (2000). Al-Junun: Mental Illness in the Islamic World. *Madison, J. Nervous & Mental Disease*. 188, 475. Retrieved April 2011, from http://journals.lww.com/jonmd/fulltext/2000/07000/al_junun__mental_illness_in_the_islamic_world.21.aspx

Al-Omari, H., & Scheibmeir, M. (2009). Arab Americans' acculturation and tobacco smoking. *Journal of Transcultural Nursing, 20*, 227–233.

Al-Shamma, K. J., Ismall, D. K., & Jamil, H. (1985). Chromium concentrations in Iraqi tanneries. *Journal of the Faculty of Medicine Baghdad, 28*, 9–19.

Al-Shammary, M. A., & Jamil, H. (1992). Mercury exposure in Chloralkali Factory. *Journal of Community Medicine, 5*, 25–30.

Al-Tawil, N. G., Al-Shamma, K. J., Ismal, D. K., Fakhre, Z. M., & Jamil, H. (1988). Chromium dermatitis among workers in the tanning industry in Baghdad. *Journal of the Faculty of Medicine Baghdad, 30*, 307–311.

Al-Timimi, D. J., Jamil, H., & Abu-Tommam, A. K. (1988). Effect of traffic and lead absorption among children. *Journal of the Faculty of Medicine Baghdad, 30*, 95–103.

American Society of Hypertension. (2003). *Public initiatives to improve the prevention, detection, and management of hypertension*. Retrieved April 2011, from http://www.ash-us.org/documents/May-2007-JCH-Leadership-Message.pdf

Apfeldorf, W. J., & Alexopoulos, G. S. (Eds.). (2003). *Late-life mood disorders* (5th ed.). New York, NY: McGraw-Hill.

Arab American Institute. (2005). *Arab American demographics*. Retrieved September 27, 2005, from http://www.aaiusa.org/demographic.htm

Arab American Institute. (2010). *Demographics*. Retrieved October 19, 2010, from http://www.aaiusa.org/pages/demographics/, http://www.sadoun.net/forums/arabic-tv/18049-arab-americans-demographics.html

Arab American Institute. (2011). *Arab American demographics*. Retrieved December 10, 2011, from http://en.wikipedia.org/wiki/Arab_American & http://www.aaiusa.org/pages/census-2010

Arif, A. A., Delclos, G. L., & Serra, C. (2006). Occupational risk factors and asthma among health care. *Journal of Occupational and Environmental Medicine, 63*, 173–179.

Arnetz, J., Rofa, Y., Ventimiglia, M., Arnetz, B., & Jamil, H. (2013). Resilience as a protective factor against the development of psychopathology among refugees. *The Journal of Nervous and Mental Disease, 201*(3), 167–172.

Aswad, M. M. A. (2001). *Health survey of the Arab, Muslim, and Chaldean American communities in Michigan*. Lansing Michigan Department of Community Health. Retrieved October 20, 2010, from http://www.naama.com/pdf/arab-chaldean-muslim-michigan-health-survey.pdf

Beasley, R., Crane, J., Lai, C. K., & Pearce, N. (2000). Prevalence and etiology of asthma. *The Journal of Allergy and Clinical Immunology, 105*(2, Pt2), S466–S472.

Bhugra, D., & Mastrogianni, A. (2004). Globalization and mental disorders: overview with relation to depression. *The British Journal of Psychiatry, 184*, 10–20.

Braman, S. S. (2006). The global burden of asthma. *Chest Journal, 130*(1, Suppl), 4S–12S.

Brittingham, A., & de la Cruz, G. P. (2005). *We the people of Arab ancestry in the United States*. Washington DC: US Census Bureau. Retrieved October 12, 2010, from http://www.worldcat.org/title/we-the-people-of-arab-ancestry-in-the-united-states/oclc/63792315?referer=list_view

Brody, D. J., Pirkle, J. L., & Kramer, R. A. (1994). Blood lead levels in the US population: Phase 1 of the Third National Health and Nutrition Examination Survey (NHANES III, 1988 to 1991). *Journal of the American Medical Association, 272*, 277–283.

Bronfenbrenner, U. (1990). Five critical processes for positive development. Discovering what families do. In D. Blankenhorn, S. Bayme, & J. B. Elshtain (Eds.), *Rebuilding the Nest: A New Commitment to the American Family*, Family Services America, Retrieved from http://www.montana.edu/www4h/process.html

Bronfenbrenner, U. (1994). *Ecological models of human development. International Encyclopedia of Education* (2nd ed., Vol. 3, pp. 1643–1647). Oxford: Elsevier.

Centers for Disease Control. (2005). Blood lead levels—United States, 1999—2002.

Centers for Disease Control. (2008). *Behavioral risk factor surveillance system*. National Center for Chronic Disease and Prevention and Health Promotion. Retrieved from http://www.cdc.gov/brfss

Centers for Disease Control. (2009). *Injury research. US department of health and human services. Centers for disease control and prevention*. National Center for Injury Prevention and Control. Retrieved December 12, 2011, from http://www.cdc.gov/injury/ResearchAgenda/CDC_Injury_Research_Agenda-a.pdf

Chaudhuri, N. (2004). Interventions to improve children's health by improving the housing environment. *Review Environmental Health, 19*(3–4), 197–222.

Cohen Hubal, E. A., Sheldon, L. S., Burke, J. M., McCurdy, T. R., Berry, M. R., Rigas, M. L., et al. (2000). Children's exposure assessment: A review of factors influencing children's exposure, and the data available to characterize and assess that exposure. *Environmental Health Perspective, 108*, 475–478.

Cook, M., & Rafferty, A. (2005). *Health risk behaviors in the state of Michigan: 2004 behavioral risk factor survey* (p. 2005). Lansing: Michigan Department of Community Health, Bureau of Epidemiology, Epidemiology Services Division.

Cowie, C. C., Rust, K. F., & Byrd-Hold, D. D. (2006). Prevalence of diabetes and impaired fasting glucose in adults in the U.S. population: National Health and Nutrition Examination Survey 1999–2002. *Diabetes Care, 29*, 1263–1268.

Dallo, F. J., & James, S. A. (2000). Acculturation and blood pressure in a community-based sample of Chaldean-American women. *Journal of Immigrant and Minority Health, 2*(3), 145–153.

de la Cruz, G. P., & Brittingham, A. (2003). The Arab population 2000. US Department of Commerce; Economics and Statistics Administration. Washington, DC.

Detroit Department of Health and Wellness Promotion. (2005). *Detroit river-western Lake Erie basin indicator project*. INDICATOR: Lead Poisoning in Detroit, Michigan. Retrieved from http://www.epa.gov/med/grosseile_site/indicators/lead.html

Dorsey, S. M., Rodriguez, H. D., & Brathwaite, D. (2002). Are things really so different? A research finding of satisfaction, illness and depression in rural South African elderly. *Journal of the Association of Black Nursing Faculty, 13*, 41–44.

Dwairy, M. (2002). Foundations of psychosocial dynamic personality theory of collective people. *Clinical Psychology Review, 22*, 343–360.

Eggleston, P. A. (2000). Environmental causes of asthma in inner city children. The National Cooperative Inner City Asthma Study. *Clinical Reviews in Allergy and Immunology Journal, 18*, 311–324.

El-Islam, F. (1984). Some trans-cultural aspects of depression in Arab patients. *Medical Journal of Islamic Word Academy of Sciences, 1*, 48–49.

El-Khawaldeh, A. S., & Jamil, H. (1994). The association between blood presure, pulse rate & noise exposure. *Journal of the Faculty of Medicine Baghdad, 36*, 657–663.

El-Sendiony, M. (1981). *The effect of Islamic Sharia on behavioral disturbances in the Kingdom of Saudi Arabia*. Makkah: Makkah Printing and Publishing.

Environment Protective Agency (EPA). (1996). *Toxic release inventory, office of toxic substances*. Washington, DC: US Environmental Protection Agency.

Genesee County Health Department, (2003). *Reports and health data*. Arab American Health Survey Report, 2003. Michigan Genesee County Health Department. Retrieved October 11, 2010, from http://www.gchd.us/ReportsAndData/

Gilbert, P. A., & Khokhar, S. (2008). Changing dietary habits of ethnic groups in Europe and implications for health. *Nutrition Reviews, 66*, 203–215.

Glanz, K., Rimer, B. K., & Viswanath, K. (2008). *Health behavior and health education: Theory, research and practice* (4th ed.). San Francisco, CA: Jossey Bass.

Gottlieb, S. S., Khatta, M., & Friedmann, E. (2004). The influence of age, gender, and race on the prevalence of depression in heart failure patients. *Journal of the American College of Cardiology, 43*, 1542–1549.

Haddad, Y. Y., & Lummis, A. T. (1987). *Islamic values in the United States*. New York, NY: Oxford University Press.

Hart, M. (1998). *Sustainable community indicators trainer's workshop*. Retrieved December 10, 2011, from http://www.sustainablemeasures.com/Training/Indicators/Cmmunty

Hassoun, R. (1995). *A bioanthropological perspective of hypertension in Arab Americans in the metropolitan Detroit area*. Gainesville, FL: University of Florida Press.

Hatahet, W., Khosla, P., & Fungwe, T. V. (2002). Prevalence of risk factors to coronary heart disease in an Arab-American population in Southeast Michigan. *International Journal of Food Sciences and Nutrition, 53*, 325–335.

Hermis, S. R., Mohammed, S., & Jamil, H. (1993). A comparative study of mortality in Iraq, 1978–79 and 1988–89, person variables. *Journal of Community Medicine, 6*, 119–126.

Holguin, F., Mannino, D. M., Anto, J., Mott, J., Ford, E. S., & Teague, W. G. (2005). Country of birth as a risk factor for asthma among Mexican American. *American Journal of Respiratory and Critical Care Medicine, 171*, 103–108. doi:10.1164/recm.200402-143OC.

Hopps, H. C. (1976). The biologic bases for using hair and nail for analyses of trace elements. *Science of the Total Environment, 7*, 71–89.

Hussain, H. Y., Jamil, H., & Al-Sharbtti, S. (1996). Field survey on maternal health of Al-Rashidia Village, Baghdad. *Journal of Community Medicine, 9*, 90–93.

Hussien, H. A., & Jamil, H. (1992). The prevalence of contact dermatitis among male workers in an engineering factory. *Journal of Community Medicine, 5*, 75–80.

Hussien, H. A., & Jamil, H. (1993a). The prevalence of low back-pain among workers in an engineering factory. *Journal of Community Medicine, 6*, 57–62.

Hussien, H. A., & Jamil, H. (1993b). The prevalence rate of hypertension among a group of industrial population. *Journal of Community Medicine, 6*, 51–55.

Ibai, A. M., Hwalla, N., & Adra, N. (2003). Prevalence and covariates of obesity in Lebanon: Findings from the first epidemiological study. *Obesity Research, 11*, 1353–1361.

Iraqi Society of Occupational Health and Safety (ISOHS). (1992). *The Iraqi Society of Occupational Health and Safety webpage*. Retrieved April 2011, from www.ISOHS.org

Jaber, L. A., Brown, M. B., & Hammad, A. (2003). Epidemiology of diabetes among Arab Americans. *Diabetes Care, 26*, 308–313.

Jaber, L. A., Slaughter, R. L., & Grunberger, G. (1995). Diabetes and related metabolic risk factors among Arab Americans. *The Annals of Pharmacotherapy, 29*, 573–576.

Jamil, H. (1982). Occupational health & safety at workplace in fourteen govern orates. *Iraqi Science Nursing Journal, 1*(1,2,3), 7–19.

Jamil, H. (1984). Accidents due to work in Iraq for fourteen years (1968–81). *Iraqi Medical Journal, 32*, 17–42.

Jamil, H. (1985a). Accidents due to work in textile factories-1984. *Journal of the Faculty of Medicine Baghdad, 27*, 99–112.

Jamil, H. (1985b). Accident due to work in construction section. *Journal of the Faculty of Medicine Baghdad, 27*, 101–112.

Jamil, H. (1986a). Accidents due to work in the electrical, mechanical & presses sector of labor work in Iraq. *Journal of the Faculty of Medicine Baghdad, 28*, volume 2, 103–111.

Jamil, H. (1986b). Accidents due to work in the oil & petrochemical sector of labor in Iraq. *Journal of the Faculty of Medicine Baghdad, 28*, volume 4, 103–111.

Jamil, H. (1995). Field survey on health, social & environmental condition of people in Al-Buetha Village -Baghdad. *Journal of Community Medicine, 8*, 3–10.

Jamil, H. (2003). Environment & people health. *The Truth Magazine, 3*(19), 23.

Jamil, H., Abdulla, H., Al-Noorachi, I. A., & Saeed, M. K. (1983). Epidemiological study of accidents among primary school children in Baghdad during 1979–1980. *Iraqi Medical Journal, 31*, 40–52.

Jamil, H., & Ali, R. T. (1989). Work injuries in Al-Mishrak sulfur establishment. *Journal of Community Medicine, 2*, 143–152.

Jamil, H., Al-Tawil, N. G., & Radhi, A. S. J. (1989). The prevalence of nickel dermatitis among females in Iraq. *Journal of the Faculty of Medicine Baghdad, 31*(2), 209–214.
Jamil, H., Al-Timimi, D. J., Al-Ajzan, J. K., & Al-Ghabban, S. (1991). Lead absorption in printing workers. *Journal of the Faculty of Medicine Baghdad, 33*, 101–112.
Jamil, H., Al-Timimi, D. J., Al-Ghabban, S. I., & Al-Niami, M. (1987). Lead absorption in battery workers. *Journal of the Faculty of Medicine Baghdad, 29*, 211–222.
Jamil, H., Al-Timimi, D. J., Al-Ghabban, S. I., & Qasim, N. (1987). Lead absorption in petrol filling station workers in Baghad City. *Journal of the Faculty of Medicine Baghdad, 29*, 95–102.
Jamil, H., Amen, S. M., & Farhoud, N. (1986). Road traffic accidents in Saddam City. *Journal of the Faculty of Medicine Baghdad, 28*, 105–111.
Jamil, H., & Arabiat, A. A. (1999). *Driver safety and road accidents*. Amman, Jordan: Amman Press.
Jamil, H., & Aziz, M. A. (1985). Industrial contact dermatitis among textile workers in 2 factories. *Journal of the Faculty of Medicine Baghdad, 27*, 41–50.
Jamil, H., Dallo, F., Fakhouri, M., Templin, T., Khoury, R., & Fakhouri, H. (2009). The prevalence of self-reported chronic conditions among Arab-, Chaldean-, and African-Americans in Southeast Michigan. *Ethnicity & Disease Journal, 19*, 293–300.
Jamil, H., Fakhouri, M., Dallo, F., Templin, T., Khoury, R., & Fakhouri, H. (2008). Disparities in self-reported diabetes mellitus among Arab-, Chaldean-, and African- Americans in Southeast Michigan. *Journal of Immigrant and Minority Health, 10*, 397–405.
Jamil, H., Grzybowski, M., Hakim-Larson, J., Fakhouri, M., Sahutoglu, J., Khoury, R., et al. (2008). Factors associated with self-reported depression in Arab, Chaldean, and African Americans. *Journal of Ethnicity & Disease, 18*, 464–470.
Jamil, H., & Haboubi, G. (1992). Contact dermatitis among self-employed workers in Baghdad City. *Journal of the Faculty of Medicine Baghdad, 34*, 363–370.
Jamil, H., Haboubi, G., & Alrawi, Z. (1989). Prevalence of contact dermatitis among employees in Falloja Cement Plant. *Journal of Community Medicine, 2*(2), 137–141.
Jamil, H., Haboubi, G., & Al-Tikriti, S. K. (1989). Epidemiological aspects of smoking habit among fourth grade male students at (8) colleges, University of Baghdad. *Journal of Community Medicine, 2*(2), 125–130.
Jamil, H., Hakim-Larson, J., Farrag, M., Kafaji, T., Duqum, I., & Jamil, L. H. (2002). A retrospective study of Arab American mental health clients: Trauma and the Iraqi refugees. *The American Journal of Orthopsychiatry, 72*, 355–361.
Jamil, H., Hakim-Larson, J., Farrag, M., Kafaji, T., Jamil, L. H., & Hammad, A. (2005). Medical complaints among Iraqi American refugees with mental disorders. *Journal of Immigrant Health, 7*, 145–152.
Jamil, H., & Hussen, H. (1989). Work injuries & cost in an engineering establishment in Iraq over a period of six years (1980–85). *Journal of Community Medicine, 2*, 45–56.
Jamil, H., & Ismail, A. S. J. (1994). Field survey on health & environmental condition of Al-Shaha Village—Abo-Graib Baghdad. *Journal of Community Medicine, 7*, 223–229.
Jamil, H., & Jamil, L. H. (1994). Occupational diseases among hairdressers in Baghdad City. *Journal of Community Medicine, 7*, 97–104.
Jamil, H., Janisse, J., Elsouhag, D., Fakhouri, M., Arnetz, J. E., & Arnetz, B. B. (2011). Do household smoking behaviors constitute a risk factor for hookah use? *Nicotine & Tobacco Research, 13*, 384–388.
Jamil, H., Mukhlis, G. M., & Al-Tikriti, S. K. (1991). Epidemiological study on the habit of smoking among youth in Baghdad City. *Journal of Community Medicine, 4*(1), 15–24.
Jamil, H., Mukhlis, G. M., & Jamil, L. H. (1992). Epidemiological study on smoking habit among females in Baghdad City-1991. *Journal of Community Medicine, 5*, 3–10.
Jamil, H., Mukliis, G. M., & Al-Habboubi, G. (1981). Epidemiological study of road traffic accidents in Baghdad area. *Journal of the Faculty of Medicine Baghdad, 23*, 267–283.
Jamil, H., Nassar-McMillan, S., & Lambert, R. G. (2006). An epidemiological study: Health assessment of Iraqi immigrants. *Journal of Immigrant and Refugee Studies, 4*, 69–73.

Jamil, H., Nassar-McMillan, S., Lambert, R., Wang, Y., Ager, J., & Arnetz, B. (2010). Pre-and post-displacement stressors and time of migration as related to self-rated health among Iraqi immigrants and refugees in Southeast Michigan. *Medicine, Conflict and Survival, 26*, 207–222.

Jamil, H., Raymond, D., Fakhouri, M., Templin, T., Khoury, R., Fakhouri, H., et al. (2011). Self-reported asthma in Chaldean, Arab, and Blacks: Factors associated with asthma. *Journal of Immigrant and Minority Health, 13*, 568–575. doi:10.1007/s10903-010-9390-0.

Jamil, H., Simpson, C. L., Upfal, M., Blessman, J. E., & Hammad, A. (2003). Characteristics that influence occupational health and afety knowledge among Arab American workers. *The Yemeni Journal for Medical Sciences, 3*, 1–8.

Johnson, N. (1995). *Health profiles of Michigan populations of color. The Arab-American community in Detroit, Michigan*. Lansing: Michigan Department of Public Health.

Johnson, M., Nriagu, J., Hammad, A., Savoie, K., & Jamil, H. (2005). Asthma prevalence and severity in the Detroit area, Michigan. *Journal of Immigrant Health, 7*, 165–178.

Johnson, M., Nriagu, J., Hammad, A., Savoie, K., & Jamil, H. (2008). Environmental risk factors, and hypertension among Arab Americans in Metro Detroit. *Journal of Immigrant and Minority Health, 12*, 640–651. doi:10.1007/s10903-008-9205-8.

Jumaian, A., Alhmoud, N., & Al-Shunnaq, S. (2004). Comparing views of medical employees and lay people towards stigma in mental health issues. *Jordan Medical Journal, 38*, 80–83.

Junga, K. (2006). Residual risk for acute stroke in patients with type 2 diabetes and hypertension in primary care: Skaraborg Hypertension and Diabetes Project. *Diabetes, Obesity & Metabolism, 8*, 492–500.

Kayyali, R. (2006). *The Arab Americans*. Westport, CT: Greenwood Press.

Kridli, S. A., Herman, W. H., Brown, M., Fakhouri, H., & Jaber, L. A. (2005). The epidemiology of diabetes and its risk factors among Chaldean Americans. *Ethnicity & Disease, 15*(1 Suppl 1), 30–31.

Kulwicki, A., & Dervartanian, H. (1995). *Arab tobacco prevention and cessation project*. Lansing, MI: Michigan Department of Community Health.

Kulwicki, A., & Rice, V. H. (2003). Arab American adolescent perceptions and experiences with smoking. *Public Health Nursing, 20*, 177–183.

LeNoir, M. A. (1999). Asthma in inner cities. *National American Association Journals, 91*(8, Suppl), 1S–8S.

Lerner, D., Adler, D. A., Chang, H., Berndt, E. R., Irish, J. T., Lapitsky, L., et al. (2011). The clinical and occupational correlates of work productivity loss among employed patients with depression. *Research in Nursing and Health, 34*, 401–407. doi:10.1002/nur.20449.

Lethbridge-Cejku, M. R. D., & Vickerie, J. (2006). Summary health statistics for US adults: National Health Interview Survey 2004: National Center for Health Statistics.

Lewis, B. (1995). *The Middle East. A brief history of the last 2000 years*. New York, NY: Simon & Schuster.

Magnusser, H., Jorres, R., & Nowak, D. (1993). Effects of air pollution on the prevalence of asthma and allergy: Lessons from German reunification. *Thorax, 48*, 879–881.

Malvasi, M. G. (2006). *Gale encyclopedia of US history*. Arab Americans. Retrieved from http://www.answers.com/topic/arab-american

Meliker, J. R., Nriago, J. O., Hammad, A. S., Savoie, K. L., Jamil, H., & Devries, J. M. (2001). Spatial clustering of emergency department visits by asthmatic children in an urban area: Southwestern Detroit, Michigan. *Ambulatory Child Health Journal, 7*, 297–312.

MMWR/54, 513–516. Retrieved from http://www.cdc.gov/mmwr/preview/mmwrhtml/mm5420a5.htmApril

Mohammed, S., Hermis, S. R., & Jamil, H. (1993). A comparative study of mortality in Iraq 1978–79 and 1988–89, time & place variables. *Journal of Community Medicine, 6*, 127–133.

Moorman, J. E., Rudd, R. A., Johnson, C. A., King, M., Minor, P., Bailey, C., et al. (2007). National surveillance for asthma: United State, 1980–2004. *MMWR Surveillance Summaries, 56*(8), 1–54.

Naff, A. (1985). *Becoming American: The early Arab immigrant experience*. Carbondale: Southern Illinois University Press.

Norman, P. E. (2006). Peripheral arterial disease and risk of cardiac death in type 2 diabetes: The Fremantle Diabetes Study. *Diabetes Care, 29*, 575–580.

Nriagu, J. O., Robins, T., Gary, L., Liggans, G., Davila, R., Supuwood, K., et al. (1999). Prevalence of asthma and respiratory symptoms in south-central Durban South Africa. *European Journal of Epidemiology, 15*, 747–755.

Nriagu, J., Senthamarai-Kannan, R., Jamil, H., Fakhori, M., & Korponic, S. (2011). Lead poisoning among Arab American and African American children in the Detroit metropolitan area, Michigan. *Bulletin of Environmental Contamination and Toxicology, 87*, 238–244. doi:10.1007/s00128-011-0346-4.

Orfalea, G. (2006). *The Arab Americans: A history*. Northhampton, MA: Olive Branch Press.

Peele, P. B., & Tollerud, D. J. (2005). Depression and occupational injury: Results of a pilot investigation. *Journal of Occupational and Environmental Medicine, 47*, 424–427. doi:10.1097/01.jom.0000158700.50594.

Petrus, N. P., & Jamil, H. (1993). Fluoride absorption among workers of lamp factory. *Journal of the Faculty of Medicine Baghdad, 35*, 223–230.

Rana, J. S., Nieuwdorp, M., Jukema, J. W., & Kastelein, J. J. (2007). Cardiovascular metabolic syndrome—An interplay of, obesity, inflammation, diabetes and coronary heart disease. *Diabetes, Obesity & Metabolism, 9*, 218–232. doi:10.1111/j.1463-1326.2006.00594.x.

Refugee Council US. (2011). *Reports on asylum seekers, refugees, and IDPs*. Retrieved April 2011, from http://www.rcusa.org/index.php?page=reports-on-asylum-seekers-refugees-and-idps

Rice, V. H. (2006). Nursing interventions for smoking cessation: Meta-analysis update. *Heart & Lung: The Journal of Acute and Critical Care, 35*, 147–163.

Rice, V. H., & Kulwicki, A. (1992). Cigarette use among Arab American in the Detroit metropolitan area. *Public Health Reports, 107*, 589–594.

Rice, V. H., Weglicki, L. S., Templin, T., Hammad, A., Jamil, H., & Kulwicki, A. (2006). Predictors of Arab American adolescent tobacco use. *Merrill-Palmer Quarterly, 52*, 327–342.

Riolo, S. A., Nguyen, T. A., & Greden, J. F. (2005). Prevalence of depression by race/ethnicity: Findings from the National Health and Nutrition Examination Survey III. *American Journal of Public Health, 95*, 998–1000.

Rottem, M., Szyper-Kravitz, M., & Shoenfeld, Y. (2005). Atopy and asthma in migrants. *International Archives of Allergy and Immunology, 136*, 198–204. doi:10. 1159/000083894.

Sandel, M., & Wright, R. J. (2006). When home is where the stress is: Expanding the dimensions of housing that influence asthma morbidity. *Archives of Disease in Childhood, 91*, 942–948. doi:10.1136/adc. 2006.098376.

Savoie, K., & Nriagu, J. (1999). *Air pollution health risk assessment of the Arab American community in Dearborn, Michigan*. Dearborn, MI: US EPA, Region S, Air and Radiation Division.

Scelfo, G. M., & Flegal, A. R. (2000). Lead in calcium supplements. *Environmental Health Perspective, 108*, 309–313.

Shafey, O. (2007). Health issues in the Arab American community. Global epidemiology and health hazards of tobacco use: Arab world patterns. *Ethnicity & Disease, 17*(2 Suppl 3), S3–S13. S13-15.

Sherina, M. S. (2002). The prevalence of depression among elderly patients attending a government primary care clinic. *Asia-Pacific Journal of Public Health*, Special issue, 52–53.

Sibai, A. M., Hwalla, N., Adra, N., & Rahal, B. (2003). Prevalence and covariates of obesity in Lebanon: Findings from the first epidemiological study. *Obesity Research, 11*, 1353–1356.

Slotnck, M. J., Nriagu, J. O., Johnson, M. M., Jamil, H., & Hammad, A. (2005). Profiles of trace elements in toenails of Arab Americans in the Detroit Area Michigan. *Biological Trace Element Research, 107*, 113–126.

Steenland, K., Johnson, J., & Nowlin, S. (1997). A follow-up study of job strain and heart disease among males in the NHANES1 population. *American Journal of Industrial Medicine, 31*, 256–260.

Tsutsumi, A., Kayaba, K., Theorell, T., & Siegrist, J. (2001). Association between job stress and depression among Japanese employees threatened by job loss in a comparison between two complementary job-stress models. *Scandinavian Journal of Work, Environment and Health, 27*, 146–153.

Von Mutius, E., Martinez, F. D., Fritzsch, C., Nicolai, T., Roell, G., & Thiemann, H. H. (1994). Prevalence of asthma and atopy in two areas of West Germany and East Germany. *American Journal of Respiratory Critical Care, 149*, 358–364.

Weglicki, L. S., Templin, T. N., Rice, V., Jamil, H., & Hammad, A. (2008). Comparison of cigarette and water-pipe Smoking by Arab and Non–Arab-American youth. *American Journal of Preventive Medicine, 35*, 335–339.

Whooley, M. A., Kiefe, C. I., Chesney, M. A., Markovitz, J. H., Matthews, K., & Hulley, S. B. (2002). Depressive symptoms, unemployment, and loss of income: The CARDIA Study. *Archives of Internal Medicine, 162*, 2614–2620.

World Health Organization. (1948). Preamble to the Constitution of the World Health Organization as adopted by the International Health Conference, New York, 19–22 June, 1946; signed on 22 July 1946 by the representatives of 61 States (Official Records of the World Health Organization, no. 2, p. 100) and entered into force on 7 April 1948.

World Health Organization. (2002). *The world health report 2002—reducing risks, promoting healthy life*. Retrieved from http://www.who.int/whr/2002/en/

World Health Organization. (2005). *Why is tobacco a public health priority*? Retrieved January 10, 2010, from http://www.who.int/tobacco/health_priority/en/index.html

World Health Organization. (2009). *Global status report on road safety: Time for action*. Geneva: 2009. ISBN 978-92-4-156384-0. Department of Violence & Injury Prevention & Disability (VIP). Retrieve from http://whqlibdoc.who.int/publications/2009/9789241563840_eng.pdf

World Health Organization. (2010). *Tobacco free initiative*. (2006). Retrieved from http://www.who.int/tobacco/global_data/country_profiles/emro/en/

World Health Organization (2011). *Global status report on road safety*. Retrieve April 2011, from http://www.who.int/violence_injury_prevention/road_safety_status/en/

World Health Organization (2012). Environmental health. Retrieved from http://www.who.int/topics/environmental_health/en/

Wylie-Rosett, J., Mossavar-Rahmani, Y., & Gans, K. (2002). Recent dietary guidelines to prevent and treat cardiovascular disease, diabetes, and obesity. *Heart Disease, 4*, 220–230. doi:10.1097/001325 80-200207000-00005.

Yadav, J. S., & Thakur, S. (2000). Genetic risk assessment in hookah smokers. *Cytobios Journal, 101*, 101–113.

Part III
Health and Disease: Risks and Resilience

Sylvia C. Nassar-McMillan

The greatest mistake in the treatment of disease is that there are physicians for the body and physicians for the soul, although the two cannot be separated. (Plato)

Introduction

The Middle East and North Africa region is currently undergoing rapid and vast urbanization processes, with major impacts on the physical health and well-being of its inhabitants. These impacts, coupled with the assimilation and acculturative adaptations of new diets and lifestyles, synergistically impact, then, the lives of Arab Americans, particularly those who have most recently immigrated to the United States. A second set of parallel phenomena are the environmental risks identified in the recent decade within MENA regions, along with those found domestically in the United States, particularly those in underresourced or otherwise marginalized communities, such as those described in Jamil's chapter on environmental health in Part II of this text. This additional array of risks, for example, exposures of Iraqis during the Gulf War, could result in both higher levels of psychological distress as symptomized by posttraumatic stress disorder, anxiety, and depression (Jamil, Nassar-McMillan, Lambert, & Hammad, 2007) as well as, simultaneously, maladies of fibromyalgia and chronic fatigue (Nassar-McMillan, Jamil, & Lambert, 2010) and the like (Jamil, Nassar-McMillan, Lambert, & Hammad, 2006).

S.C. Nassar-McMillan (✉)
Department of Curriculum, Instruction, and Counselor Education,
North Carolina State University, 2310 Stinson Dr., Poe 520, Campus Box 7801,
Raleigh, NC 27695-7801, USA
e-mail: snassar@ncsu.edu

Because of the limited data sources available to examine the specific diseases in question, the populations of focus within this part do tend to be more on the newer immigrant populations and their offspring. However, it is clear that, due to the biobehavioral components of these diseases, the intergenerational effects and cumulative risks in years to come are perhaps even more critical than the current vulnerabilities facing Arab American immigrants and communities. In our selection of key health issues for Arab American communities, we sought to identify both key areas of focus for national (Arab American and non Arab American populations) such as child and maternal health and cancer, as well as those areas which seem to have particular salience for Arabs and Arab Americans such as substance abuse (specifically, tobacco and water pipe smoking) and diabetes, for which Arabs and Arab Americans face substantially higher risk. In both kinds of chapters, we focus on the etiology and prevalence of the specific biobehavioral health risk as manifest within the Arab American community. We identify mitigating factors and provide evidence-based practice recommendations. We close the part with a chapter on health disparities and the corresponding need for advocacy and public policy efforts at local and national levels. The five chapters in this part are summarized below.

In their chapter on substance abuse, Hammad and his Colleagues provide a background on substance abuse within the Arab culture and contemporary Arab American communities. While Arab countries are beginning to develop an awareness of the pitfalls associated with smoking tobacco, tobacco use has long been an integral cultural behavior and a means of expressing hospitality. Accurate data are difficult to ascertain but studies conducted within the Greater Detroit area (i.e., large Arab American ethnic enclave) suggest somewhat higher rates of cigarette smoking among Arab Americans as compared to non-Arab American populations. Moreover, water pipe smoking statistics, particularly among Arab American youth represent alarmingly high rates. Because this latter custom is specifically linked to and supported within the Middle East and North African region, it is inherently supported by the Arab American community, as well. Regarding alcohol use and abuse, rates among Arab American appear to be somewhat lower than those within the mainstream populations, reportedly due to the Islamic prohibition of alcohol use. Other drug use also appears to be prevalent at somewhat lower rates among Arab Americans as compared to non-Arab Americans. Conversely, for those who do suffer from alcohol and drug abuse, treatment is more challenging. Again, due to cultural stigmas, those who may recognize their need for treatment or who may otherwise wish to seek treatment, such as in court mandated cases, the fear of stigma negatively impacts retention and other metrics of successful treatment programs. Thus, the current need and focus are in the realm of public health prevention and education.

In the chapter on diabetes, Jaber and her Colleagues make a compelling case for diabetes as a primary health concern within the Arab American community. Specifically, among the top ten developing countries with the highest cases of diabetes, six are Arab countries—United Arab Emirates, Saudi Arabia, Bahrain, Kuwait, Oman, and Egypt. Moreover, there is a projected increase in prevalence of diabetes of 80 % in the Middle East North Africa region as compared to the rest of the world. This staggering prevalence rate is associated with the rapid increases in urbanization and socioeconomic status and their associated lifestyle shifts in nutritional and psychical activity patterns. Within the Arab American community, there have been some studies conducted within the past decade or so that have shed light onto some of the key issues related to effective diagnosis and treatment. The patterns in the urban MENA communities as described, coupled with changes in lifestyle and other acculturative impacts of immigration, appear to create similar, or perhaps even more alarming risk factors among Arab American populations in the United States. For example, obesity, another by-product of these described lifestyle shifts, creates an array of concomitant diabetes risks. Smoking does, as well, and as characterized in the substance abuse chapter of this part, occurs at higher rates within this population. Barriers to effective treatment of diabetes are significant in working with Arab American populations, particularly immigrants. Linguistic and cultural barriers inhibit effective education and monitoring of dietary practices. Misconceptions and knowledge deficits do, as well. Unfortunately, deficits in health care system delivery create a great need for cultural competent health care professionals who can more effectively navigate and circumvent these barriers, along with engage in advocacy efforts and local and national levels.

Within the arena of child and maternal health (CMH), Dallo and Colleagues examine the current state of affairs with regard to Arab Americans as compared to the overall US population, accessing the small amount of actual research available along with their expertise about risks and resiliencies for CMH, and finally, drawing compelling conclusions and recommendations for urgently needed research and policy change. Within the few studies available, a few metabolic and a hereditary blood disorder were implicated as being significantly higher for Arab American newborns as compared to others. Another study indicated higher prevalence of preterm births and lower birth weights post 9-11, while another similar study yielded no differences. Several risk factors within the CMH arena include exposure to environmental toxins and obesity. While neither of these actual risks and effects have been examined among Arab Americans within the CMH research and clinical literature, other related research, as reviewed in Jaber's diabetes chapter and Jamil's environmental health chapter has indicated that these risks (i.e., obesity and exposures, respectively) are significantly prevalent within the population. Clearly, these represent areas of priority for scientific inquiry and policy changes to support it. Moreover, another understudied area is the factors related to low acculturation rates, such as lack of information or lack of engagement in westernized practices such as immunizations or physical activity regimens during child-bearing years and pregnancy, along with potentially being under-insured as is not atypical for new immigrants in particular. Finally, issues related to both immigration as well as the troubled relationship within the host US culture, such as profiling and discrimination and stress and mental health issues in general, might well impact child and maternal health issues. It behooves our nation to support the examination of these issues for the sake of overall societal good.

In her chapter on cancer, Schwartz and her colleagues provide a description of cancer as manifest within the Arab American community. Incidence and mortality rates are overviewed, naming the top five cancers in Arab American men as lung, bladder, prostate, non-Hodgkin lymphoma and liver, and the top five in Arab American women as breast, colorectal, cervical, non-Hodgkin lymphoma, and ovary; as compared to the top five cancers in the overall United States for men and women as, respectively, prostate, lung, colorectal, bladder, and skin melanoma; and breast, lung, colorectal, uterine, and thyroid. While there do appear to be some differences in these comparisons, they are based on estimates due to the lack of population identification of Arab Americans in the US Census and medical data sources. This challenge poses a barrier to fully elucidating the effects of migration versus genetics. The limited research that has been conducted provides implications for further study. For example, like with CMH, multiple risk factors have been identified within this community that also serve as risk factors for cancer, such as smoking and obesity, both of which have been alluded to within related research on Arab Americans. As yet, however, direct linkages have been elusive at best due to the limitations of population identification within national efforts to measure cancer burden. Moreover, some of the challenges in effective diagnosis and treatment identified in the other chapters in this part hold true for cancer services, as well. Screening services are not fully utilized, presumably due to similar stigmas and misconceptions relative to health behaviors and help seeking.

In a final chapter on health disparities and advocacy issues relevant to Arab Americans, Hammad and his Colleagues highlight some of the key areas of need among Arab Americans (such as higher prevalence rates and risk factors in environmental exposures, smoking, obesity, diabetes, and certain cancer burdens), underscoring the increasing need for both education and advocacy efforts at local and national policy levels (such as culturally relevant education on nutrition, prevention, and other health care; health care access and the need for ethnic identification in national and local statistical databases and research initiatives). As key personnel representing Arab Center for Economic and Social Services (ACCESS), arguably the largest full-service human service agency in the world serving this population, they are well qualified to discuss both national and ethnographic local scenarios. Their compelling stance is both personal and evidence based. Their examples of advocacy efforts, including public health efforts to various levels of stakeholders, serve as models for other agencies and professionals across the country. Moreover, they underscore the importance of collaborative care efforts between health care professionals across a broad spectrum of services, from medical to mental health.

References

Jamil, H., Nassar-McMillan, S. C., Lambert, R. G., & Hammad, A. (2006). An epidemiological study: Health assessment of three waves of Iraqi immigrants. *Journal of Immigrant & Refugee Studies, 4*, 69–74.

Jamil, H., Nassar-McMillan, S. C., Lambert, R. G., & Hammad, A. (2007). Medical complaints of Iraqi American people before and after the 1991 Gulf War. *Ethnicity & Disease, 17*(Suppl 3), S3-77–S3-78.

Nassar-McMillan, S. C., Jamil, H., & Lambert, R. G. (2010). Chemical, environmental, and trauma exposures and corresponding health symptoms among Iraqi American women. *Journal of Applied Biobehavioral Research, 15*(2), 88–102.

Chapter 13
Substance Abuse

Adnan Hammad, Cynthia L. Arfken, Virginia Hill Rice, and Manal Said

This chapter addresses substance abuse among Arab Americans. For general information and history about Arab Americans, the reader is referred to the Culture section of this text. The following sections focus on tobacco use (i.e., cigarettes and waterpipe smoking), alcohol, and other drug use. The end of the chapter includes a discussion regarding current community-based activities targeting tobacco and substance use led by the Arab Community Center for Economic and Social Services (ACCESS), a large social, health and advocacy organization located in metropolitan Detroit, Michigan.

Background on Substance Abuse

The use of tobacco, alcohol or other drugs differs from other health behaviors or diseases in that access to the substance is by definition required and potential consequences of use include death, development of chronic diseases such as cancer or cirrhosis, development of psychiatric disorders of abuse or dependence, acute injury,

---

A. Hammad, Ph.D. (✉) • M. Said
ACCESS Community Health and Research Center, 6450 Maple Street, Dearborn, MI 48126, USA
e-mail: ahammad@accesscommunity.org; msaid@accesscommunity.org

C.L. Arfken, Ph.D.
Department of Psychiatry and Behavioral Neuroscience, Wayne State University, 3901 Chrysler Drive, Detroit, MI 48201, USA
e-mail: carfken@med.wayne.edu

V.H. Rice, Ph.D.
Wayne State University, College of Nursing and Karmanos Cancer Institute, 5557 Cass Avenue, OFC 366, Detroit, MI 48202, USA
e-mail: vrice@wayne.edu

S.C. Nassar-McMillan et al. (eds.), *Biopsychosocial Perspectives on Arab Americans: Culture, Development, and Health*, DOI 10.1007/978-1-4614-8238-3_13,

social problems, and legal complications. To reduce the access and consequences, researchers have looked at environmental interventions such as banning the substance (e.g., heroin), restricting sales (e.g., alcohol), taxation (e.g., cigarettes), and point of sales interventions (e.g., verifying age before purchase). Additionally, researchers have investigated psychological and social risk and protective factors. Importantly, these risk and protective factors can differ along the continuum of use from first experimentation with the substance to those associated with problematic use or development of abuse/dependence. Moreover, there may be unique risk and protective factors for relapse after successful quit attempts. With that caution, risk factors in general for substance abuse include genetic and environmental influences within a developmental framework, a theoretical framework known as developmental psychopathology (Cicchetti & Toth, 2009) and protective and resilience factors (Masten, 2007). Although smoking, drinking, and taking drugs at any age can cause problems, earlier use is more likely to progress to more serious abuse than use that is initiated later (Breslau, Fenn, & Peterson, 1993; Grant, Stinson, & Harford, 2001). Unfortunately because adolescents' brains are still developing in the areas of judgment and self-control, they are especially likely to try something risky and be susceptible to pressure from their peers to smoke, drink and use drugs (US Department of Health and Human Services, 2007). Protective factors include high self-esteem, involvement in meaningful activity, educational achievement, ethnic pride, and religiosity (i.e., external behaviors and internalized motivation to behave according to an individual's religious affiliation independent of religious doctrine) (Ghandour, Karam, & Maalouf, 2009; Gorsuch, 1995; Mason & Windle, 2002). The selection of potential risk and protective factors thus depend on what stage of continuum of substance abuse is examined and what level of analysis is specified—is the focus on the person, family, peers, schools, community, or nation?

Consequence of Substance Abuse

Substance abuse and dependence, whether it is from tobacco, alcohol, illegal drugs, prescription drugs, or over-the-counter drugs, is a major public health and medical problem in the USA (Horgan, 2001). Importantly it exists among every racial and ethnic group examined to date, including Arab Americans. Estimates of the costs of substance abuse, covering health- and crime-related costs as well as losses in productivity vary but one estimate from 1995 was $110 billion for illicit drugs and $167 billion for alcohol (Harwood, 2000). In terms of health care dollars and productivity losses, cigarette smoking costs the USA more than $193 billion dollars (Centers for Disease Control and Prevention [CDC] 2008). These costs include lost wages due to premature mortality and illness, and hospitalizations.

In the USA tobacco use is responsible for about one in five deaths annually (i.e., about 443,000 deaths per year). Tobacco use causes about 85 % of all lung cancers in the USA. In addition to cancer, low levels of smoke exposure, including exposure to second hand smoke, can lead to a rapid and sharp increase in dysfunction and inflammation of the lining of the blood vessels, which are implicated in heart attacks and strokes. Chemicals in tobacco smoke also interfere with the functioning of fallopian tubes thus increasing the risk for adverse pregnancy outcomes such as ectopic pregnancy, miscarriage, and low birth weight. They can also damage the sperm DNA that reduces fertility and harms fetal development Both the risk and the severity of smoking-related diseases are directly related to how long a person has smoked and the number of cigarettes smoked per day (Centers for Disease Control and Prevention [CDC], 2012; National Cancer Institute, 2012).

Substance Use Disorder Is a Chronic Brain Disease

Apart from the medical consequences, substance use disorder (either abuse or dependence) is a chronic brain disease that causes compulsive drug seeking and use despite harmful consequences to the individual, family and society. It is often relapsing, similar to other chronic diseases, but like other chronic diseases can be managed successfully (McLellan, Lewis, O'Brien, & Kleber, 2000). Research has repeatedly shown that medications for tobacco, alcohol and opiate dependence, and therapy for all substances are effective for most patients (Anton et al., 2006; Fiore, Hatsukami, & Baker, 2002; National Institute on Drug Abuse, 2009; Tobacco Use and Dependence Guideline Panel, 2008). However, treatment approaches should be tailored to the culture and substance abuse patterns of the individual and any co-occurring medical, psychiatric, and social problems. Prevention efforts including both school-based and environmental interventions such as taxes have also been shown repeatedly to lower the incidence of substance abuse (e.g., Botvin, Baker, Dusenbury, Botvin, & Diaz, 1995).

Tobacco Use

Currently over 20 % of the US adults smoke cigarettes (Dube et al., 2010). The Monitoring the Future Study, which has tracked teen substance use for over 36 years, has reported that the prevalence of current smoking almost doubled between eighth graders and tenth graders (Johnston, O'Malley, Bachman, & Schulenberg (2011), emphasizing that prevention activities need to be implemented prior to high school. Risk factors for youth tobacco use include easy availability of cigarettes, low socioeconomic status, low academic performance, poor self-esteem and self-efficacy, and aggressive behavior, lack of skills to resist the peer pressure to smoke, peer pressure to smoke, and smoking in the home and community (Skinner, Haggerty, & Catalano, 2009).

Beyond cigarettes, another source of tobacco exposure is through waterpipe smoking. In fact, the American Lung Association (2007) described "waterpipes (also known as Hookahs or Argilehs) as the first new tobacco trend of the twenty-first century." The waterpipe has four fundamental parts: (1) A head where the tobacco is placed and heated (usually with charcoal); (2) A bowl or smoke chamber which is partially filled with water; (3) a pipe or body connecting the head to the bowl by a tube that carries the smoke down into the water; and (4) A hose with a mouthpiece through which the smoke is drawn from the bowl. As the smoker inhales, the tobacco smoke is sucked down into the bowl and then bubbles up through the water into the air of the smoke chamber and then through the hose to the smoker (Cobb, Ward, Maziak, Shihadeh, & Eisenberg, 2010). Water cools the smoke but does not filter much out (Eissenberg & Shihadeh, 2009; Hadidi & Mohammed, 2004; Shafagoj, Mohammed, & Hadidi, 2002).

Contrary to users' perception, waterpipe use is not safe. Use by adults has been shown to be associated with poor lung function (Kiter, Uçan, Ceylan, & Kilinç, 2000) malignant and nonmalignant lung disease (Al-Fayez, Salleh, Ardawi, & Zahran, 1988), cancers of the mouth (El-Hakim & Uthman, 1999), coronary heart disease (Jabbour, El-Roueiheb, & Sibai, 2003), perinatal risks (Nuwayhid, Yamout, Azar, & Kambris, 1998), and various other health problems (Knishkowy & Amitai, 2005). A comparative study of human toxicant exposure of waterpipe and cigarette smoking, under controlled laboratory conditions found peak carbon monoxide levels bound to red blood cells were three times higher in waterpipe smokers compared to cigarette smokers and the number and volume of each puff indicated waterpipe smokers inhaled about 48 times more smoke than cigarette smokers (Cobb et al., 2010). A recent meta-analysis summarized the harmful effects of waterpipe smoking (Akl et al., 2010).

Smoking the waterpipe is a ceremonial activity governed by rules for each stage in the process of preparing, lighting, sharing, and smoking (Hammal, Mock, Ward, Eissenberg, & Maziak, 2008). Major reasons for its growing popularity worldwide include migrations of people from regions where use of the waterpipe is common, flavored tobacco mix (maassel), public restaurants and cafes that host waterpipe use, and publicity (WHO Study Group on Tobacco Product Regulation, 2005). There many web sites to learn about waterpipes purchase elements for use. Importantly, it is a social event (Maziak, 2011) as opposed to cigarette smoking. Not surprisingly, waterpipe smokers report that it is "cool" and less harmful/addictive than cigarette smoking.

Tobacco Use in the Arab Countries

Many Arab Americans come to the USA from countries where tobacco use is a part of the culture and a means of showing hospitality (World Health Organization, 2011). Unfortunately, Arab countries are only beginning to develop smoking prevention and cessation programs (WHO Study Group on Tobacco Product Regulation, 2005). Recent tobacco control programs implemented have included banning indoor smoking and meeting with faith leaders (El Awa, 2004). This latter effort lead to

Islamic scholars in some Arab countries declaring tobacco use was prohibited because of the harm it does to the body. Unfortunately, not all Arabs believed that these declarations of prohibition applied to waterpipe smoking (Singh et al., 2010), possibly due to the perceived safety from the water filtration and use of flavored tobacco (maassel).

The World Health Organization reports adult smoking rates in Arab countries range from 23 to 61 % (Shafey & Musa, 2010). Countries with the highest male smoking rates include Jordan (61.7 %), Tunisia (51 %), and the Syrian Arab Republic (42 %). Prevalence is also high among adolescents (Al-Faris, 1995). These statistics do not include waterpipe smoking. In Arab countries, the waterpipe is a symbol of social sharing and cultural identity and is a centuries old form of tobacco use traditionally engaged in by older men in Arab countries (Hammal et al., 2008).

Tobacco Use Among Arab Americans

There is limited national data on tobacco use among Arab Americans. However, in the Detroit metropolitan area which has a high concentration of people of Arab heritage (de la Cruz & Brittingham, 2003), a series of studies have examined cigarette and waterpipe use among Arab Americans. The first study was a population survey of the area with the largest concentration of Arab Americans which found 40.6 % of Arab American men smoke and 38.2 % of Arab American women smoke (Rice & Kilwicki, 1994). A survey 2 years later in the same Detroit area confirmed the high rates of smoking: 35 % among Arab American men and a 31.5 % among Arab American women (Gold, 1994).

Using these high rates of smoking as motivation, several studies were launched to identify the protective and risk factors for tobacco use, with an emphasis on Arab American youth. In one study that extended over an 8 year period, tobacco use information was collected from thousands of Arab American and other high school students (14–18 years). Some of the findings included identifying risk and protective factors for different tobacco use outcomes. Peer use was especially potent as a risk factor. Youth with one or more close friends who smoke were 3.72 times more likely to contemplate smoking in the future, 6.08 times more likely to have smoked cigarettes in the past 30 days, and 3.23 times more likely to have experimented with cigarettes (Rice, Templin, & Kulwicki, 2003).

This study was also one of the first to report the growing use of waterpipe smoking (Rice et al., 2006). Experimentation with waterpipe smoking increased from 23 % among 14 year olds to 40 % among students who were 18 years old. In contrast, experimentation with cigarette smoking increased from 15 % at 14 years to 44 % at 18 years. The strongest predictor of experimenting with cigarettes was waterpipe use.

Arab American youth reported significantly higher percentages of ever waterpipe smoking (38 % vs. 21 %) and current waterpipe smoking (17 % vs. 11 %) than other youth. If one or more family members smoked the waterpipe in the home, youth were 6.3 times more likely to be current waterpipe smokers (Weglicki, Templin, Rice, Jamil, & Hammad, 2008). The influence of the family among Arab Americans was also by Jamil et al. (2011).

To investigate in greater detail waterpipe smoking, all students were surveyed (N=2,454) in two high schools during the fall of 2002 (Templin et al., 2005). Arab Americans and males were significantly more likely to smoke the waterpipe than other ethnicities or females. Age of first using the waterpipe was predictive of regular waterpipe use, but not of regular cigarette use. The age of first smoking a whole cigarette was predictive of both regular waterpipe use and cigarette smoking. Contrary to expectations, these asymmetric results suggest that cigarette smoking rather than waterpipe smoking is a gateway behavior for Arab American youth.

These studies were conducted with predominately Lebanese, Syrian, and Palestinian American youth. As the Arab American population includes diverse countries of origin and ethnic groups within them, tobacco use might vary between them. To assess tobacco use among Yemeni Americans, an adolescent sample (N=297) of Yemeni-Americans were surveyed with 39.1 % having tried cigarettes but only 17 % reporting having tried waterpipe smoking (Baker & Rice, 2008). In this survey, both gender and peer smoking influence increased the risk of experimenting with tobacco.

Another ethnicity within the Arab American population is Chaldean, an ethnicity predominately from Iraq who are members of the Chaldean Catholic Church. A survey of 1,919 adults (30 % self-identified as Chaldean, 60 % as Arab American, and 10 % as White Americans) found relatively high rates of cigarette smoking among White adults and a high rate of waterpipe smoking by those with a Chaldean or Arab American heritage (Jamil et al., 2009). Being male, older, unmarried and not Chaldean or Arab American predicted cigarette smoking; being Arab or Chaldean and having less formal education predicted waterpipe smoking.

Together these studies indicate that tobacco use among Arab Americans is a health concern and efforts should be addressed to prevention. Responding to this need, a quasi-experimental design was used to evaluate a tobacco use prevention program delivered to ninth graders (Rice, Weglicki, Templin, Jamil, & Hammad, 2010). It consisted of four 1-h interventions on preventing cigarette smoking delivered in schools as part of health education classes. The three cohorts consisted of 2,097 students enrolled in two high schools in an ethnically diverse, but predominantly Arab community in the Greater Detroit area. Although in the direction of reducing the initiation of cigarette smoking, the program had no impact on waterpipe smoking.

These studies were seminal in addressing tobacco use among Arab Americans with other researchers now starting to examine it elsewhere in the USA (Virginia Commonwealth University, 2012) as well as waterpipe use among college students. However, no information has been published on national estimates. Additionally, qualitative studies are needed to guide prevention programs as well as quantitative studies examining risk and protective factors among Arab Americans for the transition to nicotine dependence, quit attempts and relapse.

Alcohol and Other Drugs

Alcohol and Other Drug Use in the Arab Countries

Arab Americans originate from one of the areas with the lowest per capita consumption of alcohol in the world, a fact directly attributable to the majority religion, Islam, which prohibits the consumption and trafficking of alcohol (Michalak & Trocki, 2006). The low per capita consumption, however, does not mean that alcohol misuse is absent. There is documented alcohol dependence in Arab countries measured by hospital admissions among both male and female Arabs (AbuMadini, Rahim, Al-Zahrani, & Al-Johi, 2008; Hasan et al., 2009). The hospital admission data also documents dependence on other substances, including heroin, cocaine, stimulants and marijuana.

According the United Nations Office of Drugs and Crime, marijuana is the most commonly used illegal drug across the Arab countries as measured by drug demand and law enforcement seizure data (Maalouf, 2008). However, heroin, cocaine and methamphetamine are also increasingly present in drugs seized by law enforcement. As of 2008, cocaine was becoming more popular in Lebanon in particular, mirroring the growth in Europe. The Arab countries are also participating in the worldwide trends of younger age of onset for substances and increasing polydrug use. This latter phenomenon is troubling because polydrug use complicates treatment. Finally, injecting drug use is increasingly being detected in Arab countries. Due to the overall lack of needle exchanges and illegal status associated with possession of syringes in some countries, needles are believed to be frequently reused and shared. This behavior may be behind localized epidemics of infectious diseases, including HIV. Exacerbating the increase in drug demand is the limited treatment capacity in many countries, especially the lack of aftercare (i.e., organized support for abstinence when the person leaves formal treatment) (Maalouf, 2008).

Other reports support the United Nations Office on Drugs and Crime's findings on alcohol and drug use increasing in Arab countries (Karam, Maalouf, & Ghandour, 2004). The reports point to possible influences of changing economic and social environmental, but these influences have not been well-investigated due to extreme stigmatization of alcohol and drug use constraining community surveys (Bilal, Makhawi, Al-Fayez, & Shaltout, 1990). In the past, entry to substance abuse treatment or pathway by Arabs to alcohol and drug treatment was reported to be motivated by outside forces (e.g., family, criminal justice) (Al-Krenawi, 2005).

Lebanon was the only Arab country to conduct a population-based community survey as part of the World Health Organization World Mental Health Survey Initiative (Karam et al., 2006). They reported 1.2 % of the population had substance use disorders. Their report also highlighted the association of war with the prevalence of mental health disorders. As the Arab Americans are disproportionately from areas with conflict (i.e., Lebanon, Iraq, and Yemen), US mental health clinics see many Arab Americans patients with PTSD or traumatic symptoms (Jamil et al., 2002).

Although not specifically addressed in the report, it is possible that some Arab Americans use alcohol and other substances to cope or self-treat traumatic symptoms.

Smaller surveys of targeted populations (e.g., female university students; Soueif et al., 1987) have been conducted over time in Egypt. They documented the use of alcohol and drugs in these groups. Less is known about the initiation and development of problems. Also community mental health surveys in the United Arab Emirates have been conducted which either deleted substance use disorders (Ghubash, Hamdi, & Bebbington, 1992) or found them unrealistically low (Abou-Saleh, Ghubash, & Daradkeh, 2001). In the later study, they found that when they asked about alcohol or drugs causing problems in the household, the prevalence of possible substance use disorder *quadrupled.*

Drinking patterns have also been investigated in Arab men and women living in Israel (Neumark, Rahav, Teichman, & Hasin, 2001). They found very low reported drinking by women. Both Arab men and women showed great difference in drinking prevalence by religiosity. Other research in Israel also documented that Arabs, while less likely to drink, were more likely to binge drink (Neumark, Rahav, & Jaffe, 2003). This pattern of drinking is receiving more attention as it is tied to acute problems and increased mortality.

Substance Abuse Among Arab Immigrants to Other Regions

Substance abuse research on Arabs immigrating to other regions is quite limited (Maalouf & Arfken, 2009). One study found a very low but increasing prevalence of drinking in college students with number of years in Belarus (Razvodovsky, 2004). Drinking was mostly confined to social occasions. The students were unanimous that they intended to stop drinking entirely when returning to their country of origin because it would interfere with work. These findings suggest experimentation with alcohol but continued stigmatization, especially when surrounded by other Arabs.

Substance Abuse Among Arab Americans

There is limited information on substance abuse among Arab Americans. A major barrier to collecting data is that Arab Americans are not generally identified in surveys measuring substance use. However, the limited information does not mean that abuse is absent. As highlighted above, abuse is found among all races and ethnicities. Instead it may reflect the general expectation that substance abuse would be low among Arab Americans. As stated above, per capita consumption of alcohol is very low in Arab countries. The low consumption reflects that Arab countries have both religious prohibition on and social discouragement of drinking, especially by women, as it can bring shame to the family. Although the majority of Arab Americans are Christians (Baker & Howell, 2009) and do not have doctrinal prohibition on alcohol use unless they belong to certain proscriptive Protestant denominations, their alcohol use in Arab countries may be moderated by social pressure as has been shown with other cultures (Amundsen, Rossow, & Skurtveit, 2005). Proscriptive religion, combined with high religiosity, has been shown to be associated with abstinence in Lebanon (Ghandour et al., 2009). Religious affiliation by itself, however, does not result in abstinence from drinking. For example, a national survey conducted in the USA in 2000 yielded self-reports of alcohol consumption within the past year by 10 out of 45 Muslim Americans (although not exclusively Arab Americans) (Michalak, Trocki, & Bond, 2007). Moreover, in a 2001 survey, 46.6 % of US Muslim American college students (also not exclusively Arab Americans) reported some alcohol consumption within the past year (Abu-Ras, Ahmed, & Arfken, 2010). Within the USA, Muslim and Christian Arab immigrants may be drawn to different geographic areas, as detailed extensively in section I of this text. The resulting clustering may translate to a "dry" vs. "wet" environment for social tolerance of drinking alcohol (Cahalan & Room, 1974).

Arab Americans and Substance Abuse Treatment

In the state of Michigan, Arab Americans have the option to self-identify on alcohol and drug abuse admission forms. According to these data, Arab Americans account for a disproportionately small percentage of admissions to alcohol and drug treatment programs compared to their proportion in the general population (Arfken, Kubiak, & Farrag, 2008). Supporting the validity of the self-response, approximately 80 % of the Arab-American admissions were in the metropolitan Detroit area, similar to the 2000 Census. This geographic clustering of admissions was higher for Arab Americans than for any other racial or ethnic group.

As part of an empirical investigation to identify additional information about these dynamics, interviews were conducted with regional assessors (who *must* screen all applicants for publicly funded treatment) in the metropolitan Detroit area. They reported no problems in identifying Arab Americans or reluctance by Arab Americans to identify themselves (Arfken, Berry, & Owens, 2009). Additionally, the proportion of admissions by Arab Americans has increased over time, consistent with the influx of Arab immigrants. The increase is also consistent with acculturation of Arab Americans to an environment with high levels of alcohol and drug.

Further analysis of the substance abuse treatment admission indicated that alcohol was the most common primary drug of abuse among the Arab Americans (34.8 %) and that over half had alcohol listed as primary, secondary or tertiary drug of abuse (Arfken et al., 2008). This high level of alcohol abuse is similar to that of African Americans but below those found for other racial/ethnic groups. Interestingly, African Americans also show clustering in the metropolitan area so their lower prevalence of alcohol abuse may be due to religious proscription or to the availability of alternative drugs of abuse, such as heroin or cocaine, in the metropolitan area.

The above analysis examined admissions to substance abuse treatment. For discharges, Arab Americans had low treatment completion and retention rates, similar to those of other racial and ethnic groups (Arfken, Kubiak, & Farrag, 2007). The variables predictive of treatment completion by Arab Americans included alcohol as a primary drug, criminal justice involvement, and not speaking English. Thus, Arab Americans who did not speak English, had alcohol as the primary drug of abuse, and had criminal justice pressure to enter treatment were more likely to complete their treatment than other Arab Americans who entered treatment.

Two explanations for the high percentage of Arab Americans who have alcohol as the primary drug abuse are acculturation, and not being Muslim. To explore these explanations, medical charts of Arab-American clients at one Arab-centric substance abuse clinic in the predominately Muslim local area were examined (Arfken, Kubiak, & Farrag, 2009). The charts include information on history of having at least one alcohol drink, religious affiliation, country of birth and origin, length of time in the USA, and English language proficiency. Significant risk factors for polysubstance abuse were residing in the USA, more than 10 years and fluency in English, both of which are crude measures of acculturation. Of those patients who appeared to have low acculturation in that they had been in the USA for fewer than 10 years and not proficient in English, 73.2 % had alcohol use disorders. The prevalence increased to 90.5 % for those who had lived more than 10 years in the USA and were fluent in English. This finding supports acculturation as increasing the rate of substance abuse among Arab Americans but it also underscores the notion that alcohol abuse can be present in Arab Americans who have been in the USA for a relatively short period of time.

Among the Arab American patients, 76.0 % of Muslims and 88.9 % of Christians had a diagnosis of alcohol abuse (Arfken, Kubiak, & Farrag, 2009). Almost no religious differences were evident in history of having at least one alcohol drink. Of the Muslims, 91.9 % had a history of drinking and of the Christians, 94.4 % had a history of drinking. These analyses do not support the idea that religious affiliation by itself explains the distribution of alcohol abuse among Arab Americans.

The low prevalence of Arab Americans in substance abuse treatment may be due to denial of problems by the individual and family. This denial would mean that Arab Americans would not seek out treatment. Instead, they might use different pathways to treatment. To examine these possible pathways to treatment, we reviewed descriptions of presenting problems or chief complaints for people seeking substance abuse treatment (Arfken, Kubiak, & Farrag, 2009). This analysis was limited to the region encompassing the predominately Muslim area of metropolitan Detroit (Baker & Howell, 2009). The recorded descriptions were reviewed for content by independent reviewers blinded to ethnicity. It was hypothesized that Arab Americans would be more likely to state that coercive elements (e.g., criminal justice system or family) motivated them to enter treatment than other ethnicities. The results confirmed that 43.2 % of the Arab American did mention criminal justice involvement (the highest of all racial and ethnic groups). They were the only ethnicity to mention substance use conflicting with religion as a motivation for seeking treatment.

The above analyses, while instructive, failed to include Arab Americans' perspectives. To obtain these, in-depth interviews were conducted with ten Arab Americans who were or had been in substance abuse treatment (Arfken, Berry, & Owens, 2009). The diverse sample included five with co-occurring mental disorders (emphasizing that having a co-occurring mental disorder is common in substance abuse); eight men and two women; nine Muslims and one Orthodox Christian; seven treated for alcohol use disorder and three for drug use disorders; and a range of countries of origin, generation and language proficiency. All the participants reported intense Arab-American community stigmatization of drinking and marijuana use: for example, "In the Arabic-speaking Muslim community, they would be looked down upon." and "They would look down on them. Laugh at him probably." Participants currently clean and sober seemed to perceive the community as more supportive than those who were still using alcohol or drugs: for example, "As getting help, a good thing, but still they would look at him as a bad person." and "They would say 'He must go.' They would encourage." Families and friends, once convinced of the need for treatment, were supportive but were not knowledgeable enough to recognize the need for treatment: for example, "I know they thought it was shame but no, they did not demean me, just like 'You need to get better; really, you need some help.'" The lack of knowledge is particularly discouraging as half of the participants had a family history of substance abuse, although none of them had a history of treatment. All but one of the participants reported drinking as an adolescent with friends, suggesting that community values and behavior were not identical. Criminal justice involvement and mental health referrals were major pathways to treatment. Cultural barriers to accessing and staying in treatment were common; counselor ethnic-matching did not eliminate this barrier. The study concluded that stigma in the community may discourage substance use but it also may contribute to delay in treatment seeking for those with problems. Cultural competency of programs and counselors appeared to influence both access to treatment and retention.

Substance Abuse Among Arab Americans in the Community

The above analyses were based on Arab Americans in treatment for substance abuse. As not all people who abuse substances enter formal substance abuse treatment, community-based data are needed to plan prevention and intervention targeted services. Developing these targeted approaches builds upon basic information of substance use patterns. This basic information includes estimates for the prevalence of: lifetime use (ever used), past month use (current use), misuse (e.g., heavy drinking, binge drinking), and abuse/dependence. This information is currently available for major racial/ethnic groups in the USA through special and ongoing national and state level population-based surveys.

Currently, the only national survey that can provide detailed information on alcohol and drug use is the National Survey of Drug Use and Health (NSDUH), an ongoing annual population-based survey of alcohol and drug use among community-dwelling people in the USA 12 years or older. This survey fortunately has a question on place of birth that can be used to identify immigrant Arab Americans. Arab Americans born in the USA would not be identified. From this survey, Arab immigrants nationally had lower rates of lifetime alcohol use (50.8 %), past month use (26.4 %) and binge drinking (10 %) than non-Hispanic US born White Americans (Arfken, Arnetz, Fakhouri, Ventimiglia, & Jamil, 2011).

Currently, the only statewide survey in the USA with alcohol use data for Arab Americans is the Michigan Behavioral Risk Factor Surveillance System (MiBRFSS), an ongoing population-based telephone survey of Michigan adults 18 years or older. Starting in 2007, this survey added a question asking if the respondent was of Arab or Chaldean origin. As such, the responses include both immigrants and later generations of Arab Americans. Michigan added this question in 2007 to obtain health information on Arab American as the state has the highest concentration of Arab Americans in the USA. The statewide estimates for Arab/Chaldean Americans also show lower rate of past month alcohol use (45.6 %) than the non-Hispanic Whites (59.4 %). However, there was no difference for binge drinking (17.0 % vs. 18.7 %). When the analysis was limited to those who reported drinking in the past month, the rate of binge drinking was 38.2 % among Arab Americans who drink compared to 31.8 % among the comparison group who drink (Arfken et al., 2011).

Three conclusions stand out from these analyses from community-based surveys. First, there are few databases available to estimate alcohol or drug use among Arab Americans. Second, binge drinking is a problem among Arab Americans. Third, Arab Americans have a lower prevalence of alcohol use than the majority group of non-Hispanic White Americans. It can also be inferred, although not directly tested, that immigrants are less likely to drink than all self-identified Arab Americans. Unfortunately, the information on gender-specific alcohol use pattern is limited to immigrants but consistent with the cultural expectation that among Arab Americans, men would be more likely to drink than women. The lack of gender difference in age of onset and the later mean age of first use for both men and women, although still under-aged, as compared to the majority group, suggests that there may be cultural factors influencing age of onset of drinking among Arab Americans. A limitation of the available data is that information on alcohol use among Arab American who did not participate in survey, especially due to language barriers, is lacking.

An additional source of health data on Arab Americans is the ongoing population-based national survey called the National Household Interview Study (NHIS). The NHIS collects data on a range of health topics through personal household interviews, including country of birth, but does not have detailed alcohol questions. In the public access database, Immigrant Arab Americans are grouped under "Middle East"—along with people born in Iran, Turkey, Israel and other countries in the Eastern Mediterranean region or under "African" for Arab Americans born in Egypt and other Northern African countries. Although use of this regional code has been advocated for examining Arab American's health (El-Sayed & Galea, 2009), its accuracy is unknown but should be investigated.

Perception of Arab Americans who drink is required to develop interventions. From 12 focus groups conducted in the metropolitan Detroit area with young Muslims from Lebanon, Syria, and Palestine, Muslims from Yemen, Orthodox Christians and Chaldeans, similar themes of social pressure to conform to what their friends were doing and having fun with friends were found when talking about why their peers binged on alcohol (Arfken, Owens, & Said, 2012). Some differences were found by religion in that the Yemeni youth said that no Yemeni women drank and that drinking occurred in basements and other nearby isolated areas where the Yemeni youth could not be observed. The young Muslims for Lebanon, Syria, and Palestine said women did drink but they had to hide it for their parents and other older adults. For them, drinking occurred far from home where they could not be observed and at parties/clubs. Among the young Chaldeans, drinking among men was a status symbol but not permitted among women. These gender based prohibitions appeared to be loosening with time in the USA but were still respected. Among the Orthodox Christians, there was no gender difference in drinking. One example from a Chaldean group was: "Your dad's neighbor from back home will say 'oh look at his daughter, she had a drink' or even if you have a Shirley Temple and it looks like it's a drink, you know it brings the possibility of shame." An example of peer pressure from a Muslim Lebanese youth: "If I'm going to do something stupid, I'm not going to do it alone. I'll try to get people to do it with me." An example of avoiding parental disapproval was: "Yeah, I was going to a party at a hookah lounge with a friend and he spent the night in the hookah lounge after it closed because he was really drunk and he knew someone who worked there and he didn't want his parents to found out."

The above community-based studies examined alcohol use. Less is known about use and abuse of other drugs among Arab Americans and whether detected differences were due to immigration effects or general cultural effects. Similar to the analysis on alcohol, marijuana use and misuse of prescription medications was examined among Arab immigrants (Arfken, Jamil, & Arnetz, 2012). This analysis used *Immigrant Canadian Americans* as a control group for immigration effects and *immigrant Other Middle Eastern Americans* (from Iran, Afghanistan and Pakistan) as a control group for general cultural effects. Using pooled data from 2002 to 2010 NSDUH, Arab Americans were less likely to have used marijuana and prescription drugs for nonmedical reasons than White non-Hispanic US-born group or the group of immigrant Canadian Americans. However, the pattern of drug use among Arab Americans was similar to that of immigrant Other Middle Eastern Americans. Furthermore, these results were consistent across gender, age, education and religiosity levels. However, there was no detected difference in marijuana use disorder or prescription drug use disorder between immigrant Arab Americans and the other three groups, suggesting that drug use disorder among immigrant Arab Americans is a problem. The lower prevalence of marijuana and nonmedical prescription drug use among Arab Americans (similar to lower levels of alcohol use) appears to be more influenced by cultural as opposed to general immigration factors.

These studies, similar to the ones listed for tobacco use, are mostly descriptive and rely heavily on data already available. There is a need for additional studies, especially those that will address the multiple levels of analysis as explicated in developmental psychopathology (Cicchetti & Toth, 2009). The qualitative analyses and even the secondary data on drug use patterns suggest more attention should be paid to cultural protective factors of family and friends. However, while these factors may be protective for alcohol and drug use, they may be risk factors for waterpipe use.

Conclusion

Tobacco, alcohol and drug abuse extracts a substantial societal and personal cost (Horgan, 2001). As more information on substance use patterns are documented for different racial and ethnic groups and then translated into prevention and intervention tailored services, we need to ensure that no minority group is left out. Unfortunately, there is limited data on substance use patterns among Arab Americans and no data on substance abuse prevention. The studies described and discussed highlight the concern that substance use and misuse does occur among Arab Americans, with waterpipe smoking representing a growing problem. It is not clear how much of the difference in prevalence is due to stigma. Tobacco, especially waterpipe smoking, carries lesser stigma than alcohol use among Arab Americans, especially among immigrant Arab Americans. In contrast, denial of drug and alcohol abuse may be very high among immigrant Arab Americans due to stigma. The data highlights that Arab Americans are entering substance abuse treatment for alcohol and drug abuse, but almost half of them under criminal justice pressure. This exceptionally high prevalence is similar to other ethnicities with strong stigma against drug and alcohol abuse (Arfken, Said, & Owens, 2012). Little is known about quit attempts, either from tobacco, alcohol or other drugs, among Arab Americans. Unfortunately, nothing is known about tailoring substance abuse prevention efforts to Arab Americans beyond the general risk and protective factors for tobacco use. From a public health perspective, the high level of binge drinking and waterpipe smoking especially need to be addressed.

The above information provides background on the prevalence of use and possible risk and protective factors. It does not address what interventions need to be taken to lower the societal and personal cost from tobacco, alcohol, and other drug use. One organization that has taken action is the Arab Community Center for Economic and Social Services (ACCESS) (discussed in more detail in Chap. 17). Located in Southeastern Michigan, ACCESS worked with tobacco coalitions to raise awareness among legislators and policy makers. This coalition work was instrumental in the passing of the Michigan Smoke-Air Law.

Local action has also been initiated. Tobacco vendors were and are still be contacted to educate and remind them of the legal responsibility to restrict tobacco, whether in the form of cigarettes or maassel (the pre-mix flavored tobacco used in waterpipes), to minors. Pamphlets and billboards have been designed and employed to reach out to the community. Other community based effects included establishing a community coalition with law enforcement personnel, youth, school officials, and parents with the goal of reducing substance use. To promote recovery from alcohol and drug abuse, a self-help group for Arab Americans was initiated. As this self-help or 12-step program is based upon active participation by people to accept and work on their alcohol and/or drug abuse, each person has to speak and be heard by others at the meetings. For Arab Americans who do not feel comfortable speaking English, the language barrier can be formidable. As 12-step programs have been shown to promote recovery (Fiorentine & Hillhouse, 2000) and court judges can order defendants to attend, there was a gap in service for some Arab Americans. To address this gap, Alec Berry at ACCESS created the first 12-step program that was bilingual. This program ran for several years and assisted many Arab Americans on their recovery path. Alec Berry in this role served as a translator, connection to the larger recovery community, and role model of a Muslim Arab American accepting and working on his recovery.

Other local actions include community and school presentations. These presentations are conducted to educate the public and especially the Arab American youth about the effects of waterpipe and demystify its exotic appeal. These educational efforts are complemented by a community-wide waterpipe tobacco billboard campaign as well as a bilingual brochure highlighting the adverse consequences of waterpipe and tobacco smoking.

Finally, alcohol and drug abuse are targeted through life skills curriculum at schools. This curriculum builds upon cultural values to enhance protective factors and improve familial relationships. It also addresses denial of the problem by families and to date provides a culturally accepted approach to prevent substance abuse.

References

Abou-Saleh, M., Ghubash, R., & Daradkeh, T. (2001). Al Ain community psychiatric survey. I. Prevalence and socio-demographic correlates. *Social Psychiatry and Psychiatric Epidemiology, 36*(1), 20–28.

AbuMadini, M., Rahim, S., Al-Zahrani, M., & Al-Johi, A. (2008). Two decades of treatment seeking for substance use disorders in Saudi Arabia: Trends and patterns in a rehabilitation facility in Dammam. *Drug and Alcohol Dependence, 97*(3), 231–236.

Abu-Ras, W., Ahmed, S., & Arfken, C. (2010). Alcohol Use among US Muslim college students: Risk and protective factors. *Journal of Ethnicity in Substance Abuse, 9*(3), 206–220.

Akl, E. A., Gaddam, S., Gunukula, S. K., Honeine, R., Jaoude, P. A., & Irani, J. (2010). The effects of waterpipe tobacco smoking on health outcomes: A systematic review. *International Journal of Epidemiology, 39*(3), 834–857.

Al-Faris, E. (1995). Smoking habits of secondary-school boys in rural Riyadh. *Public Health Reports, 109*, 47–55.

Al-Fayez, S. F., Salleh, M., Ardawi, M., & Zahran, F. M. (1998). Effects of sheesha and cigarette smoking on pulmonary function of Saudi males and females. *Tropical and Geographical Medicine, 40*(2), 115–123.

Al-Krenawi, A. (2005). Mental health practice in Arab countries. *Current Opinion in Psychiatry, 18*(5), 560.

Association, A. L. (2007). *Tobacco policy trend alert. An emerging deadly trend: Waterpipe tobacco use*. Washington, DC: ALA.

Amundsen, E., Rossow, I., & Skurtveit, S. (2005). Drinking pattern among adolescents with immigrant and Norwegian backgrounds: A two-way influence? *Addiction, 100*(10), 1453–1463.

Anton, R. F., O'Malley, S. S., Ciraulo, D. A., Cisler, R. A., Couper, D., Donovan, D. M., et al. (2006). Combined pharmacoptherapies and behavioral interventions for alcohol dependence. The COMBINE study: A randomized controlled trial. *Journal of the American Medical Association, 295*(17), 2003–2017.

Arfken, C., Arnetz, B. B., Fakhouri, M., Ventimiglia, M. J., & Jamil, H. (2011). Alcohol use among Arab Americans: What is the prevalence? *Journal of Immigrant and Minority Health, 13*(4), 713–718.

Arfken, C., Berry, A., & Owens, D. (2009). Pathways for Arab Americans to substance abuse treatment in Southeastern Michigan. *Journal of Muslim Mental Health, 4*(1), 31–46.

Arfken, C. L., Jamil, H., & Arnetz, B. B. (2012). Marijuana and non-medical prescription drug use among immigrant Arab Americans. *New Iraqi Journal of Medicine, 8*, 7–13.

Arfken, C. L., Kubiak, S. P., & Farrag, M. F. (2007, October 23). *Retention of Arab Americans in publicly-financed substance abuse treatment*. Paper presented at the International Society for Addiction Medicine, Cairo Egypt.

Arfken, C., Kubiak, S., & Farrag, M. (2008). Arab Americans in publicly financed alcohol/other drug abuse treatment. *Alcoholism Treatment Quarterly, 26*(3), 229–240.

Arfken, C., Kubiak, S., & Farrag, M. (2009). Acculturation and polysubstance abuse in Arab-American treatment clients. *Transcultural Psychiatry, 46*(4), 608.

Arfken, C. L., Owens, D., & Said, M. (2012). Binge drinking among Arab/Chaldeans: Exploratory study. *Journal of Ethnicity in Substance Abuse, 11*(4), 277–293.

Arfken, C. L., Said, M., & Owens, D. (2012). Racial and ethnic differences in reported criminal justice referral at treatment admission. *Journal of Psychoactive Drugs, 44*(5), 428–433.

Baker, W., & Howell, S. (2009). *Citizenship and crisis*. New York: Russell Sage Foundation.

Baker, O., & Rice, V. H. (2008). Predictors of narghile (water-pipe) smoking in a sample of American Arab Yemeni adolescents. *Journal of Transcultural Nursing, 19*(1), 24–32.

Bilal, A., Makhawi, B., Al-Fayez, G., & Shaltout, A. (1990). Attitudes of a sector of the Arab-Muslim population in Kuwait towards alcohol and drug misuse: An objective appraisal. *Drug and Alcohol Dependence, 26*(1), 55.

Botvin, G. J., Baker, E., Dusenbury, L., Botvin, E. M., & Diaz, T. (1995). Long-term follow-up results of a randomized drug abuse prevention trial in a white middle-class population. *Journal of the American Medical Association, 273*, 1106–1112.

Breslau, N., Fenn, N., & Peterson, E. L. (1993). Early smoking initiation and nicotine dependence in a cohort of young adults. *Drug and Alcohol Dependence, 33*(2), 129–137.

Cahalan, D., & Room, R. (1974). *Problem drinking among American men*. New Haven, CT: Publications Division, Rutgers Center of Alcohol Studies; distributed by College & University Press.

Centers for Disease Control and Prevention [CDC]. (2008). Smoking-attributable mortality, years of potential life lost, and productivity losses—United States, 2000–2004. *Morbidity and Mortality Weekly Report, 57*(45), 1226–1228.

Centers for Disease Control and Prevention [CDC]. (2012). *Fact Sheets*. Retrieved August 27, 2012, from http://www.cdc.gov/tobacco/data_statistics/fact_sheets/fast_facts/

Cicchetti, D., & Toth, S. L. (2009). The past achievements and future promises of developmental psychopathology: The coming of age of a discipline. *Journal of Child Psychology and Psychiatry, 50*(1–2), 16–25.

Cobb, C., Ward, K. D., Maziak, W., Shihadeh, A. L., & Eisenberg, T. (2010). Waterpipe tobacco smoking: An emerging health crisis in the United States. *American Journal of Health Behavior, 34*(3), 275–285.

de la Cruz, G. P., Brittingham, A. (2003). *The Arab Population: 2000*. U.S. Department of Commerce. U.S. Census Bureau, Census 2000 Brief.

Dube, S. R., McClave, A., James, C., Caraballo, R., Kaufmann, R., & Pechacek, T. (2010). Vital signs: Current cigarette smoking among adults aged ≥18 years—United States, 2009. *Morbidity and Mortality Weekly Report, 59*(35), 1135–1140.

Eissenberg, T., & Shihadeh, A. (2009). Waterpipe tobacco and cigarette smoking: Direct comparison of toxicant exposure. *American Journal of Preventative Medicine, 37*(6), 518–523.

El Awa, F. (2004). The role of religion in tobacco control interventions. *Bulletin of the World Health Organization, 82*(12), 894–894.

El-Hakim, I. E., & Uthman, M. A. (1999). Squamous cell carcinoma and keratoacanthoma of the lower lip associated with "Goza" and "Shisha" smoking. *International Journal of Dermatology, 38*(2), 108–110.

El-Sayed, A., & Galea, S. (2009). The health of Arab-Americans living in the United States: A systematic review of the literature. *BMC Public Health, 9*(1), 272.

Fiore, M. C., Hatsukami, D. K., & Baker, T. B. (2002). Effective tobacco dependence treatment. *Journal of the American Medical Association, 288*(14), 1768–1771.

Fiorentine, R., & Hillhouse, M. P. (2000). Drug treatment and 12-step program participation: The additive effects of integrated recovery activities. *Journal of Substance Abuse Treatment, 18*(1), 65–74.

Ghandour, L., Karam, E., & Maalouf, W. (2009). Lifetime alcohol use, abuse and dependence among university students in Lebanon: Exploring the role of religiosity in different religious faiths. *Addiction, 104*(6), 940–948.

Ghubash, R., Hamdi, E., & Bebbington, P. (1992). The Dubai community psychiatric survey: I. Prevalence and socio-demographic correlates. *Social Psychiatry and Psychiatric Epidemiology, 27*(2), 53–61.

Gold, S. (1994). *Report on the Arab community in Wayne County, Michigan*. Lansing, MI: Institute for Public Policy and Social Research.

Gorsuch, R. L. (1995). Religious aspects of substance abuse and recovery. *Journal of Social Issues, 51*(2), 65–83.

Grant, B. F., Stinson, F. S., & Harford, T. C. (2001). Age at onset of alcohol use and DSM-IV alcohol abuse and dependence: A 12-year follow-up. *Journal of Substance Abuse, 13*(4), 493–504.

Hadidi, K. A., & Mohammed, F. I. (2004). Nicotine content in tobacco used in hubble-bubble smoking. *Saudi Medical Journal, 25*(7), 912–917.

Hammal, F., Mock, J., Ward, K. D., Eissenberg, T., & Maziak, W. (2008). A pleasure among friends: How narghile (waterpipe) smoking differs from cigarette smoking in Syria. *Tobacco Control, 17*(2), e3.

Harwood, H. (2000). *Updating estimates of the economic costs of alcohol abuse in the United States: Estimates, update methods, and data. National Institute on Alcohol Abuse and.* Rockville, MD: Alcoholism.

Hasan, N. M., Loza, N., El-Dosoky, A., Hamdi, N., Rawson, R., Hasson, A. L., et al. (2009). Characteristics of clients with substance abuse disorders in a private hospital in Cairo, Egypt. *Journal of Muslim Mental Health, 4*(1), 9–15.

Horgan, C. (2001). *Substance abuse: The nation's number one health problem: Key indicators for policy update*. Princeton, NJ: The Robert Wood Johnson Foundation.

Jabbour, S., El-Roueiheb, Z., & Sibai, A. M. (2003). Nargileh (water-pipe) smoking and incident coronary heart disease: A case–control study. *Annals of Epidemiology, 13*(8), 570.

Jamil, H., Hakim Larson, J., Farrag, M., Kafaji, T., Duqum, I., & Jamil, L. H. (2002). A retrospective study of Arab American mental health clients: Trauma and the Iraqi refugees. *The American Journal of Orthopsychiatry, 72*(3), 355–361.

Jamil, H., Janisse, J., Elsouhag, D., Fafhouri, M., Arnetz, J. E., & Arnetz, B. B. (2011). Do household smoking behaviors constitute a risk factor for hookah use? *Nicotine & Tobacco Research, 13*(5), 384–388.

Jamil, H., Templin, T., Fakhouri, M., Rice, V. H., Khouri, R., & Fakhouri, H. (2009). Comparison of personal characteristics, tobacco use, and health states in Chaldean, Arab American, and Non-Middle Eastern White Adults. *Journal of Immigration and Minority Health, 11*(4), 310–317.

Johnston, L. D., O'Malley, P. M., Bachman, J. G., & Schulenberg, J. E. (2011). *Monitoring the future: National results on adolescent drug use: Overview of key findings, 2010. University of Michigan Institute for Social.* Ann Arbor, MI: Research.

Karam, E., Maalouf, W., & Ghandour, L. (2004). Alcohol use among university students in Lebanon: Prevalence, trends and covariates the IDRAC University Substance Use Monitoring Study (1991 and 1999). *Drug and Alcohol Dependence, 76*(3), 273–286.

Karam, E., Mneimneh, Z., Karam, A., Fayyad, J., Nasser, S., Chatterji, S., et al. (2006). Prevalence and treatment of mental disorders in Lebanon: A national epidemiological survey. *The Lancet, 367*(9515), 1000–1006.

Kiter, G., Uçan, E. S., Ceylan, E., & Kilinç, O. (2000). Water-pipe smoking and pulmonary functions. *Respiratory Medicine, 94*(9), 891–894.

Knishkowy, B., & Amitai, Y. (2005). Water-pipe (narghile) smoking: An emerging health risk behavior. *Pediatrics, 116*(1), e113–e119.

Maalouf, W. (2008). *Overview of the drugs and related HIV/AIDS situation. Emphasis on the MENA region.* Paper presented at the The Role of Schools in Promoting Drug Prevention, Beirut, Lebanon.

Maalouf, W., & Arfken, C. L. (2009). Guest Editors' introduction: Assessing the problem of substance abuse in the Arab world. *Journal of Muslim Mental Health, 4*(1), 5–8.

Mason, W. A., & Windle, M. (2002). A longitudinal study of the effects of religiosity on adolescent alcohol use and alcohol-related problems. *Journal of Adolescent Research, 17*(4), 346–363.

Masten, A. S. (2007). Resilience in developing systems: Progress and promise as the fourth wave rises. *Development and Psychopathology, 19*, 921–930.

Maziak, W. (2011). The global epidemic of waterpipe smoking. *Addictive Behavior, 36*(1–2), 1–5.

McLellan, A. T., Lewis, D. C., O'Brien, C. P., & Kleber, H. (2000). Drug dependence, a chronic medical illness. Implications for treatment, insurance, and outcomes evaluation. *Journal of the American Medical Association, 284*(13), 1689–1695.

Michalak, L., & Trocki, K. (2006). Alcohol and Islam: An overview. *Contemporary Drug Problems, 33*, 523.

Michalak, L., Trocki, K., & Bond, J. (2007). Religion and alcohol in the US national Alcohol Survey: How important is religion for abstention and drinking? *Drug and Alcohol Dependence, 87*(2–3), 268–280.

National Cancer Institute. (2012). *Tobacco facts.* Retrieved August 27, 2012 from http://www.cancer.gov/cancertopics/tobacco/statisticssnapshot

National Institute on Drug Abuse. (2009). *Principles of drug addiction treatment: A research-based guide.* Rockville, MD: U.S. Department of Health and Human Services.

Neumark, Y., Rahav, G., & Jaffe, D. (2003). Socio-economic status and binge drinking in Israel. *Drug and Alcohol Dependence, 69*(1), 15–21.

Neumark, Y., Rahav, G., Teichman, M., & Hasin, D. (2001). Alcohol drinking patterns among Jewish and Arab men and women in Israel. *Journal of Studies on Alcohol, 62*(4), 443–447.

Nuwayhid, I. A., Yamout, B., Azar, G., & Kambris, M. A. (1998). Narghile (Hubble-Bubble) smoking, low birth weight, and other pregnancy outcomes. *American Journal of Epidemiology, 148*(4), 375–383.45.

Razvodovsky, Y. (2004). Influence of culture on attitudes towards alcohol of Arab Muslim university students. *Adicciones, 16*(1), 53–62.

Rice, V. H., & Kilwicki, A. (1994). Cigarette use among Arab Americans in the Detroit metropolitan area. *Public Health Reports, 107*, 589–594.

Rice, V. H., Templin, T., & Kulwicki, A. (2003). Arab American adolescent tobacco use: Four pilot studies. *Preventive Medicine, 37*(5), 492–498.

Rice, V. H., Weglicki, L., Templin, T., Hammad, A., Jamil, H., & Kulwicki, A. (2006). Predictors of Arab American adolescent tobacco use. *Merrill-Palmer Quarterly, 52*(2), 327–342.

Rice, V. H., Weglicki, L. S., Templin, T., Jamil, H., & Hammad, A. (2010). Intervention effects on tobacco use among Arab and non-Arab American Adolescents. *Addictive Behaviors, 35*(1), 46–48.

Shafagoj, Y. A., Mohammed, F. I., & Hadidi, K. A. (2002). Hubble bubble (water pipe) smoking: Levels of nicotine and cotinine in plasma, saliva and urine. *International Journal of Clinical Pharmacology and Therapeutics, 40*(6), 249–255.

Shafey, O., & Musa, D. (2010). Tobacco use: Global perspective, Arab world, and Arab Americans. *ACCESS Health, 1*(1), 37–43.

Singh, P. N., Neergaard, J., Job, J. S., Setouhy, M. E., Israel, E., Mohammed, M. K., et al. (2010). Differences in health and religious beliefs about tobacco Use among waterpipe users in the rural male population of Egypt. *Journal of Religion and Health, 51*(4), 1216–1225.

Skinner, M. L., Haggerty, K. P., & Catalano, R. F. (2009). Parental and peer influences on teen smoking: Are white and black families different? *Nicotine & Tobacco Research, 11*(5), 558–563.

Soueif, M., Hannourah, M., Darweesh, Z., El-Sayed, A., Yunis, F., & Taha, H. (1987). The use of psychoactive substances by female Egyptian university students, compared with their male colleagues on selected items. *Drug and Alcohol Dependence, 19*(3), 233–247.

Templin, T., Rice, V. H., Gadelrab, M. A., Weglicki, L. S., Hammad, A., Kulwicki, A., et al. (2005). Trends in tobacco use among Arab/Arab American adolescents: Preliminary findings. *Ethnicity & Disease, 15*(Suppl 1), S1-65–S1-68.

Tobacco Use and Dependence Guideline Panel. (2008). *Treating tobacco use and dependence: 2008 update*. Rockville, MD: U.S. Department of Health and Human Services.

U.S. Department of Health and Human Services. (2007). *The Surgeon General's call to action to prevent and reduce underage drinking*. Rockville, MD: Office of the Surgeon General.

Virginia Commonwealth University. (2012). *VCU School of Nursing Center projects*. Retrieved August 27, 2012 from http://www.nursing.vcu.edu/research/centers/cbcr/projects.html

Weglicki, L., Templin, T., Rice, V. H., Jamil, H., & Hammad, A. (2008). Comparison of cigarette and water pipe smoking by Arab and non-Arab American youth. *American Journal of Preventive Medicine, 35*(4), 334–339.

WHO Study Group on Tobacco Product Regulation. (2005). *Advisory Note. Waterpipe tobacco smoking: Health effects, research needs and recommended actions by regulators*. Geneva: World Health Organization.

World Health Organization. (2011). *WHO report on the global tobacco epidemic, 2011: Warning about the dangers of tobacco*. Geneva: WHO.

Chapter 14
Diabetes Mellitus Among Arab Americans

Linda A. Jaber, Abdul Salam Al-Kassab, and Florence J. Dallo

Introduction

Type 2 diabetes mellitus is a metabolic disorder characterized by defects in insulin secretion and action and is triggered by multiple genetic, environmental, and behavioral factors, including smoking, physical inactivity, and nutrition (Ekoe, Zimmet, & Williams, 2001). Over the past two decades, there has been an explosive global increase in the prevalence of diabetes particularly in the developing countries (King, Aubert, & Herman, 1998). In 2011, the worldwide prevalence of diabetes mellitus was 366 million. By 2030, it is projected that the prevalence will reach 552 million. This increase has been attributed to adoption of advanced industrialization lifestyles.

Diabetes is an emerging clinical and public health challenge in the Arab world. Six of the ten developing countries with the highest cases of diabetes are Arab countries (Lancet, 2009). These countries are the United Arab Emirates, Saudi Arabia, Bahrain, Kuwait, Oman, and Egypt. Furthermore, it is projected that diabetes prevalence will have the largest increases, estimated at about 80 % over the next 15 years across the Middle East compared to other regions of the world.

L.A. Jaber, Pharm.D. (✉)
Department of Pharmacy Practice, Wayne State University,
259 Mack Avenue, Detroit, MI 48201, USA
e-mail: ljaber@wayne.edu

A.S. Al-Kassab, M.D., Ph.D., M.R.C.P., F.A.C.E.
Wayne State University, 2970 Crooks Road, Suite A,
Rochester Hills, MI 48309, USA
e-mail: alkassab@usa.com

F.J. Dallo, Ph.D., M.P.H.
Wellness, Health Promotion and Injury Prevention, School of Health
Sciences, Oakland University, Rochester, MI 48309, USA
e-mail: dallo@oakland.edu

S.C. Nassar-McMillan et al. (eds.), *Biopsychosocial Perspectives on Arab Americans: Culture, Development, and Health*, DOI 10.1007/978-1-4614-8238-3_14,

Rapid economic development resulting from oil discovery in the region leading to progressive urbanization and modernization is likely responsible for the increased prevalence of diabetes in the Arab countries (Alwan & King, 1995). This is supported by the consistent observation of higher estimates of glucose intolerance in urban areas characterized by higher socioeconomic status resulting in lifestyle transformation involving changes in nutritional and physical activity patterns compared to rural areas of the Arab countries (Alwan & King, 1995; Herman et al., 1995).

There is a scarcity of published research regarding the health status of the Arab American population. Differences in their health status in general and diabetes in particular are limited. A systematic review of the literature published by El-Sayed and Galea (2009) suggests that relative disease burden and determinants of diseases among Arab Americans may differ from that of other ethnic/racial populations of the USA (El-Sayed & Galea, 2009). For a disease such as diabetes, issues related to healthcare access and utilization, health beliefs and behaviors, and other cultural characteristics represent risk factors for developing diabetes. This chapter highlights key research relative to diabetes epidemiology and risk factors in the Arab American community. Issues related to barriers and strategies for providing effective diabetes care in this community are also reviewed.

The largest concentration of Arabs is in Michigan with an estimated population of over 200,000 (Zogby, 2011). Approximately 80 % of the Arab Americans in the Detroit Metropolitan identify as Lebanese/Syrian, Iraqi, Palestinian/Jordanian, or Yemeni. Approximately 75 % are foreign born, 58 % are Christian, and 42 % are Muslim. Finally, 80 % say they speak English well or very well. The following review of the literature includes numerous studies conducted within this specific community.

Epidemiology

Diabetes

To date, a total of nine studies have examined the prevalence of diabetes among Arab Americans (Hassoun, 1995; Jaber, Slaughter, & Grunberger, 1995; Genesee County Health Department, 2003; Aswad, 2001; Jaber et al., 2003; Jadalla & Lee, 2012; Jamil et al., 2008; Kridli, Herman, Brown, Fakhouri, & Jaber, 2006; Dallo & Borrell, 2006). None of the identified studies used a prospective cohort design and three of which were non-peer-reviewed (Hassoun, 1995; Genesee County Health Department, 2003; Aswad, 2001). These studies have yielded diabetes estimates ranging from 4.8 to 33.0 %.

The lack of consensus as to burden of diabetes reported in these studies is likely due to differences in the research methodologies utilized and the population studied. Of the nine studies, six used convenience samples (Hassoun, 1995; Jaber et al., 1995; Genesee County Health Department, 2003; Aswad, 2001; Jadalla & Lee, 2012; Jamil et al., 2008), two are cross-sectional analyses with randomly selected individuals from a computer-generated list (Jaber, Brown, Hammad, Nowak et al., 2003; Kridli et al., 2006), and one has utilized probability sampling from the National Health Interview Study (Dallo & Borrell, 2006). Only three of these studies utilized the oral glucose tolerance test (OGTT) for the diagnosis of diabetes. The remaining studies reported diabetes estimates based on either self-report or random glucose determinations and thus fail to detect the presence of undiagnosed diabetes. All studies were carried out in the Detroit Metropolitan area with the exception of the study by Jadalla and Lee (2012) that was conducted in southern California and the study by Dallo and Borrell (2006) that used a national dataset. As a result, it should be noted here that thus far the majority of the participants studied have been immigrants and none of the studies have systematically examined whether differences in diabetes prevalence exist between US-born and immigrant Arab Americans. Additionally, the lower prevalence estimate from the national data suggests that Arab Americans in Michigan may not be representative of the entire Arab American population across the USA.

The prevalence of self-reported diabetes among Arab Americans ranged between 7 and 20 % for those living in metropolitan areas in Michigan (Hassoun, 1995; Genesee County Health Department, 2003; Aswad, 2001; Jamil et al., 2008), 7 % for those in California (Jadalla & Lee, 2012), and 4.8 % in the lone study using national dataset (Dallo & Borrell, 2006). With the exception of the latter, all these studies used convenience samples thus limiting the validity and generalizability of the findings. In addition, the prevalence rates reported by these studies represent physician-diagnosed diabetes and therefore underestimate the actual prevalence rates.

In the two similarly designed, cross-sectional studies using the OGTT and random sampling, the age- and sex-adjusted prevalence of diabetes (either diagnosed or undiagnosed) is 18 % (Jaber, Brown, Hammad, Nowak et al., 2003) and 31 % (Kridli et al., 2006). The rate of undiagnosed diabetes was high in both studies. Undiagnosed diabetes affected 10 % (Jaber, Brown, Hammad, Nowak et al., 2003) and 14 % (Kridli et al., 2006) of the participants. It is plausible that the difference in prevalence rates reported in these two studies stems from the fact that the later has exclusively focused on Chaldean Americans.

The study by Jaber and colleagues (2003) lends support for lifestyle transformation in regard to nutritional and physical activity patterns as increasing the risk of diabetes in Arab Americans. In this study, socioeconomic characteristics (including ethnic background, education, and employment history) and behavioral factors (such as smoking habits, nutritional status, and physical activity patterns) were assessed using standardized questionnaires. The sampled community was homogeneous with striking uniformity in cultural identity based on commonality of the spoken Arabic language, the Muslim faith, and adherence to traditional values and practices. The majority (i.e., 95 %) of the study population were immigrants with a mean length of stay in the USA of 11 years. Approximately 69 % of men and 49 % of women had completed a high school education. About 80 % of men were employed compared to 19 % of women. Engagement in regular physical activity was generally low in both men and women. Analysis of nutritional intake revealed consumption of mostly traditional calorie dense Middle-Eastern foods.

The mean daily caloric intake was 2,347 ± 77 kcal, at least 150 kcal above the upper limit of daily recommended intake. The highest daily caloric intake was seen in individuals less than 35 years of age. Low intake of required vitamins and minerals such as calcium, vitamin D, biotin, copper, and chromium was also noted.

It is clear that interpretation of the findings of studies examining the burden of diabetes in this community is a challenge. A majority of these studies have used convenience sampling of Arab American immigrants in southeast Michigan and the quality of data collected is quite variable. However, the collective evidence suggests that diabetes is prevalent in the Arab American community and it is likely that the risk for the development of diabetes will continue to increase as will be demonstrated in the subsequent section.

Prediabetes

Prediabetes is defined as having impaired fasting glucose (IFG) and/or impaired glucose tolerance (IGT). IFG and IGT represent intermediate states of glucose intolerance and are known risk factors for the development of diabetes. In the Jaber et al. (2003) study of Detroit area Arab Americans, prediabetes was common, affecting about 24 % of the population. Its prevalence was much higher among men than women regardless of age. The prevalence rate of prediabetes was 30 % (95 % CI 23.4–35.9 %) in men compared to 17 % (95 % CI 12.8–20.8 %) in women ($P = 0.0007$). The mean A1C level was 5.3 % in those with prediabetes.

The Metabolic Syndrome

The metabolic syndrome is a constellation of metabolic abnormalities that has been associated with an increased risk of developing diabetes and cardiovascular disease, as well as an increase in mortality (Malik et al., 2004; Meigs et al., 2006). The metabolic syndrome is defined by the Adult Treatment Panel III diagnostic criteria as having three or more of the following: large waist circumference (>102 cm in men and >88 cm in women), high blood pressure (≥130/85 mmHg), high serum triglycerides (≥150 mg/dl), low serum HDL concentrations (<40 mg/dl in men and <50 mg/dl in women), and high fasting plasma glucose (FPG) defined at the time of the study as ≥110 mg/dl (Adult Treatment Panel III [ATPIII], 2001). The metabolic syndrome is also defined by the World Health Organization (WHO) criteria where an individual with diabetes, IFG, IGT, or insulin resistance plus two or more abnormalities (e.g., blood pressure ≥160/90, triglyceride ≥150 mg/dl, and/or HDL <35 mg/dl in men and <39 mg/dl in women, obesity with waist-to-hip ratio, WHR, >0.9 in men and >0.85 in women, and/or BMI >30 kg/m^2) is considered to have the metabolic syndrome (Alberti & Zimmet, 1998). Insulin resistance was estimated by the homeostasis model assessment (Mathews et al., 1985).

The prevalence of the metabolic syndrome and its association with insulin resistance was examined in the Arab American community (Jaber, Brown, Hammad, Zhu, & Herman, 2004). The age-adjusted prevalence of the metabolic syndrome was 23 % by the ATPIII standards and 28 % by the WHO guidelines. The prevalence rose significantly with increasing age and BMI in both sexes. Age-specific rates were similar for men and women aged 20–49 years but significantly higher in women ≥50 years of age compared to men. Low HDL cholesterol concentration was the most common component of the metabolic syndrome in both men and women. A strong association between insulin resistance (estimated by the homeostasis model assessment described by Mathews et al., 1985) and the individual components of the metabolic syndrome was observed. After fitting a model with insulin resistance as the outcome, associations remained significant for waist circumference, serum triglycerides, and FPG levels.

Diabetes Risk Factors

Several factors have been associated with increased future risk of developing diabetes. These risk factors appear to differ among different populations. The contribution of multiple risks to the progression of diabetes in Arab Americans has been systematically examined and these risk factors are reviewed below (Jaber, Brown, Hammad, Nowak et al., 2003; Jaber, Brown, Hammad, Zhu, & Herman, 2003; Pinelli, Jaber, Brown, & Herman, 2010).

Age and Sex

Higher rates of dysglycemia were associated with older age in men and women (Jaber, Brown, Hammad, Nowak et al., 2003). However, there were age- and sex-related differences in diabetes prevalence patterns. In men, diabetes prevalence was higher than in women aged 20–49. It reached a plateau in the group 40–50 years of age and then remained relatively unchanged afterwards. In women, diabetes prevalence was low below the age of 40 years old and rose steadily afterwards, affecting 54 % of women above the age of 60 years old.

Family History of Diabetes

The presence of a paternal history of diabetes was not associated with diabetes (Jaber, Brown, Hammad, Nowak et al., 2003). However, a positive association between reported maternal histories of diabetes was noted in men but not in women.

Whether the greater maternal transmission of diabetes observed in Arab American men represents a genetic predisposition or is the result of a difference in reporting recall is not known.

Physical Activity

Physical inactivity represents a major risk factor for diabetes. Patterns of physical activity were assessed in Arab Americans (Jaber, Brown, Hammad, Nowak et al., 2003). Individuals were considered to be physically active if they reported to regularly engage in activities that made them breathe hard and sweat, to walk for ≥15 min at a time, or to perform non-strenuous physical activity for ≥150 min/week. Individuals who did not engage in any of these activities were considered inactive. The majority of Arab Americans studied (72 %) were classified as inactive. More women (81 %) were inactive than men (58 %). No association between diabetes and physical inactivity was noted in this population.

Obesity

About 34 % of the Arab Americans studied were obese with BMI ≥30 kg/m^2 (Jaber, Brown, Hammad, Nowak et al., 2003). Individuals with central obesity (defined as WHR ≥0.8 for women and ≥0.9 for men) comprised 52 %. Positive and significant associations were noted between diabetes and BMI and WHR. Patients with diabetes had higher mean BMI and WHR than those with normal glucose tolerance.

Smoking

An association between smoking and incident diabetes has been established in US adults (Foy, Bell, Farmer, Goff, & Wagenknecht, 2005). Smoking is quite common among Arab Americans (Jaber, Brown, Hammad, Nowak et al., 2003). The majority (78 %) reported being either current or former smokers. To date, however, no direct relationship between smoking status and diabetes has been noted in this population.

Acculturation

Acculturation has been associated with increased risk of diabetes in some but not all migrant populations. In one study, the length of stay in the USA was shown to be negatively associated with diabetes prevalence in Arab Americans (Dallo & Borrell, 2006).

Jaber and colleagues have systematically assessed the impact of acculturation in Arab Americans using a variety of markers and scales measuring integration into the American society (Jaber, Brown, Hammad, Zhu, & Herman, 2003). These markers included the type of area an individual lived in as a child, age at immigration to the USA, duration of residence in the USA, Arabic language use and proficiency, and individual preferences as to personal ethnic identification and ethnicity of friends. This study demonstrated that less acculturated Arab Americans were generally at greater risk for diabetes than those with greater acculturation. In men, dysglycemia was associated with older age at the time of immigration (mean age was 34 years in those with diabetes and 24 years in those with normal glucose tolerance), not having employment, speaking Arabic with friends, being less active in Arabic organizations, more frequently consuming Arabic food, and being less integrated into American society. For women, dysglycemia was associated with being raised in rural areas of the Middle East, being older at the time of immigration (mean age was 40 years in those with diabetes and 26 years in those with normal glucose tolerance), having a longer length of stay in the USA (mean length of stay being 15 years in those with diabetes and 9 years with those with normal glucose tolerance), not being employed outside the home, being educated below a high school level, not attending Arabic or American schools, and not being able to read Arabic (or English).

Vitamin D Status

Low vitamin D levels are associated with diabetes in some populations. Vitamin D insufficiency was documented in 87 Arab American women. Lower levels were noted in those with the traditional Muslim clothing (Hobbs et al., 2009). Another study by Pinelli and colleagues has shown that the prevalence of vitamin D deficiency as assessed by 25-hydroxyvitamin D levels (25-OH-D) is quite high in a representative cross-sectional sample of Arab Americans (Pinelli et al., 2010). Vitamin D insufficiency (serum 25-OH-D levels, 5 to <20 ng/ml) was detected in 75 % and hypovitaminosis (serum 25-OH-D levels, 20 to <40 ng/ml) in 24 % of individuals. Lower 25-OH-D levels were associated with insulin resistance and diabetes in men but not in women.

Quality of Diabetes Care

Arab Americans face serious disparities in health compared to White Americans and receive suboptimal healthcare. The quality of care received by Arab American patients with diabetes was examined by assessing the adherence to ADA standard of care guidelines and by utilizing the Diabetes Quality Improvement Project (DQIP) quality performance measures (Berlie, Herman, Brown, Hammad, & Jaber, 2008).

Study participants were less aggressively treated with pharmacological therapies than recommended by the ADA. The majority were maintained on oral hypoglycemic agents (81 %), 18 % received insulin, and only 9 % were on combined insulin and oral agents. Daily aspirin intake was reported by 23 %, statin use by 30 %, and a majority of those with hypertension were receiving antihypertensive monotherapy. The ADA-recommended goal for A1C of <7 % was only met by 30 %. Over one quarter had worse glycemic control compared to the national population with A1C levels of ≥10 %. The goals for LDL of <100 mg/dl were met by 36 % and for blood pressure of <130/85 by 16 % of individuals studied. In general, the Arab American patients had better lipid control but worse blood pressure control than the general public.

Barriers and Strategies to Effective Diabetes Care: Implications for Practice

Unlike other illnesses, medical nutrition therapy, exercise, healthy lifestyle, and diabetes self-management education are integral components of diabetes management. It is well known that health beliefs and health behaviors are influenced, at least partly, by cultural factors. This relationship of culture to health beliefs and behaviors is especially important in diabetes treatment strategies that target lifestyle modification and often involve changing patterns of eating, physical activity, and other culturally embedded behaviors. In addition, the chronic nature of the illness often requires lifelong compliance with multiple medications. In the absence of these components, the management of the disease and its devastating complications become almost impossible. Consequently, any management plan for diabetes should take into consideration the individual's lifestyle, eating and physical activity patterns, and cultural factors, without which the expected compliance with the treatment plan becomes compromised. In this section, the barriers to effective diabetes care for Arab Americans and strategies to overcome those barriers will be addressed.

Barriers

Linguistics and Communication

Despite the fact that Arab Americans have been an important demographic component of the wider American fabric, it is surprising that few resources pertinent to Arab Americans exist. Dietary plans, for example, which are the foundation of diabetes care, are difficult to find in Arabic. Those which exist present a simple translation of the American diabetic diets. Very few Arabic patients follow such a diet and the majority instead opt for a traditional Arabic diet. Furthermore, the Arab American population is a heterogeneous group who migrated from different

Arab countries and they tend to maintain their traditional foods and meals. Therefore, it is hard to find a single universal Arab American diet as various Arab countries have diets which differ in carbohydrate contents. For example, the gulf area and Iraq principally consume rice and red meat-based foods, while countries such as Jordan, Syria, and Lebanon regularly consume foods that are vegetable- and legume-based. Although diets in general are getting more cosmopolitan, a significant number of first-generation immigrants maintain their original homeland dietary habits. Also since Arab immigrants may lack good English language skills, it becomes even more important to have culturally appropriate resources on dietary plans in Arabic. These resources must be simple to understand and follow. In addition to diet, other aspects of education relevant to diabetes, such as exercise and foot care, are also overlooked in educational materials and services available for Arab American patients.

Another major barrier is the communication with healthcare providers. Diabetes management requires a physician-coordinated team that includes nurses, dieticians, social workers, and other healthcare providers. Few physicians speak Arabic and relatively fewer mid-level providers who are likely to deliver diabetes education to patients speak Arabic. The linguistic barrier combined with cultural differences between the Arabic patient and the providers result in ineffective communication and in turn negatively impact care.

Cultural Factors

The Arabic culture promotes certain health behaviors that will adversely affect the care of the Arab American patients with diabetes. Cultural practices such as the habit of eating late and having heavy dinners are acceptable among community members and are not consistent with diabetes management principles. This widespread practice tends to promote obesity and contribute to extended periods of postprandial hyperglycemia. In addition, socialization that centers around food is quite common in the Arab American community. Different types of food are offered in plenty during regular visitation and this tradition is considered a sign of generosity. Refusal to eat is not culturally acceptable and may be viewed by some hosts as an insult.

Another major barrier to healthcare is the concept of routine visits to the healthcare providers. There is often a strong "sense of the present" within the Arab American community. Orientation toward the future is not consistent with the cultural pattern. As a result, routine health maintenance visits are not common among Arab Americans. Instead, most people seek the healthcare provider only if they are sick. The fear of uncovering serious medical problem like diabetes also contributes to the delay in seeking medical care.

Another cultural barrier is the way a diagnosis of genetically related diseases such as diabetes is viewed. A diagnosis of diabetes is commonly recognized as a stigma. While this practice is slowly fading with the increasing prevalence of diabetes in the community, it is still present and will impact medical care. This stigma often results in a reluctance to disclose information except within the family and also deters individuals from obtaining knowledge about treatment and prevention. In those patients who are maintained on insulin, there is a tendency to skip the lunchtime injection.

Myths and Misconceptions

Diabetes is a chronic condition that affects the entire body and leads to multiple complications. This complexity lends itself to a myriad of myths and misconceptions. These are reviewed below by categories revolving around the disease itself or its treatment.

Myths around the disease diabetes are plentiful. Jaber and colleagues conducted focus groups to explore myths and misconceptions relevant to diabetes in a representative sample of 71 (38 % males) community members (unpublished data). The perception of diabetes prevalence in Arabs was high among study participants. Myths and misconceptions identified included the belief that diabetes results from being upset, anxious, worried, under stress, or experiencing emotional shock or surprise. Few associate diabetes with lifestyle, dietary intake, or other environmental factors. The inability to conceive children among diabetic females is another myth.

On the treatment side, there are many myths and misconceptions about insulin. Traditionally, insulin being an injectable drug is not viewed very favorably in Arab American patients. Some believe insulin is addictive, and therefore it is impossible to get off of it. "Once on insulin you will always be on insulin" is a common belief. There are also misconceptions about hypoglycemia and weight gain resulting from insulin therapy. Many avoid insulin because of the fear of hypoglycemia. While these latter concerns are justified, they are usually exaggerated. This results in delaying early initiation and timely intensification of insulin at the expense of poor metabolic control and the advent of complications. With the plethora of oral antidiabetic agents, this phenomenon is becoming worse. A good deal of these misconceptions stems from the use of older insulin products which are more likely to cause hypoglycemia. Additionally, older insulin products are not available in pens. The availability of pens has made insulin use more convenient. Still, myths circulate regarding diet and insulin use. Some patients on insulin believe that they can eat anything without restrictions.

Regarding oral agents, it is commonly believed that these agents work the same for all patients with diabetes and therefore sharing is a relatively common practice. Food, on the other hand, is generally not regarded as harmful. Certain foods such as honey and dates are considered healthy and are usually consumed in large quantities. On the other hand, sugar substitutes are believed to be carcinogenic and are usually avoided. This is one of the reasons for the common use of complementary and alternative medicine in the Arab American community. Herbal remedies are viewed as accepted means to treat diabetes and its complications. Similar to many cultures, there is a common belief that these agents are safe since they are natural.

Knowledge Deficits

Focus groups conducted by Jaber and colleagues have demonstrated that deficits in knowledge regarding diabetes represent a major barrier for diabetes care among Arab Americans (unpublished data). Perhaps most important is the failure to understand the devastating long-term consequences of diabetes. This problem is compounded by the fact that diabetes is a silent disease until its immediate and complicated effects become quite advanced. The asymptomatic nature of diabetes combined with erroneous and inadequate knowledge about diabetes and its complications impede adherence to diet and medications and effective, long-term behavioral changes. Patients report feeling fine and do not see the immediate benefit of restrictions on diet and using any intensification of diabetic control known to be associated with hypoglycemia which can be quite symptomatic. Another common misunderstanding revolves around proper treatment of hypoglycemia; patients often overeat to treat or to prevent hypoglycemia which leads to weight gain and poor glycemic control.

Healthcare System

Deficits in the healthcare system such as gaining access to and receiving quality of healthcare represent major barriers to care particularly among minority groups including the Arab Americans. In this area, there is a difference between the first- and the second-generation Arab Americans. To the first-generation less acculturated immigrant patients, accessing the healthcare system is a challenge. They also tend to seek medical care when they feel sick which is inappropriate for effective diabetic control. Second-generation younger and more acculturated Arab Americans, on the other hand, may have better understanding of the healthcare system and health needs; however, the lack of or having limited medical insurance hinders their ability to access the healthcare system.

Cultural differences between healthcare providers and Arab patients impede medical care. Stereotyping and clinical uncertainty are common among providers. There is a lack of understanding of Arab American traditions, health beliefs and practices, family structure and role, gender considerations, and dietary and physical activity preferences. Female patients may feel more comfortable with female health providers, but there is a shortage of such providers who speak the language and understand the culture. There are instances where the provider may be perceived to be insensitive or unsympathetic to the needs of the Arab American diabetic patient. Examples of these instances include the desire to fast during the month of Ramadan for the Muslim patients or insisting on washing the feet of a person who has a foot ulcer. The perception toward the healthcare system is an important barrier that needs to change to be able to attract more patients.

Additionally, there is a lack of interpretation services or bilingual education programs that specifically target the Arab American patients with diabetes.

Strategies

Given the barriers outlined above, one can devise strategies to overcome these barriers.

If diabetes strategies are to be effective, they must be sensitive and relevant to the culture of the persons who are expected to carry them out. From the findings of focus groups conducted by Jaber and colleagues, one may conclude that any model of diabetes care adapted to the Arab American community must approach the issues of gender, religion, family, and community, as well as dispel health myths in a culturally sensitive manner (unpublished data). The cultural adaptations must include family involvement, reference to ethnic foods and cooking techniques, and culturally acceptable physical activities. Education is the key point in devising these strategies.

Increased Awareness

This is a universal strategy which can be equally applied to patients and providers. On the patients' side, increased awareness of the devastating consequences of uncontrolled diabetes may ultimately reset the mentality of seeking help only during crises. Educational efforts targeting the importance of complying with diet and medical therapies in achieving metabolic control are urgently needed. On the other hand, education to eliminate and dissipate the social stigma and many of the myths related to diabetes, such as infertility in females being attributed to diabetes, are also essential.

On the providers' side, education and increased awareness of the Arab American patients' cultural and social issues are the foundation to providing quality care. Increased awareness about the dietary habits, compliance issues, culturally driven health behaviors, the role and dynamic of family, and gender considerations are all important steps to overcome the barriers to quality healthcare.

Correcting Knowledge Gaps

Education on both the individual and community levels is needed. A common practice is to translate medical information into Arabic for more widespread use. This is especially important for diet and insulin administration instructions. Equally important is providing translation of authentic information on diabetes, diabetes complications, and dealing with hypoglycemia. Translation, in and of itself, is a challenge, as one needs professional translators who are fluent in both the language and the medical content. Very often the translation work relies on volunteers due to the limited community resources. In addition, translation should not be merely linguistic. Relevant medical information may not simply be translated into Arabic, rather it must be culturally rewritten for the use by this community in ways that reflect its cultural norms. Thus, necessary resources need to be committed to such efforts.

Additionally, the utilization of mass media is an effective tool to promote education and increase awareness. In the past, targeted media campaigns coinciding with diabetes awareness week have been useful. Culturally appropriate lectures, posters, literature, and community-based approaches are instrumental. Another target of education is to tackle the epidemic of type 2 diabetes mellitus in the country as a whole as well as in the Arab American population by addressing the risk factors of inappropriate eating habits, lack of physical activity, and obesity.

Culturally Competent Care

It is well known that culture plays an integral part in shaping health beliefs and behaviors and marginalization of culture is a barrier to care. Cross-cultural education should be integrated into the training of healthcare providers. The availability of a healthcare system of providers who understand the cultural dimensions of diabetes is needed in order to improve health outcomes, provide a better and more accepted delivery of clinical services, and reduce health disparities in the Arab American patients with diabetes. To this end, patients should feel that they are receiving compassionate care from their healthcare providers and realize the value of connecting to their providers. A good model in the Detroit and Southeastern Michigan area is the Arab Community Center for Economic and Social Services (ACCESS) clinic, which is located in the heart of the Arab American population and run by healthcare providers from the community who have an understanding of the cultural needs of the community.

Pharmacologic Therapy

In this section, the pharmacologic therapies of diabetes will be summarized in the cultural context reflecting on specifics for the Arab American community.

Insulin

Insulin is perhaps the most controversial issue from the Arab American perspective when it comes to agents used to treat diabetes because of the aforementioned myths and misconceptions. This is changing, however, with the introduction of newer insulin analogues, especially the long-acting products such as detemir and glargine which allow once-daily administration. The challenge remains when an intensive insulin therapy program is introduced where three or four injections are needed to achieve metabolic control. Such regimen is often difficult for patients to accept and follow. Since almost 50 % of patients with type 2 diabetes will need insulin, more work needs to be done to improve insulin acceptance rate. A common strategy of prescribing a once-a-day long-acting insulin (preferably using pens) in combination with one or more oral agents is potentially a good starting point. Proper education is needed regarding the prevalence of insulin-associated side effects in particular hypoglycemia and weight gain and strategies to deal with them.

Injectable Incretin Mimetics

These agents are relatively newer and have the appeal, besides being agents to lower blood glucose, of reducing body weight which is a desired outcome by a majority of patients with diabetes. Despite being injectable products, which are generally perceived as negative, the existence of pens and the use of one or two times per day and more recently, once per week, make them attractive options in the management of diabetes. In the Arab American community, their use is similar to that of the general population and is relatively low with cost posing a major issue.

Oral Agents

All oral agents are acceptable in principal to patients with type 2 diabetes. In general, compliance improves when drugs are used one to two times per day versus agents that require three or more usages per day. In the following paragraphs, an evaluation is presented in brief about each class of oral agents.

Sulfonylureas can be used once per day and are thus convenient to take. However, the risk of hypoglycemia exists. Therefore, they are not suitable for the Arab American patient who eats erratically or misses or delays meals.

Metformin, on the other hand, is a well-tolerated agent which is widely used in the Arab American community, especially due to its low risk of hypoglycemia and cost. However, the incidence of GI upset and diarrhea, especially in the immediate release version, is high. Moreover, the need for routine (though infrequent) monitoring of serum creatinine makes metformin unsuitable for individuals with advanced diabetes (hence nephropathy) and in those with unreliable track record of office visits and laboratory testing.

Meglitinides (repaglinide, nateglinide) are best described as short-acting insulin releasing agents and are useful agents with a lower risk of hypoglycemia than sulfonylureas but need to be used multiple times per day before meals. This is a downside for non-adherent patients. Other patients tend to use it as an "oral" insulin form by taking extra pills when extra food is consumed.

The oral dipeptidyl peptidase-4 inhibitors (or the gliptins) such as saxagliptin and sitagliptin are well-tolerated, can be taken once a day, and carry a low risk of hypoglycemia. However, cost remains an issue. Other newer agents such as bromocriptine and colvaslam have been recently approved for use in diabetes, but their regimen for use remains quite complicated and compliance is expected to be low. Thiazolidinediones are falling out of favor in general due to the associated risks of cardiovascular disease and weight gain.

Special Management Considerations: Guidelines

Although religiously diverse, most Arab Americans in the Detroit Metropolitan area are Muslims. The role of Islam is inseparable from the fabric of the culture with daily prayers, dietary prescriptions and proscriptions, and religious fasts. The Islamic religion requires its followers to observe five pillars that include fasting during the month of Ramadan and pilgrimage to the kingdom of Saudi Arabia. These Islamic requirements may substantially influence healthcare behaviors and practices.

Ramadan

Ramadan is the lunar month during which Muslims refrain from any oral intake including foods, fluids, and medications from dawn to dusk. Depending on the season and the geographical location, the fasting period may extend for an average of 12 to more than 18 h per day. In addition, many Muslims voluntarily fast 1–2 days per week throughout the year. During fasting, the typical daily eating pattern consists of a large meal at sunset, referred to as Iftar, and a lighter meal before dawn, known as Suhur with relatively varying amounts of sweets, dates, fruits, and juices in between the two meals. Most Muslim patients with diabetes fast during Ramadan against medical advice and despite religious exemption.

Several potential risks are associated with fasting during Ramadan especially among those with poor glycemic control and in those with type 1 diabetes. The Epidemiology of Diabetes and Ramadan study, a population-based study that included over 12,000 patients from 13 different Islamic countries, has reported increased rates of acute complications, including severe hypoglycemia requiring hospitalization and hyperglycemia with or without ketoacidosis (Salti et al., 2004). Increased risks of dehydration and thrombosis have also been reported. The practices and complications among 27 Arab American patients with diabetes observing fasting during Ramadan have been examined (Pinelli & Jaber, 2011). Consultation with their healthcare providers was reported by 67 % of patients. However, information regarding medications, fasting risks, indications for breaking fast, meal planning, or engaging in physical activity was not provided to most patients. A majority reported less physical activity (73 %). About half modified home blood glucose testing with 25 % reducing the frequency of testing and 17 % not testing at all. About half reported therapeutic modification mainly involving the timing of the dose.

The lack of education regarding safe fasting during Ramadan contributes to the suboptimal practices and the fasting-related morbidity reported in patients with diabetes. By the same token, the scarcity of research limits the development of evidence-based guidelines for the management of diabetes during Ramadan. An updated set of recommendations based on expert opinion has been published and represents a lone and valuable source for the practicing clinicians providing care for the Muslim patients with diabetes (Al-Arouj et al., 2010). In general, these guidelines emphasize the need for individualized management plans; frequent monitoring of blood glucose; performing medical assessment prior to Ramadan; providing education detailing the risks and the indications to breakfasting, in addition to specific instructions related to meal planning, time, and intensity of physical activity and modifications in therapeutic regimens. Future research examining the potential complications of fasting, the identification of high-risk groups prone to these complications, and the management approaches to minimize these complications is essential.

Islamic Pilgrimage

Pilgrimage or Haj is the journeying to the two holy cities of Mecca and Medina in the Kingdom of Saudi Arabia (where Islam was revealed to the Prophet Muhammad), at least once in the person's lifetime. To Muslims, Haj is a blessed journey that absolves all sins. However, the performance of Haj is associated with a number of potential risks for the patients with diabetes (Ahmed & Jaber, 2003). Over two million people descending on these cities leads to overcrowding, close contacts, poor hygiene, and spread of illnesses. Haj rituals are physically and mentally strenuous resulting in neglect of health and medical care. Other factors include irregular meals, altered diets, and lack of sleep. A study of pilgrims with diabetes reported increased risks of hypoglycemia, hyperglycemia, cut wounds, heat exhaustion, and coma (Baomer & El Bushra, 1998).

A set of recommendations has been published and provides guidelines aimed at minimizing the risks associated with Haj for patients with diabetes (Ahmed & Jaber, 2003). In summary, these recommendations include consultation with the primary care provider prior to travel, receiving the quadrivalent meningococcal vaccine, travel with a guided group that includes a physician, packing all diabetes care-related products in sufficient quantities, avoiding large crowds, and strictly following meal planning and therapeutic regimen.

Implications

This chapter provides clear evidence of the paucity of research related to diabetes in Arab Americans. Most studies reviewed have notable limitations precluding the validity and generalizability of their findings. Critical gaps in knowledge exist in several key areas including whether there are differences in diabetes burden and consequences among Arab Americans as a group or compared to other ethnic groups of the USA, and their response to diabetes therapies and management strategies. One of the main obstacles to research involves the fact that Arab Americans are classified as "White" by federal agencies; hence there are no numerator or denominator data available to calculate disease prevalence or incidence rates.

A change in ethnic/racial classification for this population will allow embarking on national prospective cohort studies to define diabetes burden in this population and address gaps in knowledge as to most successful approaches for the implementation of diabetes management strategies. Such research endeavors will form the foundation for a shift in healthcare policies to improve diabetes outcomes in this population.

Summary

A systematic analysis of the current knowledge clearly reveals that Arab Americans are disproportionately affected by diabetes. It is further projected that the burden of diabetes will continue to increase thus imposing a substantial public health burden and a major challenge to healthcare providers. Despite these growing concerns regarding diabetes and the cultural uniqueness of this community, critical gaps in knowledge in regard to diabetes exist. Culture shapes health behaviors relevant for diabetes and marginalization of culture is a barrier to care while incorporating cultural preferences is the foundation for effective intervention strategies. Educational programs for the Arab American patients with diabetes and for healthcare practitioners are emphasized. The scarcity of published research is also alarming and highlights the need for well-designed, prospective, population-based research studies.

References

Ahmed, A. M., & Jaber, L. A. (2003). Islamic pilgrimage (HAJ): Care of diabetic pilgrims. *Practical Diabetology, 22*, 41–43.

Al-Arouj, M., Assaad-Khalil, S., Buse, J., Fahdil, I., Fahmy, M., Hafez, S., et al. (2010). Recommendations for management of diabetes during Ramadan. *Diabetes Care, 33*, 1895–1902.

Alberti, K. G., Zimmet, P. Z. (1998). Definition, diagnosis, and classification of diabetes mellitus and its complications. Part 1: Diagnosis and classification of diabetes mellitus provisional report of a WHO consultation. *Diabetic Medicine, 15*, 539–553.

Alwan, A., & King, H. (1995). Diabetes in the Eastern Mediterranean (Middle East) Region: The World Health Organization responds to a major public health challenge. *Diabetic Medicine, 12*, 1057–1058.

Aswad, M. (2001). *Health survey of the Arab, Muslim, and Chaldean American communities in Michigan*. Dearborn, MI: ACCESS. Retrieved from http://www.accesscommunity.org/site/DocServer/health_and_research_cente_19.pdf.

Baomer, A. A. S., & El Bushra, H. E. (1998). Profile of diabetic Omani pilgrims to Mecca. *East African Medical Journal, 75*, 211–214.

Berlie, H. D., Herman, W. H., Brown, M. B., Hammad, A., & Jaber, L. A. (2008). Quality of diabetes care in Arab Americans. *Diabetes Res Clin Pract, 79*, 249–255.

Dallo, F. J., & Borrell, L. N. (2006). Self-reported diabetes and hypertension among Arab Americans in the United States. *Ethnicity & Disease, 16*(3), 699–705.

Ekoe, J.-M., Zimmet, P., & Williams, R. (Eds.). (2001). *The epidemiology of diabetes mellitus: An international perspective*. England: John Wiley and Sons.

El-Sayed, A. M., & Galea, S. (2009). The health of Arab-Americans living in the United States: A systematic review of the literature. *BMC Public Health 9*, 272. Retrieved from http://www.biomedcentral.com/1471-2458/9/272

Foy, C. G., Bell, R. A., Farmer, D. F., Goff, D. C., & Wagenknecht, L. E. (2005). Smoking and incidence of diabetes among U.S. adults. *Diabetes Care, 28*, 2501–2507.

Genesee County Health Department. (2003). *Arab American health survey*, pp. 1–24. Retrieved from http://www.gchd.us/pdf/AAHS.pdf

Hassoun, R. (1995). *A bioanthropological perspective of hypertension in Arab Americans in the metropolitan area*. Gainesville: University of Florida.

Herman, W. H., Ali, M. A., Aubert, R. E., Engelgau, M. M., Kenny, S. J., Gunter, E. W., et al. (1995). Diabetes mellitus in Egypt: Risk factors and prevalence. *Diabetic Medicine, 12*, 1126–1131.

Hobbs, R. D., Habib, Z., Alromaihi, D., Idi, L., Parikh, N., Blocki, F., et al. (2009). Severe vitamin D deficiency in Arab-American women living in Dearborn, Michigan. *Endocrine Practice, 15*, 35–40.

Jaber, L. A., Brown, M. B., Hammad, A., Nowak, S. N., Zhu, Q., Ghafoor, A., et al. (2003). Epidemiology of diabetes among Arab Americans. *Diabetes Care, 26*, 308–313.

Jaber, L. A., Brown, M. B., Hammad, A., Zhu, Q., & Herman, W. H. (2003). Lack of acculturation is a risk factor for diabetes in Arab immigrants to America. *Diabetes Care, 26*, 2010–2014.

Jaber, L. A., Brown, M. B., Hammad, A., Zhu, Q., & Herman, W. H. (2004). The prevalence of the metabolic syndrome among Arab Americans. *Diabetes Care, 27*, 234–238.

Jaber, L. A., Slaughter, R. L., & Grunberger, G. (1995). Diabetes and related metabolic risk factors among Arab Americans. *The Annals of Pharmacotherapy, 29*, 573–576.

Jadalla, A., & Lee, J. (2012). The relationship between acculturation and general health of Arab Americans. *Journal of Transcultural Nursing, 23*, 159–165.

Jamil, H., Fakhouri, M., Dallo, F., Templin, T., Khoury, R., & Fakhouri, H. (2008). Disparities in self-reported diabetes mellitus among Arab, Chaldean, and black American in Southeast Michigan. *Journal of Immigrant and Minority Health, 10*, 397–405.

King, H., Aubert, R. E., & Herman, W. H. (1998). Global burden of diabetes, 1995-2025: Prevalence, numerical estimates, and projections. *Diabetes Care, 9*, 1414–1431.

Kridli, S. A.-O., Herman, W. H., Brown, M. B., Fakhouri, H., & Jaber, L. A. (2006). The epidemiology of diabetes and its risk factors among Chaldean Americans. *Ethnicity & Disease, 16*, 351–356.

Lancet. (2009). Diabetes – A global threat [Editorial]. *Lancet, 373*(9677), 1735. doi:10.1016/S0140-6736(09)60954-5.

Malik, S., Wong, N. D., Franklin, S. S., Kamath, T. V., L'Italien, G. J., Pio, J. R., et al. (2004). Impact of the metabolic syndrome on mortality from coronary heart disease, cardiovascular disease, and all causes in United States adults. *Circulation, 110*, 1245–1250.

Mathews, D. R., Hosker, J. P., Rudenski, A. S., Naylor, B. A., Treacher, D. F., & Turner, R. C. (1985). Homeostasis model assessment: Insulin resistance and β-cell function from fasting plasma glucose and insulin concentrations in man. *Diabetologia, 28*, 412–419.

Meigs, J. B., Wilson, P. W., Fox, C. S., Vasan, R. S., Nathan, D. M., Sullivan, L. M., et al. (2006). Body mass index, metabolic syndrome, and risk of type 2 diabetes or cardiovascular disease. *Journal of Clinical Endocrinology and Metabolism, 91*, 2906–2912.

National Heart, Lung, and Blood Institute. (2001). Executive summary of the third report of the National Cholesterol Education Program (NCEP) Expert Panel on detection, evaluation, and treatment of high blood cholesterol in adults (Adult Treatment Panel III). *Journal of the American Medical Association, 285*, 2486–2497.

Pinelli, N. R., & Jaber, L. A. (2011). Practices of Arab Americans with type 2 diabetes mellitus during Ramadan. *Journal of Pharmacy Practice, 24*(2), 211–215. doi:10.1177/0897190010367432.ed.

Pinelli, N. R., Jaber, L. A., Brown, M. B., & Herman, W. H. (2010). Serum 25-hydroxy vitamin D and insulin resistance, metabolic syndrome, and glucose intolerance among Arab Americans. *Diabetes Care, 33*, 1373–1375.

Salti, I., Benard, E., Detournay, B., Bianchi-Biscay, M., Brigand, C. L., Voinet, C., et al. (2004). A population-based study of diabetes and its characteristics during the fasting month of Ramadan in 13 countries. *Diabetes Care, 27*, 2306–2311.

Zogby, J. [Arab American Institute]. (2011). *Demographics*. Retrieved from http://www.aaiusa.org/arab-americans/22/demographics

Chapter 15
Maternal and Child Health

Florence J. Dallo, Carolyn Archer, and Dawn P. Misra

Introduction

Maternal and child health (MCH) is a field that defines its focus by the growth and developmental stage of the individual. Studying and addressing the health needs of the MCH population require an appreciation of the unique nature of this population with regard to its dynamic growth and development (Zadrozny, Power, Nishimi, & Kizer, 2004). Children are not small adults, but rather, have unique vulnerabilities as well as resilience that may relate to their stage of growth and/or development. The health of the MCH population has long been well established as pivotal to the health of the adult population. At its most basic, life expectancy is strongly determined by the infant mortality rate. However, more recently, evidence has been accumulating that the in utero environment as well as early childhood exposures and experiences may influence health in adulthood (Smith et al., 2006; Xue & Michels, 2007). It appears that effects on health may result from exposures in critical periods (e.g., in utero) or from accumulation of exposures over the life course beginning in childhood (Gustafsson, Janlert, Theorell, Westerlund, & Hammarstrom, 2010; Misra, Astone, & Lynch, 2005). This is a burgeoning area of research that promotes even greater emphasis on the health of the MCH population.

Traditionally, the MCH population has encompassed pregnant women, infants, children, and adolescents (Kotch, 2005; Wallace, Green, & Jaros, 2003). More recently, preconceptional and overall women's health has been integrated into

F.J. Dallo, Ph.D., M.P.H. (✉)
Wellness, Health Promotion and Injury Prevention, School of Health Sciences, Oakland University, Rochester, MI 48309, USA
e-mail: dallo@oakland.edu

C. Archer • D.P. Misra
Department of Family Medicine and Public Health Sciences, Wayne State University School of Medicine, 3939 Woodward Avenue, Detroit, MI 48201, USA
e-mail: carche@med.wayne.edu; dmisra@med.wayne.edu

S.C. Nassar-McMillan et al. (eds.), *Biopsychosocial Perspectives on Arab Americans: Culture, Development, and Health*, DOI 10.1007/978-1-4614-8238-3_15,

MCH, and there has also been a renewed emphasis on the role of fathers and addressing the needs of families more broadly in contrast to the focus being solely on the child or pregnant woman. All issues of importance in the MCH population are theoretically of importance for Arab-American families. This chapter is not a comprehensive review of all health issues for MCH populations. We have focused this section of the chapter on those issues for which there is a particular cause for concern (data or research indicating its particular importance for the Arab-American community) or for which data either currently exist or could feasibly be reported separately for Arab Americans. While there is considerable racial-/ethnic-specific data for African-Americans, Hispanics, and children from families with low socio-economic status, national data are often unavailable for the Arab-American MCH population. One of the reasons is, according to the Office of Management and Budget, Arab Americans are classified as white (Revisions to the Standards for the Classification of Federal Data on Race and Ethnicity). Therefore, any differences in their health, disease, or behaviors are masked under the white category. Furthermore, those topics covered at length in other chapters of this volume have not been included due to space limitations. These topics include domestic violence (see Part II, Contemporary Issues), smoking and substance abuse (see Part III, Smoking and Substance Abuse), and gestational diabetes (see Part III, Diabetes).

For each of these selected topics, we provide context by describing data available for the US population as a whole. We then provide information relative to these topics specific to the Arab-American MCH population. In the area of mental health and stress, we provide an extended discussion of two key issues for this population: (1) migration and acculturation and (2) discrimination. We follow with a discussion that first reviews the dearth of research and then the possible data sources that could be considered in the future for enhanced surveillance and monitoring of health for the Arab-American MCH population. Finally, we provide an overview of programs and policies relevant to the Arab-American MCH population.

Perinatal Health

The health of a population is often said to be reflected by the health of its children and even more so by morbidity and mortality in the perinatal period. Life expectancy is intrinsically linked to the infant mortality rate. But beyond the logical relationships, there is a general consensus that infants are the most vulnerable members of the population (Kotch, 2005; Wallace et al., 2003).

Data on perinatal outcomes are easily available for the general population as births and deaths are registered in the US vital statistics system. Outcomes that are routinely reported and tracked include rates of birth (number of live births per 10,000 women of childbearing age), low birth weight (percent of live births weighing less than 2,500 g at birth), preterm birth (percent of live births delivered at less than 37 completed weeks gestation), and infant mortality (number of deaths in first year of life per 1,000 live births). Preterm birth and low birth weight are strongly associated with an increased risk of morbidity and mortality in childhood and adulthood (Swamy, Ostbye, & Skjaerven, 2008). Birth defects, or congenital anomalies, are recorded on the birth certificate, but this source of data is often incomplete as many of these conditions are not recognized at delivery. Therefore, birth defect registries are relied upon for the best estimates.

While all of these perinatal outcomes are reported by race and ethnicity, such reports are generally limited to differentiating non-Hispanic whites, non-Hispanic Blacks, Hispanics, Asians, and Native Americans. Reports identify these groups to parallel the OMB racial and ethnic classifications. No national data on outcomes for Arab Americans have been reported. Two studies have examined birth outcomes for Arab Americans with regard to the impact of the September 11, 2001, terrorist attacks in the United States. An increased risk of low birth weight (relative risk 2.25; 95 % CI 1.29–3.90) and preterm births (relative risk 1.50; 95 % CI 1.06–2.14) was seen among Arab-American women living in California (Lauderdale, 2006). However, a similar analysis based on Michigan vital statistics data reported no difference in the risk of adverse birth outcomes for Arab-American women giving birth after compared to before September 11, 2001 (El-Sayed, Hadley, & Galea, 2008).

While surveillance data reported for the United States or specific states with regard to perinatal health for Arab Americans are limited, such data could be derived by using variables from birth and death certificates such as ancestry, nationality, or place of birth or merging the original data with Arabic surname lists to identify Arab Americans. Surveillance is defined as the ongoing, systematic collection, analysis, and interpretation of health data essential to planning, implementing, and evaluating public health practice, closely integrated with the timely dissemination of these data to those who need to know (McGraw-Hill Concise Dictionary of Modern Medicine, 2002) The Michigan Department of Community Health has been an important stakeholder in this area. Table 15.1 provides data from Michigan specific to Arab Americans. Michigan uses a question on ancestry to identify the population in the vital statistics data. This is one approach that states could use to report Arab-American data.

In a recent analysis of data from the Michigan Birth Defects Registry (MBDR), data on parents' country of birth and ancestry were analyzed to compare birth defects of Arab-American children to those of non-Hispanic white children. Twenty-one major categories of birth defects and twelve congenital endocrine, metabolic, and hereditary disorders were tabulated. For a subset of structural birth defects, Arab-American children had similar or lower birth prevalence estimates when compared with non-Hispanic whites. However, for three types of metabolic disorders and one hereditary blood disorder, Arab-American children had higher estimates: maple syrup urine disease and other branched-chain aminoacidopathies, medium chain acyl-CoA dehydrogenase deficiency and other specified metabolic disorders, organic acidemias and other acidoses, and glucose-6-phosphate dehydrogenase deficiency, thalassemia (Yanni, Copeland, & Olney, 2010).

Risk factors for adverse birth outcomes more broadly (infant mortality, preterm birth, low birth weight) include social factors (e.g., poverty, low education, segregation), psychosocial factors (e.g., stress, depression), and biomedical (smoking, infection, chronic disease) factors. Many of these factors are also risk factors for

Table 15.1 Michigan Arab-American maternal and child perinatal health, 2009

Variable	*N*, *n*	Description	%
Live births[a]	*N*=3,766	–	–
Infant mortality[b,c]	*n*=22	5.8 (±2.4) per 1,000 live births	–
Live births with prenatal care[d,e]	*n*=2,533	–	67.3
Birth weight[f]		Mean=3,623 g Median=3,289 g	–
Birth weight distribution[g]	*n*=15	<750 g	0.4
	n=20	750–1,499 g	0.5
	n=230	1,500–2,499 g	6.1
	n=3,500	≥ 2,500 g	92.9
Low birth weight[h]	*n*=265	<2,500 g	7.0
Gestational diabetes[i,j]	*n*=196	–	5.2
Previous preterm births[k,l]	*n*=63	–	1.7

Note: All information gathered from www.michigan.gov/mdch

[a](Table: Number of live births by birth weight race and ancestry of mother Michigan residents, 2009) (http://www.mdch.state.mi.us/pha/osr/natality/tab1.9.asp)

[b](Table 8-AB: Number of Hispanic and Arabic infant deaths by selected county and Michigan residents, 2009) (http://www.mdch.state.mi.us/pha/osr/InDxMain/HispInfantDeaths.asp)

[c](Table 9: Infant hebdomadal fetal and perinatal death rates by specified race and ancestry Michigan residents, 2009) (http://www.mdch.state.mi.us/pha/osr/InDxMain/Table2pt23.asp)

[d](Table: Number of live births with prenatal care beginning in the first trimester by age race and ancestry of mother Michigan residents, 2009) (http://www.mdch.state.mi.us/pha/osr/natality/tab1.6.asp)

[e](Table: Percent of live births with prenatal care beginning in the first trimester by age race and ancestry of mother Michigan residents, 2009) (http://www.michigan.gov/mdch/0,1607,7-132-2944_4669_4681---,00.html)

[f](Table: Number of live births by birth weight race and ancestry of mother Michigan residents, 2009) (http://www.mdch.state.mi.us/pha/osr/natality/tab1.9.asp)

[g](Table: Number of live births by birth weight race and ancestry of mother Michigan residents, 2009) (http://www.mdch.state.mi.us/pha/osr/natality/tab1.9.asp)

[h](Table: Numbers and percent of low-birth-weight live births by prenatal care index by race and ancestry of mother Michigan residents, 2009) (http://www.mdch.state.mi.us/pha/osr/natality/tab1.10.asp)

[i](Table: Number of live births by maternal risk factors in pregnancy by race and ancestry of mother Michigan residents, 2009) (http://www.mdch.state.mi.us/pha/osr/natality/RisksRaceNo.asp)

[j](Table: Percent of live births by maternal risk factors in pregnancy by race and ancestry of mother Michigan residents, 2009) (http://www.mdch.state.mi.us/pha/osr/natality/RisksRacePer.asp)

[k](Table: Number of live births by maternal risk factors in pregnancy by race and ancestry of mother Michigan residents, 2009) (http://www.mdch.state.mi.us/pha/osr/natality/RisksRaceNo.asp)

[l](Table: Percent of live births by maternal risk factors in pregnancy by race and ancestry of mother Michigan residents, 2009) (http://www.mdch.state.mi.us/pha/osr/natality/RisksRacePer.asp)

birth defects, but many birth defects have a very specific set of factors that have been identified. For example, neural tube defects are strongly associated with folic acid levels, and risk has been reduced by dietary changes, including supplementation of the grains in the US food supply (Mersereau et al., 2004). Occupational and environmental exposures to toxicants, including lead and other heavy metals, have also been linked to a number of specific birth defects. Information on these risk factors in the Arab-American population is again very limited. Given the importance of social and behavioral risk factors for all of the birth outcomes described here (infant mortality, preterm birth, low birth weight, birth defects), it is certainly plausible that Arab Americans as a group may be at more or less risk and that interventions to address risk factors may need to be targeted if they are to effect change. For example, one strategy undertaken to reduce neural tube defects has been to fortify the breads in the United States. If Arab Americans consume less of the fortified bread products, they may be more at risk. As we gain an understanding of these issues, we may be able to determine what will be the best strategies to assure healthy birth outcomes for the Arab-American population in particular.

Immunization

More and more vaccines have become available to prevent diseases of childhood. Over the past several decades in the United States, deaths from vaccine-preventable diseases have declined substantially. There are a number of reasons why timely and complete vaccination is a public health goal. First, mortality and morbidity from vaccine-preventable diseases (e.g., measles, Haemophilus influenza B, polio) was high prior to development of effective childhood immunization schedules. Second, the cost to society in lost work by parents is substantial even if morbidity does not result in lifelong disability (e.g., varicella, measles). Third, in contrast to many other methods of prophylaxis or treatment, vaccines are usually a quick and easy intervention to deliver to the population with little need for follow-up care (Rodewald & Santoli, 2003). Unfortunately, achievement of timely and complete vaccination for all children has remained elusive, and there are disparities by race, ethnicity, and socioeconomic status. While there is considerable data on disparities for African-Americans, Hispanics, and children from families with low socioeconomic status, national data on vaccinations have not been reported for Arab-American children. As mentioned in the introduction for this chapter, one of the reasons is Arab Americans are classified as white in these data sources (Revisions to the Standards for the Classification of Federal Data on Race and Ethnicity). Therefore, any differences in their vaccination behaviors are subsumed under the white category. For 2020, the Public Health Service has set an objective of 80 % for children aged 19–35 months to receive the recommended doses of diphtheria-tetanus-polio (DTaP), measles-mumps-rubella (MMR), Haemophilus influenza B (HiB), hepatitis B, varicella, and pneumococcal conjugate vaccine (PCV). Only 68 % of children had achieved this target in 2008. These data are derived from reports of state registries. None of the states to our knowledge have identified Arab-American children separately. Risk factors for failure to immunize can be categorized as system, provider, and family factors. Some of these risk factors may disproportionately play a role in Arab-American families. Among Arab-American families, there may be cultural, religious, language, and other barriers that affect whether or not they choose to immunize their children. However, these factors have not been studied. If disparities are identified in achieving complete and timely immunizations, there may be a need for targeted outreach to this community.

Obesity

The prevalence of overweight and obesity among women of childbearing age as well as among children has increased dramatically in the last several years for the US population overall. Obesity in children has been associated with a higher risk of morbidity, including type 2 diabetes and asthma (Daniels et al., 2005). Maternal overweight and obesity influences a number of physiologic systems that can affect fetal development and the course of pregnancy (Misra & Trudeau, 2011). There has been growing concern about the impact of these trends on maternal and child health across the generations. Again, studies focused on overweight and obese for the Arab-American maternal and child population are sparse. In general, it is estimated that some 30.6 % of the US population is obese (Hedley et al., 2004) and 65.7 % are overweight (25 $kg/m^2 \leq$ body mass index <30 kg/m^2) or obese (Hedley et al., 2004). In the above study, Mexican Americans and blacks (72 %) have higher estimates compared to whites (63 %). Studies of Arab Americans have not primarily focused on assessing overweight or obesity; but most of these studies include adiposity measurements. In two probability sample studies, one-third (33.9 %) of Arab Americans were obese (Jaber, Brown, Hammad, Zhu, & Herman, 2004) and 31 % had a high waist circumference (Jaber et al., 2004). Studies using convenience samples report 46 % (Genesee County Health Department, 2003) and 81 % (Jamil et al., 2009) of Arab Americans were overweight or obese. Another study found 26 % were obese (Genesee County Health Department, 2003). The National Health Interview Survey reports that 51 % of Arab Americans and 57 % of whites were overweight or obese (Dallo & Borrell, 2006). Compared to both national and Michigan data, it appears that the percentage of *self-reported* overweight or obesity is slightly lower for Arab Americans as compared to whites or other minority groups. However, Arab Americans have a higher percentage (33.9 %) of *measured* obesity levels in comparison to the estimated national prevalence (30.6 %) of *measured* obesity levels in the study by Hedley and colleagues (Hedley et al., 2004). There is just one paper, published more than 10 years ago, that provides data on Arab-American children and obesity; this study measured whole body bone, fat, and lean mass of third-grade children in a suburban public school district adjacent to Detroit. Findings indicate that among 71 Chaldeans, 437 blacks, and 226 whites, Chaldeans and blacks had significantly more lean mass and height than whites. The average whole body bone mineral content (BMC) of Chaldean and black children were not dissimilar from each other but were significantly greater than whites ($p<0.05$). Compared with whites, the ratio of BMC to height was also significantly higher in Chaldeans and blacks. Finally, weight and fat mass were significantly greater in Chaldeans than either the black or white children, and a significantly smaller amount of physical activity was reported among Chaldeans than either the black or the white children (Nelson & Barondess, 1997).

Risk factors for obesity are complex. While obesity may be thought to simply reflect an imbalance between intake and activity, research has yet to characterize the reasons why this occurs. Furthermore, prevention in childhood and adolescence is far more effective than are attempts at change in adulthood. No single lifestyle (non-pharmacologic, nonsurgical) strategy appears to be effective in the long term for weight loss in adulthood, although a number of studies on exercise and diet appear to have benefits within the short period of follow-up (Shaw, Gennat, O'Rourke, & Del Mar, 2006). A lack of data on the prevalence of obesity for Arab-American mothers and children creates a knowledge gap in the baseline from which prevention and interventions can be identified as needed (or not) and their effects evaluated.

To date, intervention studies to reduce or delay the onset of overweight and obesity have not been conducted among Arab Americans. Cultural factors may be a barrier to physical activity for women of childbearing age. Strategies to address obesity can broadly be categorized as information, administrative, financing, provider, nongovernmental (e.g., religious community, neighborhood children's programs), and environmental (e.g., safe playgrounds, walkable neighborhoods) (Misra & Grason, 2006). Each of these areas may present unique challenges in effectively addressing the needs of the Arab-American MCH population around this health concern.

Mental Health and Stress

The importance of mental health for children has long been overlooked. Mental health can affect other health issues, and these disorders (e.g., depression, attention-deficit hyperactivity disorder, generalized anxiety disorders) as well as their treatments may also interfere with growth and development in childhood and lead to lasting sequelae. Data on children's mental health are difficult to obtain. While a number of studies have recently focused on the rise in use of medications to treat children for these conditions, reliable and valid data on prevalence nationally or by state is largely lacking. Except for questions on suicidal thoughts in the Youth Risk Behavior Survey (YRBS), none of the data sources described in preceding pages specifically consider mental health and the US surveys that focus on mental health do not include children. The Epidemiologic Catchment Area program (a community-based survey based on five catchment areas designed to estimate prevalence of mental disorders) includes only adults 18 years and older, and the National Comorbidity Survey (nationally representative sample survey that was designed to study the comorbidity of psychiatric disorders and substance use disorders in the United States) uses a sampling frame of 15–54 years of age, so adolescents are partially included. As limited as data are on the other health issues for Arab-American children, there are even fewer data sources and reports on their mental health. We were not able to find any reports, peer-reviewed or not, of Arab-American children's mental health. Beyond diagnosed mental health conditions, Arab-American children may be more exposed to stressors, and therefore, their physical and mental health may be impacted. In particular, children who have immigrated from war-torn countries or whose parents came to the United States from these environments may experience significant stress themselves or be stressed from exposure to parents who are experiencing these conditions.

Migration and Acculturation

More than one-half of Arab Americans are immigrants. Given that acculturation is associated with health status (Lara, Gamboa, Kahramanian, Morales, & Bautista, 2005), we briefly explore this relationship among Arab Americans. Among Arab Americans, the literature suggests that *greater* acculturation is associated with the following variables: less stress and depression (Ajrouch, 2005; Amer, 2005), except among the elderly (Wrobel, Farrag, & Hymes, 2009), and greater life satisfaction (Ajrouch, 2005); being Christian versus Muslim (Farragallah, Schumm, & Webb, 1997; Horan, 1995); better mental health and health promotion practices (Jadalia, 2007); better self-rated health (Abdulrahim & Baker, 2009); lower estimates of diabetes (Jaber, Brown, Hammad, Zhu, & Herman, 2003) and *higher* estimates of asthma (Johnson, 2005; Johnson, Nriagu, Hammad, Savoie, & Jamil, 2005); and having one or more chronic conditions (Jamil et al., 2009), having diabetes (Jamil et al., 2008a), but only for those who identified as "Arab" compared to those who identified as "Chaldean" (Catholic Iraqis), and having heart disease (Jamil et al., 2008b). These findings highlight the complexity of acculturation and the importance of comprehensively assessing migration history and health status variables.

Discrimination

Perceptions of discrimination have been shown to adversely affect a broad range of physical and mental health outcomes for multiple stigmatized groups in several countries (Ibish, 2003; Williams & Mohammed, 2009; Williams, Neighbors, & Jackson, 2003; Paradies, 2006). Given that Arab Americans belong to a stigmatized ethnic category, are not well understood by the US public (Hassoun, 2005), and suffer from discrimination (Ibish, 2003; Singh, 2002) based on their religion, race, and events related to 9/11, it is highly likely that these issues will have long-term effects on their physical and mental health. Research on Arab Americans prior to 9/11 found that 3.3 % of Christians and 2.8 % of Muslims reported they had "very often" been discriminated against. In stark contrast, after 9/11, 4.0 % of Christians and 11.9 % of Muslims reported that they had "very often" been discriminated against (Read, 2008). To our knowledge, only one study focused on adolescents. More specifically, among 240 Arab-American adolescents between the ages of 13 and 18, a strong relationship emerged between perceived discrimination and acculturative stress. Perceived discrimination and acculturative stress were positively associated with psychological distress (Ahmed, Kia-Keating, & Tsai, 2011).

With regard to perinatal health, there have been a few reports examining the effect of September 11, 2001 events on birth outcomes for Arab Americans, hypothesizing that stress from perceived discrimination might adversely affect pregnant women. Of the three recent studies (El-Sayed & Galea, 2009a; Lauderdale, 2006; Yanni et al., 2010) that examined birth-related issues, one of them provides a striking example from the record of birth weight of Arab Americans. Lauderdale used a surname list to identify Arab-American women's birth records in California and compared the levels of birth weight pre- and post-9/11. She showed that prior to 9/11, women with an Arabic surname had a risk of low birth weight similar to white women (i.e., those not having an Arabic surname). This changed in the 6 months after 9/11, when women with Arabic surnames became 34 % more likely to have a low-birth-weight infant (Lauderdale, 2006) compared to pre-9/11. The relative risk of having a low-birth-weight baby did not change for white women during these time periods (Lauderdale, 2006). The study by Lauderdale (Lauderdale, 2006) contrasts with the only other study published by El-Sayed and colleagues in Michigan (El-Sayed et al., 2008). El-Sayed and colleagues did not find a difference in birth weight of babies born to Arab-American women when comparing the periods of pre- and post-9/11. This could have been due to differences in the Arab-American populations of Michigan and California. El-Sayed and Galea also examined preterm birth using a similar analysis to that for birth weight. Using birth data from the state of Michigan from 2000 to 2005, there was no difference in preterm birth risk for babies born to Arab-American women when comparing the periods of pre- and post-9/11 (El-Sayed & Galea, 2009a). Again, more research should be conducted to analyze how these methods were both similar and different.

Access and Utilization of Health Care

Some studies have examined frequency of office visits by Chaldeans and Arabs. They found that approximately 10 % of Chaldeans and Arabs visited a doctor's office in the past 6 months compared to 1.5 % of Blacks (Jamil et al., 2008b). Also 70.5 % of Chaldeans and 67.1 % of Arabs had health insurance compared to 71.1 % of whites and 83.1 of Blacks (Jamil et al., 2008a). While health care is not the sole determinant of health in the population, poor access and utilization of preventive care and treatment can be detrimental to health. This is especially true with regard to preventive care for the maternal and child population. Prenatal care and well-child care provide the opportunity for screening for disease as well as developmental problems (e.g., spina bifida, cerebral palsy, autism). Other important preventive services in this population include immunization and counseling on a broad range of topics including smoking, and nutrition, physical activity. Treatment for conditions such as asthma and diabetes are also essential for management of these disorders in order to prevent unnecessary morbidity and mortality.

The state of Michigan, as with birth outcomes data, does report Arab-American-specific prenatal care utilization. Based on the Kessner index for prenatal care

(Kotelchuck, 1994), only about two-thirds (68.1 %) of all live births were to Michigan women with adequate prenatal care (Michigan Department of Community Health, 2010). Surprisingly, given the strong connection between prenatal care and birth outcomes and the relatively good outcomes for Arab-American women in the state, the proportion of live births with adequate prenatal care was much lower for Arab Americans (62.3 %) as compared to whites (72.3 %) (Division for Vital Records & Health Statistics & Health, 2010).

Health insurance coverage (Lasser, Himmelstein, & Woolhandler, 2006) and self-rated health (Goldman, Glei, & Chang, 2004) are associated with the health and disease status of individuals in a number of studies regardless of age, race, ethnicity, or ancestral origin. Health insurance and access to services have also specifically been identified as important influences on children's health (America's Children Health Insurance and Access to Care, 1998). Based on data in the United States for 2009 (Child Health USA, 2010), children without health insurance were almost 13 times as likely to not have a usual place of health care as children with private health insurance (25 % versus 2 %). Among children with a usual place of health care, almost 9 out of 10 with private health insurance visited a doctor's office for that care compared with 6 out of 10 with Medicaid coverage. Health insurance coverage and access specific to the Arab-American MCH population have not been reported in published research or surveillance data nationally or by state. Studies on adults have suggested that the proportion of Arab Americans with health insurance is similar to the US adult non-elderly population (using convenience samples (Aswad, 2001; Genesee County Health Department, 2003) and a probability sample (Read, Amick, & Donato, 2005)). Future research should examine how health varies by health insurance coverage and self-rated health for the MCH population.

Medicaid is an important program with regard to health insurance coverage and access for children and pregnant women in the United States. Medicaid is a partnership between the states and the federal government established in 1965 by Title XIX of the Social Security Act. While the federal government sets a minimum standard for eligibility and services covered by Medicaid, states are able to expand eligibility and services with some restrictions by the federal government. Medicaid provides coverage for children primarily on the basis of family income coupled with the child's age. However, children with documented disabilities may also be eligible for Medicaid regardless of family income. Coverage for pregnant women has expanded greatly within the past three decades; nearly two-thirds of births in the United States are to women who were covered by Medicaid during pregnancy. However, women who are undocumented immigrants still remain largely without any source of health insurance during pregnancy (DuBard & Massing, 2007). This may be a particular problem for Arab-American women. Health insurance coverage for children has increased through two separate programs that often overlap in their administration: Medicaid and the Child Health Insurance Program (CHIP). Title XXI of Social Security Act (1997) created a federal block grant to establish state CHIP programs. These programs are a federal-state partnership for health insurance for children (and, in some states, pregnant women) that provides coverage for children in families up to 200 % of the federal poverty level (FPL) or 50 % higher than the existing eligibility ceiling if it exceeds 150 % of the FPL. States may choose to expand Medicaid as a method of administering CHIP or create a new separate program. CHIP has an enhanced federal/state match compared to Medicaid. Similar to Medicaid, there is a required and optional set of covered services. Despite eligibility for either Medicaid or CHIP, many families do not enroll their children. US-born children of foreign-born parents are more likely to be uncovered even when eligible for Medicaid or CHIP (Kaiser Commission on Medicaid and the Uninsured, 2001). Finally, as with Medicaid for pregnant women, undocumented immigrants are still generally excluded.

In the overall MCH population, reduced access and utilization of health care are associated with lack of health insurance, lower education and income, and language and cultural factors {America's Children Health Insurance and Access to Care, 1998 #87}. The Arab-American MCH population may be even more likely to experience these risk factors. In addition to addressing the underlying risk factors, steps to improve access and utilization may include targeted outreach to educate families about programs (such as the Child Health Insurance Program, Medicaid) as well as health centers focused on the Arab-American population. In the Detroit metropolitan area, the Arab Community Center for Economic and Social Services (ACCESS) was created more than 40 years ago to provide assistance to the Arab immigrant population. ACCESS began a community health and research center in 1989 which is now one of the largest and most comprehensive health and mental health centers in North America to focus on the Arab-American community.

Literature and Data Sources Including the Arab-American MCH Population

The health of Arab Americans is not well understood due to the dearth of research conducted among this population. In a published literature review of the health of Arab Americans living in the US, El-Sayed and Galea (El-Sayed & Galea, 2009b) found just 34 papers in the peer-reviewed published literature with 26 of the reported studies carried out in Michigan. None of the studies used a prospective cohort design; 27 were cross-sectional and 7 were retrospective or medical chart reviews. The two areas most often studied, albeit still very sparse, were diabetes (11 papers) and tobacco use (11 papers). With regard to maternal and child health specifically, there were just three published papers, all of which focused on birth outcomes. A more recent (2011) literature review (unpublished, Dallo and Williams) included 50 studies (Dallo, Schwartz, Ruterbusch, Booza, & Williams, 2012). To identify all published and unpublished (e.g., organization reports) research and to avoid publication bias on Arab-American health, the authors searched several databases in the following ways: (1) using the keywords *Arab American*, *Arab*, *Middle East*, *Health*, *Immigrant*, *Foreign-Born*, *U.S.-Born*, *Refugee*, *Chaldean* (*Catholic Iraqis*), *Children*, *Women*, *Elder*, *Discrimination*, and *Health Care* separately and in various combinations in the PubMed and Ovid databases, without date restrictions, (2) using the keyword *Arab American* in Google to identify unpublished studies and websites that collect and report information related to health characteristics for Arab Americans, (3) searching the Digital Dissertations database using the keyword *Arab American*, and (4) searching for books on Arab Americans that contained chapters related to health or issues that affect health. Of the 50 studies, six focused on MCH (Ahmed et al., 2011; El-Sayed et al., 2008; El-Sayed & Galea, 2009a; Nelson & Barondess, 1997; Nriagu, Senthamarai-Kannan, Jamil, Fakhori, & Korponic, 2011; Ohlsson & Shah, 2011). None of these six studies were identified in the review article by El-Sayed and Galea (El-Sayed et al., 2008) because all but one was published after their review article was published. To better understand the health and disease status of the Arab-American population, continued research is imperative in the areas of immunizations rates, perinatal health, and others.

As seen in our discussions of MCH health issues, data specific to the Arab-American child health population is quite limited. The only two national data sets that include health questions and identify Arab Americans are the National Health Interview Survey (NHIS) and the decennial census, including the American Community Survey. The NHIS is an annual, face-to-face interview of the civilian, noninstitutionalized household population of the United States that uses a three-stage stratified cluster probability sampling design (National Health Interview Survey). The NHIS consists of a core set of questions (questions that are repeated yearly) and supplemental questions/modules. For the first time in 2000, the NHIS questionnaires included a question on region of birth that categorized respondents into 1 of 12 categories, based on their country of origin. One of these regions is the Middle East. While the household is the unit of sampling for the NHIS, an adult household respondent is asked about both adults and children in household. Supplemental questionnaires are given for one core adult and one core child per household. Beginning in 1980, the census included an ancestry question, which asked, "What is this person's ancestry or ethnic origin?" (US Census Bureau Population Division). The question allows respondents to provide a maximum of two attributions. This question was not included in the 2010 census count, but the question was included in the American Community Survey, which is an ongoing survey that provides data every year. The limitation with the census information is only one health-related question, and disability is included. This variable is usually used among those 65 years of age and older and is rarely used among the youth population.

To conduct studies that are more representative and reliable, we need to include an ethnic identifier for Arab Americans in national public health surveys. In addition, although Arab Americans constitute a relatively small population (3,500,000), they should be identified in national, regional, and state surveys. In 2000, the National Health Interview Survey added a question on place of birth, which allowed us to identify individuals born in the Middle East. However, a more specific identifier should be included, as has been done for many smaller ethnic populations (i.e., subgroups of Asians). Since the National Health Interview Survey contains only self-reported information (i.e., no data are available from medical examinations or laboratory results), other surveys (such as the National Health and Nutrition Examination Survey) should add an ethnic identifier for Arab Americans, using as a model the Hispanic Health and Nutrition Examination Survey, which was a one-time attempt to obtain data on a small but regionally concentrated population. Finally, such US-based studies on Arab Americans would provide us with prevalence and incidence estimates to make international comparisons. The recommendation to include Arab-American identifiers in national surveys is more urgent today than ever. The only dependable and reliable source for the Arab-American community, from 1980 to 2000, was the census (Samham, 1999). It was used to disseminate demographic, housing, and other information about Arab Americans (Brittingham & de la Cruz, 2003; Dallo, Ajrouch, & Al-Snih, 2008; de la Cruz, 2003; El-Brady, 1987; Nigem, 1986). Such information could be used for planning and program implementation purposes. Unfortunately, the ancestry question was not included in the 2010 census, because the "long form" was eliminated. The "long form" has been replaced by the American Community Survey, which is an ongoing annual survey and sent to a small (approximately three million individuals per year) sample of the population on a rotating basis (United States Census, 2010, 2009). While the American Community Survey provides immediate access to data, the undercount of Arab Americans will only be exacerbated.

In addition to including an ethnic identifier for Arab Americans, future research should rely on probability samples, include subgroups of Arab Americans, and go beyond studies conducted only in Michigan to other states with large Arab-American populations, such as California and New York (Arab American Institute). In the remaining sections of this chapter, we review the potential data sources routinely available for the US population for which data specific to Arab Americans could be extracted either through explicit identification by adding survey queries or by application of an algorithm with a list of Arab names to identify likely Arab Americans. A number of researchers have successfully used such strategies, including Schwartz (Schwartz et al., 2004), Dallo (Dallo et al., 2012), and Nasseri (Nasseri, Mills, & Allan, 2007).

In the following section, we review various sources of data from which Arab Americans could potentially be identified, but reports from these sources that do so are rare. Unless otherwise noted, the source does not identify ethnicity, country of origin, or language.

Vital Records (Birth, Death)

Beginning early in the last century, the United States began to register live birth and deaths, producing certificates and later deidentified data aggregated at the state and national level. There have been no reports of US statistics on birth outcomes or risk factors for the Arab-American population. However, in states with large number of Arab Americans, both government and academic researchers have begun to use these data to examine perinatal health for this population. In Michigan, the state has reported perinatal surveillance data (see Table 15.1) using a question on ancestry to identify the Arab-American population. Research by El-Sayed has also used this method to identify Arab Americans in the birth and infant death data (El-Sayed et al., 2008; El-Sayed & Galea, 2009a). There have been no similar official surveillance reports from other states. However, researchers have used a names algorithm (see preceding paragraph) to identify likely Arab Americans in the California vital statistics data for analysis of perinatal health outcomes (Lauderdale, 2006).

National Surveys and Databases

National Health Interview Survey (NHIS)

The National Health Interview Survey (NHIS) is the principal source of information on the health of the civilian, noninstitutionalized population of the United States and is one of the major data collection programs of the National Center for Health Statistics (NCHS). The NHIS, initiated in July 1957, is a cross-sectional household interview survey conducted throughout each year among a sample of the population selected from each state. The NHIS data are collected annually through a personal household interview currently including approximately 43,000 households including about 106,000 persons. While the household is the unit of sampling, the survey includes supplemental questionnaires for one identified core adult and one core child. The annual response rate of NHIS is greater than 90 % of the eligible households in the sample. Patients in long-term care facilities, persons on active duty with the armed forces (though their dependents are included), and US nationals living in foreign countries are excluded from the survey. Because it is an annual survey, the NHIS allows public health researchers and policy makers to monitor trends in illness and disability and track progress toward achieving national health objectives. Further information on current NHIS activities and updated fact and figures may be obtained at the CDC-maintained website located at www.cdc.gov/nchs/nhis.htm (National Health Interview Survey).

National Health and Nutrition Examination Survey (NHANES)

The National Health and Nutrition Examination Survey (NHANES) is conducted by the National Center for Health Statistics (NCHS) and is designed to collect information about the health and diet of people in the United States. Among the various surveys, NHANES is unique in that it combines a home interview with direct measures of health via physical examination and blood tests conducted on participants. The first program, the National Health Examination Survey (NHES 1960–1962), focused on estimating the total prevalence of chronic disease and the distributions of various physical and physiologic measures, including blood pressure and serum cholesterol levels, among the sample of adults aged 18–79 years surveyed. NHES II (1963–1965) and NHES III (1966–1970) focused on the growth and development of children. The first cycle of NHANES, or NHANES I (1971–1974), focused on chronic disease, specifically cardiovascular, respiratory, arthritic, and hearing conditions among adults, with the addition of the measurement of the nutritional status of the participants. In NHANES II (1976–1980), the nutritional component was expanded and focus was directed toward the measurement of diabetes, kidney and liver function, allergy, and speech pathology among the participants. The NHANES I and NHANES II focused on the general US population between 1982 and 1984, and the Hispanic Health and Nutrition Examination Survey (HHANES) focused on specific ethnic groups, namely, Mexican Americans, Cuban Americans, and Puerto Ricans. Recognizing the increasing burden of chronic disease among minority groups, NHANES III (1988–1994), included an oversampling of both black and Mexican Americans. NHANES III included participants as young as 2 months of age and adults with no upper age limit and focused on the effects of the environment upon health. Approximately 5,000 national participants are screened using sample selection, followed by detailed household interviews. Sample individuals are invited to receive physical examinations and health and dietary interviews in mobile examination centers. Various medical tests and procedures are conducted to enable analysis of the relationship between health and nutrition status and disease risk factors, to measure the prevalence and comorbidity of diseases and disorders, to establish reference standards, and to monitor secular trends in health and nutrition status. Beginning in 1999, NHANES became a continuous, annual survey that can be linked to related federal government surveys of the general US population, specifically the National Health Interview Survey (NHIS) and, in the future, the US Department of Agriculture's (USDA) Continuing Survey of Food Intakes by Individuals (CSFII). In January 2001, the USDA CSFII study will merge with NHANES to form the National Food and Nutrition Survey (NFNS). Further information on current NHANES activities and updated fact and figures may be obtained at the CDC-maintained website located at www.cdc.gov/nchs/nhanes.htm (National Health and Nutrition Examination Survey).

Youth Risk Behavior Surveillance System (YRBSS)

The Youth Risk Behavior Surveillance System (YRBSS) monitors six categories of priority health-risk behaviors among youth and young adults—behaviors that contribute to unintentional and intentional injuries, tobacco use, alcohol and other drug use, sexual behaviors that contribute to unintended pregnancy and STDs (including HIV infection), unhealthy dietary behaviors, and physical inactivity. The YRBSS includes a national, school-based survey, the Youth Risk Behavior Survey (YRBS) conducted by CDC, as well as state, territorial, and local, school-based surveys conducted by education and health agencies. The first national, school-based YRBS was completed in 1990, and repeat surveys have been conducted every other year since 1991. The national YRBS is based on a national probability sample, and the data are representative of students in grades 9 to 12 in public and private schools in the 50 states and the District of Columbia. In the 1999 YRBS, 15,349 surveys were completed by students in 144 schools across the nation, and the overall response rate was 66 %. Further information on current YRBS activities and updated fact and figures may be obtained at the CDC-maintained website located at www.cdc.gov/nccdphp/dash/yrbs/index.htm (Youth Risk Behavior Surveillance System).

National Survey of Family Growth (NSFG)

The National Survey of Family Growth (NSFG) is a multipurpose periodic survey based on personal interviews with a national sample of women 15–44 years of age in the civilian, noninstitutionalized population of the United States. The goal of the survey is to collect data on factors affecting pregnancy and women's health in the United States, such as the number of children women have had, intended and mistimed pregnancies, contraceptive use, infertility, impaired fecundity, and sterilization operations. Previous NSFG surveys were conducted in 1973, 1976, 1982, 1988, 1995, 2002, and 2006–2008. Further information on current NSFG activities and updated facts and figures may be obtained at the CDC-maintained website located at www.cdc.gov/nchs/nsfg.htm (National Survey of Family Growth).

National Longitudinal Survey of Youth (NLSY)

The Labor Department conducted this series of surveys. The most recent enrollment period was in 1997. The NLSY97 is made up of youth ages 12–16 years old as of December 31, 1996. The sample is nationally representative and has approximately 9,000 participants. In the first round of the survey, in 1997, hour-long personal interviews were administered to youth that met eligibility criteria and one parent of that youth. A two-part questionnaire was also given during the screening process. In this extensive questionnaire, demographic information on people who lived in the youth's household as well as his or her immediate family members not living in the household were collected. The NLSY97, which interviews youth annually, was created to examine the educational experiences of youth in school as well as their behavior in the labor market and over time into adulthood. The NLSY97 also contains comprehensive information in many other areas, including the relationship youths have with their parents, the contact they have with absent parents, puberty, dating, marital and fertility experiences, government assistance, time use, training, expectations, as well as alcohol and drug use. The interview was also made up of a self-administered portion where sensitive questions, such as sexual history and criminal behavior, were posed. Another part of the NLSY97 is the parent questionnaire in round 1 that produces information about the family background and history of the youths. Information generated in this questionnaire includes as follows: the parents' marital and employment experiences, the relationship they have with a spouse or partner, their ethnic background and religious beliefs, household income and assets they own, government assistance they receive, early childcare and custody arrangement for the youth, their health and the health of their child, as well as parent expectations of the youth. More information is available at the website http://www.bls.gov/nls/y97summary.htm (National Longitudinal Surveys).

National Survey of Children's Health

This is among the most recent of the national surveys. This survey addresses the paucity of reliable national and state level estimates of children's health and health-care experiences. There is a special emphasis on factors that may relate to child well-being, including medical homes, family interactions, parental health, school and after-school experiences, and safe neighborhoods. The first wave of the survey was conducted in 2003 with the second wave in 2007. The survey has sampled children from 0 to 17 years of age. Further information and data updates can be found at the website, http://www.nschdata.org/Content/Default.aspx# (National Survey of Children's Health, 2003, 2007).

Summary

The goal of this chapter has been to provide an overview of MCH health among the Arab-American population. While there is considerable racial-/ethnic-specific data for African-Americans, Hispanics, and children from families with low socioeconomic status, national data are often unavailable at a national level for the Arab-American MCH population. When such data are available, it may only be as a result of using surname and other algorithms to identify ancestry rather than directly assessment of ethnicity. In a number of areas, these data are available only for selected US states, generally those in which Arab Americans are more likely to reside (e.g., Michigan, California). The current state of data recalls earlier decades in which data on Hispanics were also unavailable and often treated as "whites."

What has emerged from this chapter is the urgent need for the following: (1) including ethnic identifiers for Arab Americans in vital statistics data (e.g., birth certificates), a key data source for MCH policy and programs; and (2) Arab-American-specific data from US national and state surveys (e.g., BRFSS, NHANES), also frequently relied upon for development and tracking of MCH policy and programs.

Beyond data limitations for the MCH population, we have reviewed how stress, migration, acculturation, and discrimination may influence the health of the Arab-American MCH population. These factors may be particularly salient for Arab Americans. Future studies of health in the Arab-American MCH population should consider studying whether such factors play a role in the pathways between ethnicity and health.

References

Abdulrahim, S., & Baker, W. (2009). Differences in self-rated health by immigrant status and language preference among Arab Americans in the Detroit Metropolitan Area. *Social Science & Medicine (1982), 68*(12), 2097–2103.

Ahmed, S. R., Kia-Keating, M., & Tsai, K. H. (2011). A structural model of racial discrimination, acculturative stress, and cultural resources among Arab American adolescents. *American Journal of Community Psychology, 48*(3–4), 181–192.

Ajrouch, K. J. (2005). Social relations and mental health among Arab-American elders. *Ethnicity & Disease, 15*(1 Suppl 1), S1–S109.

Amer, M. (2005). *Arab American mental health in the post September 11 era: Acculturation, stress, and coping*. Dissertation, The University of Toledo, Ohio.

America's Children Health Insurance and Access to Care. (1998). In M. Edmunds & M. J. Coye (Eds.), *Committee on children health insurance and access to care division of health care services*. Washington, DC: Institute of Medicine and Board on Children Youth and Families National Research Council and Institute of Medicine.

Arab American Institute. Retrieved September 1, 2011, from http://www.aaiusa.org/pages/demographics/

Aswad, M. (2001). *Health Survey of the Arab, Muslim, and Chaldean American Communities in Michigan*. Dearborn, MI: ACCESS.

Brittingham, A., & de la Cruz, G. P. (2003). *We the people of Arab ancestry in the United States* (pp. 1–24). Washington, DC: U.S. Census Bureau.

Child Health USA. (2010). Retrieved September 1, 2011, from http://mchb.hrsa.gov/mchirc/chusa/

Dallo, F., Ajrouch, K. J., & Al-Snih, S. (2008). The ancestry question and ethnic heterogeneity: The case of Arab Americans. *International Migration Review, 42*, 505–517.

Dallo, F. J., & Borrell, L. N. (2006). Self-reported diabetes and hypertension among Arab Americans in the United States. *Ethnicity & Disease, 16*(3), 699–705.

Dallo, F. J., Schwartz, K., Ruterbusch, J. J., Booza, J., & Williams, D. R. (2012). Mortality rates among Arab Americans in Michigan. *Journal of Immigrant and Minority Health, 14*(2), 236–241.

Daniels, S. R., Arnett, D. K., Eckel, R. H., Gidding, S. S., Hayman, L. L., Kumanyika, S., et al. (2005). Overweight in children and adolescents: Pathophysiology, consequences, prevention, and treatment. *Circulation, 111*(15), 1999–2012.

de la Cruz, G. P. (2003). *The Arab population: 2000* (pp. 1–12). Washington, DC: U.S. Census Bureau.

Division for Vital Records & Health Statistics, & Health, M. D. o. C. (2010). *Michigan resident birth file*, from http://www.mdch.state.mi.us/pha/osr/chi/births/frame.html

DuBard, C. A., & Massing, M. W. (2007). Trends in emergency Medicaid expenditures for recent and undocumented immigrants. *Journal of the American Medical Association, 297*(10), 1085–1092.

El-Brady, S. M. (1987). *Fitting in: An analysis of socioeconomic attainment patterns of foreign-born Arab-Americans and other nationalities in the United States*. Dissertation, The University of Texas at Austin.

El-Sayed, A. M., & Galea, S. (2009a). Explaining the low risk of preterm birth among Arab Americans in the United States: An analysis of 617451 births. [Comparative Study Research Support, N.I.H., Extramural]. *Pediatrics, 123*(3), e438–e445. doi:10.1542/peds.2008-1634.

El-Sayed, A. M., & Galea, S. (2009b). The health of Arab-Americans living in the United States: A systematic review of the literature. [Research Support, N.I.H., Extramural Review]. *BMC Public Health, 9*, 272. doi:10.1186/1471-2458-9-272.

El-Sayed, A., Hadley, C., & Galea, S. (2008). Birth outcomes among Arab Americans in Michigan before and after the terrorist attacks of September 11, 2001. [Research Support, N.I.H., Extramural]. *Ethnicity & Disease, 18*(3), 348–356.

Farragallah, M., Schumm, W., & Webb, F. (1997). Acculturation of Arab-American immigrants. *Journal of Comparative Family Studies, 28*, 182–203.

Genesee County Health Department. (2003). *Arab American health survey*. Retrieved September 1, 2011, from http://www.gchd.us/pdf/aahs.pdf

Goldman, N., Glei, D. A., & Chang, M. C. (2004). The role of clinical risk factors in understanding self-rated health. *Annals of Epidemiology, 14*(1), 49–57.

Gustafsson, P. E., Janlert, U., Theorell, T., Westerlund, H., & Hammarstrom, A. (2010). Fetal and life course origins of serum lipids in mid-adulthood: Results from a prospective cohort study. *BMC Public Health, 10*, 484.

Hassoun, R. (2005). *Arab Americans in Michigan*. Lansing, MI: Michigan State University Press.

Hedley, A. A., Ogden, C. L., Johnson, C. L., Carroll, M. D., Curtin, L. R., & Flegal, K. M. (2004). Prevalence of overweight and obesity among US children, adolescents, and adults, 1999-2002. *Journal of the American Medical Association, 291*(23), 2847–2850.

Horan, A. E. (1995). *Arab-American communities and their acculturation into the American culture and society*. Dissertation, Walden University, Minneapolis, Minnesota.

Ibish, H. (2003). *Report on hate crimes and discrimination against Arab Americans: The Post-September 11 Backlash*, September 11, 2001–October 11, 2002 (pp. 1–150).

Jaber, L. A., Brown, M. B., Hammad, A., Zhu, Q., & Herman, W. H. (2003). Lack of acculturation is a risk factor for diabetes in arab immigrants in the US. *Diabetes Care, 26*(7), 2010–2014.

Jaber, L. A., Brown, M. B., Hammad, A., Zhu, Q., & Herman, W. H. (2004). The prevalence of the metabolic syndrome among arab americans. *Diabetes Care, 27*(1), 234–238.

Jadalia, A. A. (2007). *Acculturation, health, and health behaviors of adult Arab Americans*. Dissertation, Loma Linda University, California.

Jamil, H., Dall, F., Fakhouri, M., Templin, T., Khoury, R., & Fakhouri, H. (2009). The prevalence of self-reported chronic conditions among Arab, Chaldean, and African Americans in southeast Michigan. *Ethnicity & Disease, 19*, 293–300.

Jamil, H., Fakhouri, M., Dallo, F., Templin, T., Khoury, R., & Fakhouri, H. (2008a). Disparities in self-reported diabetes mellitus among Arab, Chaldean, and black Americans in Southeast Michigan. *Journal of Immigrant and Minority Health, 10*(5), 397–405.

Jamil, H., Fakhouri, M., Dallo, F., Templin, T., Khoury, R., & Fakhouri, H. (2008b). Self-reported heart disease among Arab and Chaldean American women residing in Southeast Michigan. *Ethnicity & Disease, 18*, 19–25.

Johnson, M. (2005). *Risk factors for asthma among Arab American immigrants in the metro Detroit area*. Dissertation, University of Michigan, Detroit.

Johnson, M., Nriagu, J., Hammad, A., Savoie, K., & Jamil, H. (2005). Asthma prevalence and severity in Arab American communities in the Detroit area, Michigan. *Journal of Immigrant Health, 7*(3), 165–178.

Kaiser Commission on Medicaid and the Uninsured. (2001). Retrieved September 1, 2011, from http://www.kff.org/about/kcmu.cfm

Kotch, J. (Ed.). (2005). *Maternal and child health: Programs, problems, and policy in public health* (2nd ed.). Sudbury, MA: Jones and Bartlett.

Kotelchuck, M. (1994). An evalution of the Kessner Adequacy of Prenatal Care Index and a proposed Adequacy of Prenatal Care Utilization Index. *American Journal of Public Health, 84*, 1414–1420.

Lara, M., Gamboa, C., Kahramanian, M. I., Morales, L. S., & Bautista, D. E. (2005). Acculturation and Latino health in the United States: A review of the literature and its sociopolitical context. *Annual Review of Public Health, 26*, 367–397.

Lasser, K. E., Himmelstein, D. U., & Woolhandler, S. (2006). Access to care, health status, and health disparities in the United States and Canada: Results of a cross-national population-based survey. *American Journal of Public Health, 96*(7), 1300–1307.

Lauderdale, D. S. (2006). Birth outcomes for Arabic-named women in California before and after September 11. *Demography, 43*(1), 185–201.

McGraw-Hill. (2002). *Concise dictionary of modern medicine*. New York: The McGraw-Hill Companies.

Mersereau, P., Kilker, K., Carter, H., Fassett, E., Williams, J., Flores, A., et al. (2004). Spina bifida and anencephaly before and after folic acid mandate-United States, 1995-1996 and 1999-2000. *MMWR. Morbidity and Mortality Weekly Report, 53*, 362–365.

Michigan Department of Community Health. (2010). *Michigan maternal, infant, and early childhood home visiting program: Statewide needs assessment* (pp. Appendices).

Misra, D. P., Astone, N., & Lynch, C. D. (2005). Maternal smoking and birth weight: Interaction with parity and mother's own in utero exposure to smoking. *Epidemiology, 16*(3), 288–293.

Misra, D. P., & Grason, H. (2006). Achieving safe motherhood: Applying a life course and multiple determinants perinatal health framework in public health. *Women's Health Issues, 16*(4), 159–175.

Misra, V. K., & Trudeau, S. (2011). The influence of overweight and obesity on longitudinal trends in maternal serum leptin levels during pregnancy. *Obesity (Silver Spring), 19*(2), 416–421.

Nasseri, K., Mills, P. K., & Allan, M. (2007). Cancer incidence in the Middle Eastern population of California, 1988-2004. *Asian Pacific Journal of Cancer Prevention, 8*(3), 405–411.

National Health and Nutrition Examination Survey. Retrieved September 1, 2011, from www.cdc.gov/nchs/nhanes.htm

National Health Interview Survey. Retrieved September 1, 2011, from http://www.cdc.gov/nchs/nhis.htm

National Longitudinal Surveys. Retrieved September 1, 2011, from http://www.bls.gov/nls/y97summary.htm

National Survey of Children's Health. (2003, 2007). Retrieved September 1, 2011, from http://www.nschdata.org/Content/Default.aspx#

National Survey of Family Growth. Retrieved September 1, 2011, from www.cdc.gov/nchs/nsfg.htm

Nelson, D. A., & Barondess, D. A. (1997). Whole body bone, fat and lean mass in children: Comparison of three ethnic groups. *American Journal of Physical Anthropology, 103*(2), 157–162.

Nigem, E. T. (1986). Arab Americans: Migration, socioeconomic and demographic characteristics. *International Migration Review, 20*(3), 629–649.

Nriagu, J., Senthamarai-Kannan, R., Jamil, H., Fakhori, M., & Korponic, S. (2011). Lead poisoning among Arab American and African American children in the Detroit metropolitan area, Michigan. *Bulletin of Environmental Contamination and Toxicology, 87*(3), 238–244.

Ohlsson, A., & Shah, P. S. (2011). Effects of the September 11, 2001 disaster on pregnancy outcomes: A systematic review. *Acta Obstetricia et Gynecologica Scandinavica, 90*(1), 6–18.

Paradies, Y. (2006). A systematic review of empirical research on self-reported racism and health. *International Journal of Epidemiology, 35*, 888–901.

Read, J. G. (2008). Discrimination and identity formation in a Post-9/11 Era: A comparison of Muslim and Christian Arab Americans. In A. Jamal & N. Naber (Eds.), *Race and Arab Americans before and after 9/11* (pp. 305–317). New York: Syracuse University Press.

Read, J. G., Amick, B., & Donato, K. M. (2005). Arab immigrants: A new case for ethnicity and health? *Social Science & Medicine (1982), 61*(1), 77–82.

Revisions to the standards for the classification of federal data on race and ethnicity. Retrieved from http://www.whitehouse.gov/omb/fedreg_1997standards.

Rodewald, L., & Santoli, J. (2003). Childhood immunizations. In H. Wallace, G. Green, & K. Jaros (Eds.), *Health and welfare for families in the 21st century* (pp. 342–354). Sudbury, MA: Jones and Bartlett.

Samham, H. H. (1999). Not quite white: Race classification and the Arab American experience. In M. Suleiman (Ed.), *Arabs in America: Building a new future* (pp. 209–649). Philadelphia: Temple University Press.

Schwartz, K. L., Kulwicki, A., Weiss, L. K., Fakhouri, H., Sakr, W., Kau, G., et al. (2004). Cancer among Arab Americans in the metropolitan Detroit area. *Ethnicity & Disease, 14*(1), 141–146.

Shaw, K., Gennat, H., O'Rourke, P., &, Del Mar, C. (2006). Exercise for overweight or obesity. *Cochrane Database System Review* (4), CD003817.

Singh, A. (2002). We are not the enemy: Hate crimes against Arabs, Muslims, and those perceived to be Arab or Muslim after September 11. *Human Rights Watch, 14*, 1–41.

Smith, A. H., Marshall, G., Yuan, Y., Ferreccio, C., Liaw, J., von Ehrenstein, O., et al. (2006). Increased mortality from lung cancer and bronchiectasis in young adults after exposure to arsenic in utero and in early childhood. *Environmental Health Perspectives, 114*(8), 1293–1296.

Swamy, G. K., Ostbye, T., & Skjaerven, R. (2008). Association of preterm birth with long-term survival, reproduction, and next-generation preterm birth. *Journal of the American Medical Association, 299*(12), 1429–1436.

Table 8-AB: Number of Hispanic and Arabic infant deaths by selected county and Michigan Michigan residents. (2009). Retrieved September 1, 2011, from http://www.mdch.state.mi.us/pha/osr/InDxMain/HispInfantDeaths.asp

Table 9: Infant hebdomadal fetal and perinatal death rates by specified race and ancestry Michigan residents. (2009). Retrieved September 1, 2011, from http://www.mdch.state.mi.us/pha/osr/InDxMain/Table2pt23.asp

Table: Number of live births by birth weight race and ancestry of mother Michigan residents. (2009). Retrieved September 1, 2011, from http://www.mdch.state.mi.us/pha/osr/natality/tab1.9.asp

Table: Number of live births by maternal risk factors in pregnancy by race and ancestry of mother Michigan residents. (2009). Retrieved September 1, 2011, from http://www.mdch.state.mi.us/pha/osr/natality/RisksRaceNo.asp

Table: Number of live births with prenatal care beginning in the first trimester by age race and ancestry of mother Michigan residents. (2009). Retrieved September 1, 2011, from http://www.mdch.state.mi.us/pha/osr/natality/tab1.6.asp

Table: Numbers and percent of low birth weight live births by prenatal care index by race and ancestry of mother Michigan residents. (2009). Retrieved September 1, 2011, from http://www.mdch.state.mi.us/pha/osr/natality/tab1.10.asp

Table: Percent of live births by maternal risk factors in pregnancy by race and ancestry of mother Michigan residents. (2009). Retrieved September 1, 2011, from http://www.mdch.state.mi.us/pha/osr/natality/RisksRacePer.asp

Table: Percent of live births with prenatal care beginning in the first trimester by age race and ancestry of Mother Michigan residents. (2009). Retrieved September 1, 2011, from http://www.mdch.state.mi.us/pha/osr/natality/tab1.6perc.asp

U.S. Census Bureau Population Division. Retrieved September 1, 2011, from http://www.census.gov/population/ancestry/anc-faq.html#q02.

United States Census. (2010, 2009). Retrieved September 1, 2011, from http://www.census.gov/

Wallace, H., Green, G., & Jaros, K. (Eds.). (2003). *Health and welfare for families in the 21st century* (2nd ed.). Sudbury, MA: Jones and Bartlett.

Williams, D. R., Neighbors. H. W., & Jackson, J. S. (2003). Racial/ethnic discrimination and health: Findings from community studies. *American Journal of Public Health, 93*, 200–208.

Williams, D. R., & Mohammed, S. A. (2009). Discrimination and racial disparities in health: Evidence and needed research. *Journal of Behavioral Medical, 32*, 20–47.

Wrobel, N. H., Farrag, M. F., & Hymes, R. W. (2009). Acculturative stress and depression in an elderly Arabic sample. *Journal of Cross-Cultural Gerontology, 24*(3), 273–290.

Xue, F., & Michels, K. B. (2007). Intrauterine factors and risk of breast cancer: A systematic review and meta-analysis of current evidence. *The Lancet Oncology, 8*(12), 1088–1100.

Yanni, E. A., Copeland, G., & Olney, R. S. (2010). Birth defects and genetic disorders among Arab Americans–Michigan, 1992–2003. *Journal of Immigrant and Minority Health, 12*(3), 408–413.

Youth Risk Behavior Surveillance System. Retrieved September 1, 2011, from www.cdc.gov/nccdphp/dash/yrbs/index.htm.

Zadrozny, S., Power, E. J., Nishimi, R.Y., & Kizer K.W. (Eds.). (2004). Child healthcare quality measurement and reporting. In *Workshop Proceedings*. Washington, DC: National Quality Forum.

Chapter 16
Cancer: Cross-Roads of Ethnicity and Environment

Kendra Schwartz, Kiumarss Nasseri, and Emad Shehada

Cancer is the second leading cause of death in the United States, with an estimated 1,596,670 new cases and 571,950 deaths in 2011(American Cancer Society, 2012). Both external factors (e.g., tobacco, infectious organisms, chemicals, and radiation) and internal factors (e.g., inherited mutations, immune conditions) have been determined to be causally associated with cancer. Cancer is a general name given to a group of more than 100 distinct diseases with different etiologies characterized by uncontrolled growth of abnormal cells. Although cancer historically has been a deadly disease, cancer survival has increased in recent years, due in large part to early detection and treatment advances. The number of cancer survivors in the United States is estimated at 13.7 million in 2012, representing approximately 4 % of the population (Siegel et al., 2012). Because cancer is a reportable disease in the United States, cancer-related statistics are readily available, which allow public health officials and researchers to study cancer trends over time as well as cancer incidence and outcomes in different demographic groups.

In contrast to the United States, Arab countries often do not have compulsory reporting of cancer on a nation-wide basis and therefore reliable cancer statistics are often lacking and when present are imputed for the total population based on limited statistics. In the United States, cancer among Arab Americans cannot be easily

K. Schwartz, M.D., M.S.P.H. (✉)
Department of Family Medicine and Public Health Sciences, 3939 Woodward, Detroit, MI 48201, USA
e-mail: kensch@med.wayne.edu

K. Nasseri, D.V.M., M.P.H., Ph.D.
Department of Epidemiology and Biostatistics, School of Public Health, Medical Sciences University of Tehran, 265 Calle Esperanza, Santa Barbara, CA 93105, USA
e-mail: qnasseri@west.net

E. Shehada, M.D.
Division of Pulmonary and Critical Care Medicine, Department of Internal Medicine, 3990 John R-3 Hudson, Detroit, MI 48201, USA
e-mail: eshehad@med.wayne.edu

S.C. Nassar-McMillan et al. (eds.), *Biopsychosocial Perspectives on Arab Americans: Culture, Development, and Health*, DOI 10.1007/978-1-4614-8238-3_16,

determined because Arab Americans are not officially recognized as a separate racial/ethnic group. Therefore, describing and comparing the cancer burden among Arab countries and Arab Americans is a difficult and inexact undertaking. Nevertheless, as the population of Arab Americans continues to grow, it is important to recognize that Arab Americans, like many other immigrant populations, may experience health disparities that once identified can be addressed by prevention and early detection interventions. This chapter presents the efforts that have been made to at least estimate the cancer burden among Arab Americans, and make comparisons to their home countries as well as the general population of their adopted country in order to begin to understand the effects of external and internal factors related to cancer diagnosis in this population.

The Healthy Migrant Effect

Study of cancer in specific minority subgroups is important because it allows for identification of patterns of genetic predisposition and environmental exposures. These types of studies are further enhanced by the study of generations of migrant populations over time. First-generation immigrants often have better health, particularly for chronic diseases like cancer, than the residents of their adopted country (Fennelly, 2005; Singh & Siahpush, 2001). This difference is known as the "healthy migrant effect". However, the healthy migrant effect often diminishes over time and the health of successive generations approaches that of their US born compatriots. The healthy migrant effect has been observed in studies of immigrants to the United States, primarily Hispanic and Asian (Dey & Lucas, 2004), and among immigrants to Canada (Hyman, 2001), Australia (Australian Institute of Health and Welfare, 2000), and Western Europe (Razum, Zeeb, & Rohrmann, 2000). In the United States, the effect has been noted for overall mortality (Singh & Siahpush, 2001), heart disease (Dey & Lucas, 2004), cancer (John, Phipps, Davis, & Koo, 2005; Lee, Demissie, Lu, & Rhoads, 2007), and obesity (Barcenas et al., 2007). The pattern of successive generations becoming more similar in health to their adopted country indicates the substantial role of environmental risk factors in the etiology of cancers. As an example of the healthy migrant effect, the US-born Hispanics experience a higher breast cancer incidence than foreign-born Hispanics (John et al., 2005) indicating that migration-related changes in lifestyle factors may be associated with the increases seen in successive generations.

Such migrant studies, however, are possible only if the immigrant population is easily and uniformly identifiable in health-related databases through identification of ethnicity and nativity status. Both Hispanics and Arab Americans are heterogeneous groups originating from many different countries, but share a common language, as well as ancestry (Ennis, Rios-Vargas, & Albert, 2011), and both are included in the White/Caucasian race group in disease registries and health databases. Hispanic ethnicity, as well as Asian origin, are uniformly recorded in the US databases, which allows for specific studies of cancer in these population groups. In contrast, the US Government does not recognize Arab Americans as a distinct population subgroup; hence studies of their health and social issues pose difficult challenges and require special efforts.

In this chapter, estimates for cancer incidence and mortality in Arab countries are presented and compared with estimates for Arab Americans. Comparisons are also made to US populations to begin to make inferences about migration effects. We also present the state of knowledge on cancer prevention and control among Arab Americans. We conclude that much more research is needed to truly understand the state of the cancer burden and factors that may be influencing the findings.

Cancer in Arab Countries

For the 350 million Arabs who are living in the 22 countries of the Arab League, mostly in the Middle East and North Africa, accurate cancer statistics are rarely available. Only nine countries (Saudi Arabia, Jordan, Kuwait, United Arab Emirates, Qatar, Oman, Lebanon, Gaza Strip and West Bank, Bahrain) have national cancer registries. The most reliable estimates for the remaining countries are produced by the International Agency for Research on Cancer (IARC) (Ferley et al., 2010). The data presented here are based on official estimates for 2008 and represent all Arab countries combined.[1]

Table 16.1 presents the estimates of cancer incidence and mortality by site and sex in the Arab world for 2008. Cancers of the lung and bladder in men and breast in women are the most frequently diagnosed, and most frequently identified cause of cancer mortality (cancer death) in the Arab population. Although the population sizes of the United States of America and the Arab countries are similar, the general patterns of cancer incidence and mortality are notably different.

Incidence and Mortality Comparisons with the United States

Figure 16.1 presents cancer incidence and mortality in Arab men and US men. As noted in the figure, both the magnitude and patterns of the incidence and mortality for various cancers in the two populations are noticeably different. The incidence of

[1] Various methodologies were used to obtain these estimates. Only nine countries (Saudi Arabia, Jordan, Kuwait, United Arab Emirates, Qatar, Oman, Lebanon, Gaza Strip and West Bank, Bahrain) have national cancer registries. Statistics for these countries are based on the most recent years of rates applied to the 2008 population. For three countries (Tunisia, Egypt, Algeria) multiple local data were used to estimate the national rate. For two countries (Morocco, Libya) statistics for one cancer registry covering parts of the country were accepted as the country estimate. For three countries (Yemen, Sudan, Iraq) national estimates were based on overall statistics partitioned by sex and age based on information from some local registries. For the other five (Somali, Mauritania, Djibouti, Comoros, Syrian Arab Republic) national estimates were based on rates from neighboring countries. Cancer mortality data are available only for three countries (Bahrain, Kuwait, Gaza Strip and West Bank). For the remaining countries, mortality is estimated based on incidence data.

Table 16.1 Cancer incidence and mortality by site and sex, Arab countries, 2008[a]

	Male				Female			
	Incidence		Mortality		Incidence		Mortality	
Cancers	Number	ASR[b]	Number	ASR[b]	Number	ASR[b]	Number	ASR[b]
All cancers[c]	106,795	104.7	84,607	85.6	109,577	98.1	72,526	67.5
Bladder	11,519	12.4	7,413	8.4	2,409	2.4	1,578	1.6
Brain, nervous system	3,925	3.2	2,903	2.4	2,766	2.2	2,044	1.6
Breast	–	–	–	–	35,507	31.2	18,014	16.7
Cervix uteri	–	–	–	–	5,971	5.5	3,530	3.4
Colorectum	7,245	7.1	5,343	5.4	6,028	5.6	4,465	4.3
Corpus uteri	–	–	–	–	2,515	2.6	763	0.8
Gallbladder	814	0.9	757	0.8	1,217	1.3	1,146	1.2
Hodgkin lymphoma	2,892	2.0	2,252	1.6	1,858	1.3	1,434	1.0
Kaposi sarcoma	269	0.2	236	0.2	50	0.0	45	0.0
Kidney	2,015	1.9	1,552	1.5	1,558	1.3	1,219	1.0
Larynx	3,662	3.9	2,087	2.3	516	0.5	298	0.3
Leukaemia	5,988	4.8	5,480	4.3	4,275	3.3	3,946	3.1
Lip, oral cavity	2,402	2.4	1,028	1.1	1,976	1.9	852	0.9
Liver	6,867	7.2	6,688	7.1	2,678	2.6	2,617	2.7
Lung	11,625	12.7	10,774	11.9	2,489	2.5	2,318	2.3
Melanoma of skin	518	0.5	286	0.3	470	0.4	271	0.3
Multiple myeloma	1,597	1.6	1,442	1.5	1,110	1.1	1,002	1.0
Nasopharynx	2,156	1.9	1,324	1.2	971	0.8	602	0.5
Non-Hodgkin lymphoma	9,095	7.9	7,219	6.4	5,826	5.1	4,621	4.2
Oesophagus	2,371	2.5	2,269	2.4	1,852	1.8	1,759	1.7
Other pharynx	981	0.9	819	0.8	849	0.8	710	0.7
Ovary	–	–	–	–	5,214	4.7	3,801	3.6
Pancreas	2,279	2.4	2,211	2.4	1,606	1.6	1,560	1.6
Prostate	6,698	8.1	5,022	6.1	–	–	–	–
Stomach	3,644	3.7	3,367	3.5	2,574	2.5	2,383	2.3
Testis	1,128	0.7	586	0.4	–	–	–	–
Thyroid	1,301	1.2	764	0.8	3,779	3.1	1,772	1.7

[a]GLOBOCAN 2008, IARC

[b]Age standardised rate, world standard population. Crude and ASR per 100,000

[c]Excludes non-melanoma skin cancers

most cancers is higher in US men, while mortality for cancers of the bladder, liver, non-Hodgkin lymphoma, and stomach are higher in the Arab population.

Figure 16.2 presents the incidence and mortality of cancer in Arab women and US women. Again, incidence and mortality in US females is almost always higher, but for some cancers such as cervix uteri, liver, and stomach, the incidence and mortality rates are fairly similar. The cancers that are documented as having substantively higher incidence among US females are cancers of the breast, colon and

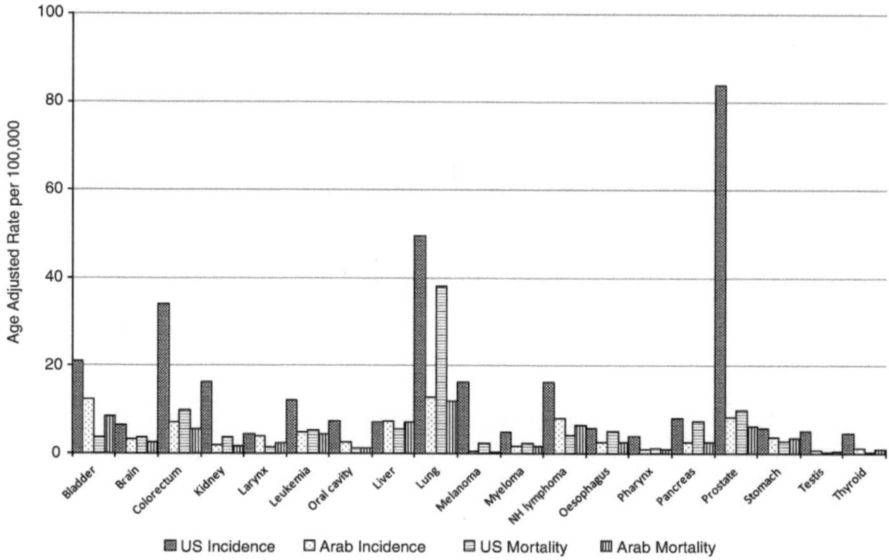

Fig. 16.1 Cancer incidence and mortality rates in men in the Arab Countries and the USA, 2008

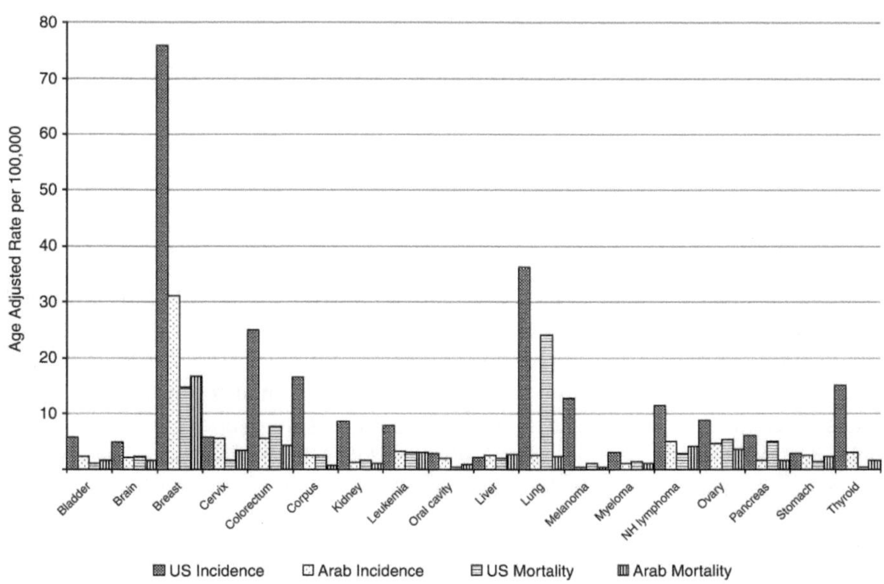

Fig. 16.2 Cancer incidence and mortality rates in women in the Arab Countries and the USA, 2008

Table 16.2 Incidence of total and the top five cancers in men, Arab Countries and USA, 2008[a]

Arab countries				United States of America (USA)			
Population[b]	176,309,000			Population[b]	153,702,000		
Cancer	Number	ASR[c]	%	Cancer	Number	ASR[c]	%
All[d]	106,795	104.7	100.0	All[d]	745,187	335.0	100.0
Lung	11,625	12.7	10.9	Prostate	186,320	83.8	25.0
Bladder	11,519	12.4	10.8	Lung	114,691	49.5	15.4
Prostate	6,698	8.1	6.3	Colon and rectum	79,271	34.1	10.6
Non-Hodgkin lymphoma	9,095	7.9	8.5	Bladder	51,231	21.1	6.9
Liver	6,867	7.2	6.4	Melanoma of skin	34,949	16.3	4.7
Top five percentage of total			42.9				62.6

[a]GLOBOCAN 2008 (IARC) section of cancer information
[b]Estimated population in 2008
[c]Age standardized rate, world standard population
[d]Excludes non-melanoma skin cancers

rectum, lung, melanoma, and thyroid. Cancer deaths for Arab and US women are fairly similar except in the case of breast and lung where US women have higher mortality.

These figures suggest that while incidence of cancer in the Arab population is generally lower than that of the United States, its impact in terms of mortality is equal or higher. This paradox of mortality rates similar between the groups despite the much higher incidence in the United States (see male and female lung, female breast, and male prostate) may be related in part to poorer access to health care, particularly both early detection and therapeutic facilities in the Arab world.

Top Five Cancers for Arab Men and Women

Overall, the patterns of cancer incidence and mortality are different in the Arab and US populations. As shown in Table 16.2, the total number of newly diagnosed cancers in 2008 in US men was seven times more than those in Arab men even though the population size of all Arab countries combined is similar to that of the United States. There also is a difference in the two populations for overall age-standardized incidence rate,[2] which is three times higher for US men. Furthermore, the top five cancers in Arab men account for less than half of all cases, while in the United

[2] Age-Standardization is a statistical method to make rates in different populations comparable. International comparisons use the World Standard Population for comparisons (Bray F. Age-standardization. In: Parkin DM, Whelan SL, Ferlay J, et al. Cancer incidence in five continents. Vol VIII. Lyon, France: International Agency for Research on Cancer, 2002. (IARC Scientific Publications No. 155.)).

Table 16.3 Incidence of total and the top five cancers in women, Arab Countries and USA, 2008[a]

Arab countries				United States of America (USA)			
Population[b]	168,800,000			Population[b]	157,963,000		
Cancer	Number	ASR[c]	%	Cancer	Number	ASR[c]	%
All[d]	109,577	98.1	100.0	All[d]	692,012	274.4	100.0
Breast	35,507	31.2	32.4	Breast	182,460	76.0	26.4
Colon and rectum	6,028	5.6	5.5	Lung	100,330	36.2	14.5
Cervix uteri	5,971	5.5	5.4	Colon and rectum	74,610	25.0	10.8
Non-Hodgkin lymphoma	5,826	5.1	5.3	Corpus uteri	40,102	16.5	5.8
Ovary	5,214	4.7	4.8	Thyroid	28,411	15.1	4.1
Top five percentage of total			53.4				61.6

[a]GLOBOCAN 2008 (IARC) section of cancer information
[b]Estimated population in 2008
[c]Age standardized rate, world standard population
[d]Excludes non-melanoma skin cancers

States, they account for almost two thirds of all cancer diagnoses. Also different are the types of cancer in the Arab countries and the United States.

Table 16.3 presents the comparison of cancer incidence for Arab and US women. The total number of newly diagnosed cancers in 2008 in the United States was almost seven times more than in the Arab countries, and the age-standardized rate (ASR) about three times higher. Breast cancer is the most frequently diagnosed cancer in women in both areas, but the ASR in Arab women is about half of US women. Among Arab women, cancers of the cervix uteri and ovary are among the top five sites, whereas in the US women, cancers of corpus uteri and thyroid are among the top cancers. Another difference between the two areas is the presence of lung cancer in US women and that of non-Hodgkin lymphoma among Arab women. The top five cancers in Arab women account for about half of all cancers, while in US women, the top five represent almost two thirds of all cancers.

Table 16.4 compares cancer mortality between Arab and US men. The total number of cancer deaths in the United States is 3.5 times more and the ASR is about 40 % higher than in Arab countries. Lung cancer is the number one killer in both areas, although the ASR among Arabs is about 70 % lower. Cancers of the bladder and non-Hodgkin lymphoma in Arab men are common causes of cancer death, while in US men cancers of the pancreas and colon and rectum are common causes of cancer death. The ASR for liver cancer as a cause of death in Arab men is about 30 % higher than in US men, while the ASR for prostate cancer is 30 % lower. Unlike the incidence, the proportion of all cancer deaths caused by the top five cancers is more similar between the two groups.

Table 16.5 compares cancer mortality between women in Arab countries and the United States. Again, the total number of cancer deaths in the United States is 3.7 times that of the Arab countries while the ASR is 34 % higher. Lung cancer is the top killer in US women but not among the top five cancer mortality causes for Arab

Table 16.4 Mortality of total and the top five cancers in men, Arab Countries and USA, 2008[a]

Arab countries				United States of America (USA)			
Population[b]	176,309,000			Population[b]	153,702,000		
Cancer	Number	ASR[c]	%	Cancer	Number	ASR[c]	(%)
All[d]	84,607	85.6	100.0	All[d]	294,115	121.4	100.0
Lung	10,774	11.9	12.7	Lung	90,809	38.2	30.9
Bladder	7,413	8.4	8.8	Colon and rectum	24,509	9.9	8.3
Liver	6,688	7.1	7.9	Prostate	28,660	9.7	9.7
Non-Hodgkin lymphoma	7,219	6.4	8.5	Pancreas	17,500	7.3	6.0
Prostate	5,022	6.1	5.9	Liver	12,569	5.5	4.3
Top five percentage of total			43.9				59.2

[a]GLOBOCAN 2008 (IARC) section of cancer information
[b]Estimated population in 2008
[c]Age standardized rate, world standard population
[d]Excludes non-melanoma skin cancers

Table 16.5 Mortality of total and the top five cancers in women, Arab Countries and USA, 2008[a]

Arab countries				United States of America (USA)			
Population[b]	168,800,000			Population[b]	157,963,000		
Cancer	Number	ASR[c]	%	Cancer	Number	ASR[c]	%
All[d]	72,526	67.5	100.0	All[d]	271,529	90.6	100
Breast	18,014	16.7	24.8	Lung	71,032	24.1	26.2
Colon and rectum	4,465	4.3	6.2	Breast	40,481	14.7	14.9
Non-Hodgkin lymphoma	4,621	4.2	6.4	Colon and rectum	26,131	7.7	9.6
Ovary	3,801	3.6	5.2	Ovary	15,519	5.4	5.7
Cervix uteri	3,530	3.4	4.9	Pancreas	16,790	5.1	6.2
Top five percentage of total			47.5				62.6

[a]GLOBOCAN 2008 (IARC) section of cancer information
[b]Estimated population in 2008
[c]Age standardized rate, world standard population
[d]Excludes non-melanoma skin cancers

women. The ASR for breast cancer mortality in Arab women is lower than in US women. In Arab women, cancers of the cervix uteri and non-Hodgkin lymphoma are replaced by cancers of the lung and pancreas in US women as among the top five causes of cancer deaths.

Some of the observed differences between the Arab countries and the United States are clearly due to better and more accurate data collection in the latter. Nevertheless, certain differences like the dominance of cancers of the bladder and liver in Arab men, and lack of lung cancer mortality in Arab women are most likely due to environmental and cultural differences. It is imperative to determine if these differences are observed among Arab Americans as compared to their US counterparts or if a new environment in the United States leads to rates similar to the US rates.

Cancer in Arab Americans

Description of the Arab Population in the United States

There have been essentially three waves of immigrants from the Arab states to the United States (El-Sayed & Galea, 2009). In the late 1800s the majority of immigrants were from current-day Syria and Lebanon and were mainly Christians. Immigrants in the more recent wave since the 1990s are often from war-torn countries such as Iraq and Lebanon and are more likely to be Muslim. Between 1990 and 2000 there also was a large influx of immigrants from Egypt and Yemen (de la Cruz & Brittingham, 2003). In between the recent and distant past, following World War II, there was migration from multiple countries of educated urbanites. In the end, most of the Arab League States are represented, with Lebanese being the largest group followed by Egyptian and Syrian (de la Cruz & Brittingham, 2003). In fact, these three ancestries combined account for about three-fifths of the Arab population in the United States.

Because "Arab" is not recognized as a distinct ethnic group within the "White" race category, it is difficult to find true population numbers for this group. Nevertheless, both California and Michigan, which are home to sizable populations of Arab Americans, both immigrants and descendants of immigrants (de la Cruz & Brittingham, 2003), have made an attempt. Both these states also have well-developed population-based cancer registry systems that are supported by the National Cancer Institute Surveillance, Epidemiology and End Results (SEER) Program. This resource provides an opportunity to begin to estimate the cancer burden among Arab Americans in these two geographic areas. Unfortunately, SEER registries are not a good source for determining whether the cancer case is foreign or US born.

Southeast Michigan has the largest proportion of Arab Americans in all of Michigan; in fact, the city of Dearborn is 29 % Arab (de la Cruz & Brittingham, 2003). Lebanese is the dominant ancestry, followed by general "Arab", based on self-report responses to the US Census. Southeast Michigan also is home to many Chaldeans, who are Iraqi Christians. In California, Lebanese also represents a large proportion of the Arab population. In contrast to Michigan, there also are large proportions of Egyptians and Syrians (de la Cruz & Brittingham, 2003), as well as Middle Easterners that are from countries outside the League of Arab States, such as Iran and Armenia.

Arab American Cancer Statistics

Since Arabs are not specifically identified in various US databases, to estimate the cancer burden among persons of Arab and Middle Eastern descent, several investigators located in geographic areas with large Arab/Middle Eastern populations have developed novel strategies. The primary strategy is development of name lists to identify cases. Such name lists have a long history in population statistics, starting with the development in the 1930s of a Spanish surname list (U.S. Immigration and Naturalization Service, 1936) and later refined by the US Bureau of the Census (Passel & Word, 1980). This Spanish surname list with additional enhancements has been used for decades by SEER and other cancer registries. The North American Association of Central Cancer Registries developed the Asian and Pacific Islander Identification Algorithm (NAPIIA), which uses birthplace and name fields (first, last, and maiden names) to assign a specific race to one of eight Asian race groups (Adamo, Johnson, Ruhl, & DIckie, 2011). In Great Britain, the South Asian Name and Group Recognition Algorithm (SANGRA) is used for health database research (Nanchahal, Mangtani, Alston, & Dos Santos Silva, 2001).

Two name lists for identification of Arab and Middle Easterners have been developed and used in the United States. In Detroit, Schwartz and colleagues (Schwartz et al., 2004) developed and validated a name database and algorithm to estimate the cancer burden in the metropolitan Detroit area. This name list was further updated and validated in 2010 and used to compare age-adjusted proportional incidence ratios between Arabs and Chaldeans (Iraqi Christians) and non-Arab Whites in the Metropolitan Detroit Cancer Surveillance System database. An age-adjusted proportional incidence ratio compares the proportion of one cancer site (e.g., breast) of all cancers between two population groups while adjusting for the age distribution of the two populations. It is important to age-adjust when comparing an immigrant population to an established population because the immigrant population, as a whole, tends to be younger, and advanced age is a risk cancer for most cancers.

Arab/Chaldean American men had proportionally more kidney, leukemia, liver, multiple myeloma, stomach and urinary bladder cancers, and less melanoma of the skin and cancers of the lung, esophagus, and testis compared to the non-Hispanic, non-Arab White men (unpublished data). For Arab/Chaldean women, the cancers with a proportionally greater incidence were leukemia, liver, stomach, and thyroid while skin melanoma and cancers of the lung and cervix were lower. Data are not available in the SEER registry to compare estimates between foreign and US born.

In California, Nasseri (2007) developed a surname database that identifies Arabs from Arab League States and other Middle Easterners from Afghanistan, Armenia, Iran, Pakistan, and Turkey. When age-adjusted incidence rates of Middle Eastern men were compared with non-Hispanic White men, Middle Eastern men had higher incidence of breast, leukemia, liver, multiple myeloma, stomach, and thyroid cancers (Nasseri, Mills, & Allan, 2007). Middle Eastern men had a lower incidence of cancers of the colon and rectum, esophagus, kidney, lung and bronchus, skin melanoma, Non-Hodgkin's lymphoma, oral cavity, prostate, and testis than non-Hispanic Whites. For Middle Eastern women, the elevated incidence occurred in leukemia, liver, stomach, and thyroid cancers, while there was decreased incidence of cancers of the breast, cervix, corpus uteri, colon and rectum, lung and bronchus, skin melanoma, oral cavity, ovary, and urinary bladder. This comparison of incidence rates is unable to provide generational information, that is, data related to foreign or US born.

Table 16.6 Comparison of metropolitan Detroit Arab Chaldean American and California middle eastern incidence to non-Hispanic Whites in same respective geographic location

	Men		Women	
Cancer site	California	Metro Detroit	California	Metro Detroit
Breast	L	–	L	–
Cervix uteri	N/A	N/A	L	–
Colon and rectum	L	–	L	–
Corpus uteri	N/A	N/A	L	–
Esophagus	L	L	–	–
Hodgkins disease	–	–	–	–
Kidney	L	H	–	–
Larynx	–	–	L	–
Leukemia	H	H	H	–
Liver	H	H	H	H
Lung and bronchus	L	L	L	L
Melanoma of skin	L	L	L	L
Multiple myeloma	–	H	–	–
Non-Hodgkins lymphoma	L	–	–	–
Oral cavity and pharynx	L	L	L	–
Ovary	N/A	N/A	L	–
Pancreas	L	–	–	–
Prostate	L	–	N/A	N/A
Stomach	H	H	H	H
Testis	L	L	–	–
Thyroid	H	–	H	H
Urinary bladder	–	H	L	–

L lower incidence compared to Non-Hispanic White, *H* higher, *N/A* Not applicable, – no significant difference in proportional incidence ratio (Detroit data) or incidence rate ratio (California data)

Table 16.6 compares the findings of Detroit and California. Although the two geographic sites defined the population of interest in a slightly different way and used different methodologies (proportional incidence ratio and incidence rate ratio), both included age-adjustment when comparing the populations of interest to the non-Hispanic, non-Arab/Middle Eastern White population in the same geographic area. There are strong and compelling similarities in the results from the two different geographic locations. Both found an elevated incidence of leukemia, liver, and stomach cancers for both men and women when compared to the White population. Both sites also found higher incidence of thyroid cancer among Arab/Middle Eastern women. Detroit and California both found decreased lung and bronchus cancers and skin melanoma among Arab and Middle Eastern men and women, as well as lower incidence in esophagus, oral cavity, and testis cancers in men.

These results suggest opportunities for further research. For instance, Arab and Middle Eastern men have lower smoking-related cancers of the esophagus, lung and bronchus, and oral cavity. Yet, as a group, Arab and Middle Easterners men are often thought to have higher rates of tobacco exposure (Aswad & Hammad, 2001;

Rice & Kulwicki, 1992) than their US counterparts, although some studies suggest that Arab American consumption may be lower (Jamil et al., 2009). An accurate picture of the types and quantities of tobacco exposure among this group is sorely needed.

The higher incidence in gastrointestinal cancers of stomach and liver among Arab/Middle Eastern men and women from Michigan and California is also compelling. The incidence of these cancers also is elevated in the Arab countries. Descriptive studies of first-, second-, and third-generation immigrants may be informative as to the etiology of these cancers and would lead to interesting genetic and epigenetic epidemiological research. For instance, if over successive generations, the incidence became more similar to the United States White population, it might then be suspected that the current higher incidence is due in large part to foreign-born cases, who may have increased risk due to infectious etiologies of *Hepatitis C* and *Helicobacter pylori,* which affect more people in developing countries, including the Arab world (Daw & Dau, 2012; Hunt et al., 2011).

Breast cancer incidence in Arab American women appears to be less common than or at least similar to US White women. Additional studies have been done to determine if there are differences in age and stage at diagnosis and survival between the two groups (Hensley-Alford et al., 2009; Nasseri, 2009). Arab American women are diagnosed with breast cancer at a younger age and higher stage than non-Hispanic White women (Hensley-Alford et al., 2009); however, Arab American women have a survival pattern that is similar to non-Hispanic White women (Hensley-Alford et al., 2009; Nasseri, 2009).

Cancer Control and Prevention in Arab Americans

The World Health Organization (WHO) estimates that at least one third of all cancer cases are preventable and prevention is the preferred and most cost-effective method for controlling cancer (World Health Organization, 2009). Primary cancer prevention focuses on health promotion and risk reduction, which involves avoiding carcinogens, using vaccines for certain cancers and considering prophylactic surgeries in individuals at high risk for certain types of cancers (Adami, Day, Trichopoulos, & Willett, 2001). Examples of this approach are abstinence from smoking and second-hand smoking exposures, adequate physical activity and healthy diet, limiting environmental pollution and occupational carcinogens and avoidance of harmful use of alcohol (World Health Organization, 2009).

There are few sources for determining cancer prevention and early detection patterns among Arab Americans. Only a handful of studies have been conducted, almost all have been done in Michigan. In 2001, 2004, 2006, and 2008, the State of Michigan oversampled minority populations, including Arab Americans, to conduct a Special Cancer Behavioral Risk Factor Survey (SCBRFS), as part of the national Behavioral Risk Factor Surveillance System annual survey and reported results of the four surveys in the 2008 report (Yassine & Galka, 2010). In 2001, the Arab Community Center for Economic and Social Services (ACCESS), in conjunction with the Michigan Department of Community Health, asked Arab and Chaldean Americans at 34 different community centers to complete a health survey (Aswad & Hammad, 2001). These data provide most of the estimates of behavioral and preventive health in this population.

Tobacco Use

Arab American smoking prevalence data have been variable over the last two decades. A study done in the early 1990s reported that 38.9 % of Arab Americans living in a dense Arab community in the Detroit area were current cigarette smokers (Rice & Kulwicki, 1992). More recent surveys have reported a much lower prevalence; however, the methodologies of data collection are different. The earlier study used in-home interviews of a random sample from a geographic area and the later studies relied on convenience sampling and telephone surveys. The 2001 ACCESS survey reported a 15 % smoking rate among Arab American participants, which was attributed to the relatively high socioeconomic status for the study participants compared to the general population (Aswad & Hammad, 2001). In a 2005 study, Jamil and colleagues (Jamil et al., 2009) reported a 28 % current smoking rate. The 2008 SCBRFS also reported a lower prevalence of smoking among Arab Americans 40 years of age and older compared to the general population (18.2 vs. 20.6 %) (Yassine & Galka, 2010). However, the 2004 SCBRFS prevalence for Arab Americans was 28.2 % (Yassine & Galka, 2010).

The difference in smoking prevalence between men and women is more pronounced among Michigan Arab Americans than among the Michigan general population (8.1 % Arab American women vs. 18.4 % general population women and 27.1 % Arab American men vs. 19.5 % general population men) (Yassine & Galka, 2006). The majority of Arab American smokers consume less than 1 pack/day (89 % vs. 53.4 % of general population) and the majority report receiving advice to stop smoking (88.2 % vs. 91.4 % of general population) (Yassine & Galka, 2010).

Smoking prevalence also has been studied in Arab American adolescents in southeast Michigan and is reported to be 18–29 % for ever-smoking and less than 5 % for regular cigarette smoking (Islam & Johnson, 2003; Rice et al., 2006; Weglicki, Templin, Rice, Jamil, & Hammad, 2008). Arab American youths are less likely than non-Arab American youths to ever smoke cigarettes (20 % vs. 39 %) or to be regular cigarettes smokers (3 % vs. 15 %). On the other hand, Arab American adolescents are more likely to smoke using a water pipe despite the majority (77 %) of these youths having the perception that it is as harmful or more harmful than cigarette smoking (Weglicki et al., 2008). Up to 40 % of Arab American youths reported having tried water pipes in the past (Rice et al., 2006).

In a 2009 study, Al-Omari and Scheibmeir (Al-Omari & Scheibmeir, 2009) reported that Arab American smokers prefer cigarettes to other tobacco products. The study also revealed a strong association between smoking and second-hand smoking exposure from family members and peers. In addition, there was a negative association between successful acculturation of Arab Americans in their new environment and nicotine dependence.

Overall, the prevalence of smoking among Arab Americans is reported to be lower than the general population. This may be surprising when taking into account that smoking prevalence is similar or higher than the United States in many Arab countries (World Health Organization, 2011). To compare directly to the WHO results; however, it would be necessary to conduct a similar survey of Arab Americans. In addition, smoking prevalence varies among the different reports. Because there were different recruitment sites and methods for the different surveys, the respondents may be quite different in their smoking habits, which could lead to discrepancies between results. Furthermore, the actual method of obtaining data, telephone or face-to-face, can lead to different responses regarding smoking. In a study of Arabs in Israel, women tended to report more often being a smoker in a face-to-face interview than a telephone interview (Baron-Epel, Haviv-Messika, Green, & Kalutzki, 2004).

Alcohol Use

Excessive alcohol use is linked to cancers of the oral cavity, digestive system, liver, and breast (Wiseman, 2008). The risk of cancer increases with the amount of alcohol consumed and if alcohol consumption is accompanied by smoking (Wiseman, 2008). Alcohol consumption among Michigan Arab Americans was reported as low compared to the general population: only 6.7 % of adults reported current alcohol use and 10.7 % of those current drinkers consumed more than 6 drinks/week (Aswad & Hammad, 2001). In comparison, 57.6 % of the general Michigan population were current drinkers in 2001 (Centers for Disease Control and Prevention, 2012b). In a national survey, Arab American immigrants reported a lower rate of lifetime alcohol use (50.8 %) compared to the majority group (87 %) (Arfken, Arnetz, Fakhouri, Ventimiglia, & Jamil, 2011). Arab American immigrants also had lower rates of past month alcohol use, past year alcohol use, binge use in past month, and heavy use in past month compared to the majority population.

Physical Activity and Diet

Participating in regular physical activity, maintaining a healthy body weight along with a healthy diet are important factors in reducing cancer risk, given that one third of cancer deaths in the United States annually can be attributed to physical activity and dietary habits (Wiseman, 2008). Obesity has been associated with many types of cancer including breast, endometrium, kidney, and some gastrointestinal tumors (Wiseman, 2008). Obesity is a prevalent problem among Arab Americans. Jaber and colleagues, in collaboration with ACCESS reported an obesity rate of 51 % in a population-based sample of 542 Arab Americans aged 20–75 years old (Jaber, Brown, Hammad, Zhu, & Herman, 2004). Hatahet and colleagues reported, based on a survey of 352 Arab Americans in southeast Michigan, the prevalence of being overweight varied for different age groups: 37.9 % for 30 years and younger, 60.9 % for ages 31–40 years, 67.8 % for ages 41–50 years, 73.3 % for ages 51–60 years, and 68.4 % for ages 61–70 years (Hatahet, Khosla, & Fungwe, 2002). The proportion of overweight varied for gender by age. In the 41–50 year group, men were more likely to overweight than women (74.2 % vs. 60 %), while in the 41–60 year group 90 % of women were overweight compared to 67.9 % of the men. The 2001 ACCESS survey indicated that 41.5 % of the respondents reported consuming "junk" food on a daily basis while only 27.5 % did not consume "junk" food in an average week (Aswad & Hammad, 2001).

In conclusion, prevalence of cancer-related risk factors among Arab Americans compared to the general population varies. Although they compare favorably to the general population with regard to smoking and alcohol consumption, they appear to have risks related to obesity and healthy diet. The overall effect of these behavioral risk factors on the incidence of cancer in Arab Americans will be difficult to determine, just as it is in other populations, because of the different interactions between these risk factors and factors such as genetics and environmental exposures.

Early Detection

Secondary cancer prevention focuses on detection of cancer at an early stage, when it is most treatable, in asymptomatic individuals (Adami et al., 2001). The U.S. Preventive Services Task Force has recommended several screening tests for different types of cancer to improve cancer mortality and morbidity (U.S. Preventive Services Task Force, 2012). In addition, benchmarks were established by the Healthy People 2020 Initiative in regard to compliance with recommended screening guidelines and are being monitored by the National Health Interview Survey (NHIS). Among immigrant populations, higher level of education, longer length of residence in the United States, and access to health care have all been associated with higher screening rates (Centers for Disease Control and Prevention, 2012a).

The reported rates of cancer screening by Arab Americans vary. In the 2001 survey conducted by ACCESS and the Michigan Department of Community Health only 26.6 % of Arab Americans were aware of undergoing a screening test for cancer in their lifetimes (Aswad & Hammad, 2001). In this study, Arab Americans were less likely to be screened for cancer compared to the general population. However, the rate of screening varied for the different types of cancer. For breast cancer, 68.9 % of Arab American women reported ever having had a mammogram in their lifetime. This was consistent with the results of a population-based survey by Schwartz and colleagues in which 70 % of Arab American women 40 years and older had a mammogram in their lifetime and 58.1 % had a mammogram every 1–2 years (Schwartz, Fakhouri, Bartoces, Monsur, & Younis, 2008). In the 2008 SCBRFS, Arab American women 40 years and older reporting a mammogram and clinical breast examination varied over the past decade, from a high of 65.2 % in 2001 to a low of 43.2 % in 2004(Yassine & Galka, 2010).

In both the SCBRFS survey and the survey by Schwartz et al., mammography uptake varied by age, with the over 65 years and older having the lowest prevalence; however, the SCBRFS data also included a 75 years and older group that had a remarkably high rate of 96.2 % (Schwartz et al., 2008; Yassine & Galka, 2010). Overall the prevalence of mammography screening is substantially higher for Arab Americans in the SCBRFS report than in the survey by Schwartz et al. (86.3 % vs. 58.1 % reporting a mammogram in past 2 years). The discrepancy could be due to differences in the surveyed populations; the Schwartz et al. sample comprised 96 % immigrant women with an average age of 53.2 years (SD 10.8). These demographic details of the SCBRFS sample are not available.

Prevalence rates for screening for cervical cancer have been fairly consistent between 2001 and 2008. In the 2001 ACCESS survey, 44.8 % of participating females, 18 years and older, reported never having a Papanicolaou (pap) smear(Aswad & Hammad, 2001). The SCBRFS data show a range of 66.6 % in 2001 to 60.4 % in 2008 of Arab American women, 40 years and older, reporting having had a pap test in the past year, and 73.3 % in 2008 reporting a pap test in the last 3 years, compared to 79.0 % in the general population (Yassine & Galka, 2010).

The rates of colon cancer screening among Arab Americans have not been historically high although screening rates have been slowly improving over the last few years. The 2001 ACCESS survey reported that 91.6 % of females and 77.8 % of men in the surveyed Arab American population did not have screening for colon cancer in the past 10 years (Aswad & Hammad, 2001). In the 2008 SCBRFS data, 45.6 % of Arab Americans, 50 years and older, reported having had some type of colon cancer screening (Yassine & Galka, 2010). Of the people who were screened, Arab Americans report having abnormal results 7.9 % of the time compared with 7.4 % of the general population (Yassine & Galka, 2010).

Although screening for prostate cancer is controversial, such screening is widespread (U.S. Preventive Services Task Force, 2012). Among Arab American men, 40 years or older, 57.6 % reported never having had a rectal exam and 37.6 % never had a prostate-specific antigen (PSA) test in 2001 (Aswad & Hammad, 2001). These numbers decreased in 2008, with 53.5 % of Arab Americans, 40 years and older, reporting ever having a PSA test compared to 56.8 % in the general population (Yassine & Galka, 2010). Sixty-eight percent of Arab American men compared to 81 % of general population men reported having ever had a digital rectal examination (Yassine & Galka, 2010). Interestingly, more Arab Americans (65.3 %) discussed the advantages and disadvantages of PSA testing with their doctors compared to the general population (57.3 %) (Yassine & Galka, 2010).

In summary, the prevalence of cancer screening among Arab Americans generally has been lower than the majority population but recent reports are indicating an upward trend with the gap becoming smaller with time.

Cancer Control and Prevention Barriers

Identifying the barriers to effective cancer prevention and screening is crucial to improving Arab American compliance with recommended guidelines. A 2008 qualitative study of Arab American immigrants in New York reported barriers that are often associated with cancer screening among immigrants: language, time, discrimination, and beliefs about illness causation that are not identified or addressed by health care providers (Shah, Ayash, Pharaon, & Gany, 2008). Barriers to breast cancer screening have been the most studied. Several factors have been positively associated with increased rate of breast cancer screening among Michigan Arab American women including age between 50 and 64 years US residency of more than 10 years, being married, having health insurance, general health motivation, and perceived seriousness of illness (Schwartz et al., 2008). Among Washington D.C. Jordanian and Palestinian women, a positive relationship between general health habits and breast cancer screening was again reported, and a belief in the value of breast cancer screening was associated with higher frequency of screening (Kawar, 2009).

Several attempts have been made to improve cancer screening rates among Arab Americans. Vicini and colleagues report that implementing a community-based participatory process model in which community leaders are mobilized and educational symposiums and forums are conducted can help in reducing the disparities in cancer screening rates between the general population and ethnic minorities (Vicini et al., 2011). In their study, 80 % of the Arab Americans and Chaldeans who completed their post-symposium survey indicated that they learned something new about cancer prevention, screening, and treatment. Although 72 % indicated that they would seek cancer screening, only 28.9 % actually underwent some type of screening within the 12 months following the intervention.

The Arab American Breast Cancer Education and Referral (AMBER) program is another program that utilizes a community-based participatory approach to design program interventions such as culturally appropriate Arabic language breast cancer education, screening coordination, and cultural competency training for healthcare professionals in New York City (Ayash et al., 2011). Almost 600 Arab American women were educated resulting in 68 women receiving breast cancer screening, which led to the identification of 1 new case and 4 cases in need of follow up. Nearly 68 % of the participating women reported having a better understanding of the importance of cancer screening as a result of the workshop.

Breast cancer screening education by in-home community health workers (CHW) is being evaluated to determine if knowledge and screening behaviors are increased (Williams et al., 2011). The Kin Keeper Cancer Prevention Intervention conducts two home visits by culturally matched CHWs, using visual aids and the language of the female family members to educate about breast cancer early detection and develop a screening plan. Comparison of pre- and post-test knowledge testing indicates an improvement in screening knowledge; screening practices post education will be assessed at the 12 month follow-up visit.

Critique

Population Estimates Are a Problem

There is no doubt that the lack of easy identification of Arab Americans in health statistics severely limits our ability to characterize the cancer burden in this population or make comparisons to other population groups. Furthermore, the lack of population-based data from Arab States leads to serious difficulty interpreting comparisons between Arab and Arab American cancer statistics. As cancer becomes a more prevalent and chronic disease in the Arab world, the need for cancer surveillance will likely become evident. As for the US statistics, until immigrants from Arab States and their descendants are recognized as a separate ethnic group by the US government, investigators and public health officials must rely on crude estimates.

Name lists may work fairly well for numerator estimation, but the denominator estimation is even less rigorous. Past and current calculations of this number have employed the US Census long-form data in the past, which was completed by only 1 in 6 households. Moving forward the denominator estimation will be even less precise, as starting with the 2010 decennial census, the long-form questions regarding ancestry, place of birth, and language spoken at home, the three questions used to estimate denominator (Read, 2007), are no longer collected. Rather, the US Census Bureau has implemented the American Community Survey, which is a year-round continuous survey of American households that samples many fewer households than the decennial long-form census. The possibility of less reliable data for estimates of the Arab American population with this new measurement is very real.

Additionally, generational information is needed for in-depth migrant studies. It is necessary to know if health data on Arab Americans is based on foreign-born or US-born. Country of birth is collected by cancer registries, but is often not available in the source data, namely the medical record. As more health records become electronic, perhaps in the future they will be standardized and include country of birth and Arab ancestry/ethnicity.

Need for More Research on Cancer Risk Factors

There has been little work done outside of Michigan on characterizing cancer risk factors among Arab Americans. Given the sizable population in other areas of the country, such as California and New York, population-based data regarding risk factors and screening habits could be easily accomplished using sampling methods that ensure a representative sample.

Furthermore, current methods employed in the BRFSS may not lead to adequate representation of the Arab American population. The BRFSS has been finding it difficult to obtain response rates of 50 % in the general population due to call screening and lack of land lines; the median response rate in 2000 BRFSS was 48 % (Schneider,

Clark, Rakowski, & Lapane, 2009). After adjustment for nonresponse, Schneider and colleagues still found underrepresentation of racial/ethnic minorities, women and younger individuals (Schneider et al., 2009). In general, representation of racial/ethnic minorities and/or women in surveys is influenced by factors such as culturally sensitive terms and material, the survey mode itself (telephone, mail, face-to-face), choice of an appropriate interviewer, or subjective sense that the survey is important (Sykes, Walker, Ngwakongnwi, & Quan, 2010). Following from this work, Arab Americans, as a group, may be more likely to participate in surveys that are face-to-face with an interviewer who is responsive to the participant's cultural norms.

Implications for Practice, Research, and Policy

In conclusion, despite the limitations of the data, there are several practice, research, and policy areas that deserve mention. First, in the area of practice, several lessons can be gleaned from the breast cancer screening literature. It certainly appears that community-based education programs improve knowledge and early detection efforts. Educational programs in the community delivered by community members in a culturally appropriate way will improve cancer prevention and screening. The evidence for this approach is based on a few studies done with breast cancer screening for women as described above in 16.3.5. It is unclear if this same approach would work as well for men or for other types of cancer.

In the area of research, there are numerous paths for investigation. There is a distinct need to glean an accurate picture of the smoking habits among Arab Americans, especially men. Although smoking is thought to be prevalent in this group, the few studies available present a wide range of estimates of smoking prevalence. Furthermore, lung cancer has high incidence and mortality in the Arab States, but when compared to US men, Arab American men have lower incidence of several smoking-related cancers, including lung, esophagus, and oral cavity. The reason for such a paradox is unclear; two possible reasons are smoking exposure is truly less among Arab American men or epigenetic influences work differently among Arab American men compared to in Arab countries.

Liver cancer is among the top five cancers for incidence and mortality among Arab men. In California and Michigan Arab American populations, the incidence of liver cancer appears to be elevated compared to non-Hispanic Whites for both men and women. This finding presents additional research opportunities to look at genetic, infectious, and environmental exposures for liver cancer, comparing the US and Arab cases.

Although the incidence of thyroid cancer appears to be lower among Arab women when comparing to the US statistics, Arab American women appear to have higher incidence than non-Hispanic white women. Again, this observation points toward a need to better understand exposure differences between the two populations. Preliminary work indicates that Arab American women with thyroid cancer have more exposure to medical radiation than non-Hispanic White women with thyroid cancer (Peterson, Soliman, Ruterbusch, Smith, & Schwartz, 2011).

The two most important policy recommendations are based on the need for accurate health statistics for the Arab American population. First is the call for this population group to be recognized as a distinct ethnic group. Without this government recognition, it always will difficult to know how accurate and/or comparable the health statistics are for this group compared to other racial/ethnic groups. Furthermore, without ongoing statistics, it will be difficult to track trends over time, which will in turn make it difficult to assess large-scale prevention and screening interventions. The second recommendation, mentioned above, is to include, at least periodically, this population as an oversampled population in nationally collected data, particularly those that collect data in the home, such as NHIS. If the first recommendation were to be observed, the second may easily follow, as the lack of and need for reliable health data for Arab Americans would be readily apparent.

References

Adami, H., Day, N., Trichopoulos, D., & Willett, W. (2001). Primary and secondary prevention in the reduction of cancer morbidity and mortality. *European Journal of Cancer, 37*(Suppl 8), s118–127.

Adamo, M., Johnson, C., Ruhl, J., & DIckie, L. (2011). *SEER Program Coding and Staging Manual 2011*. Bethesda: Department of Health and Human Services.

Al-Omari, H., & Scheibmeir, M. (2009). Arab Americans' acculturation and tobacco smoking. *Journal of Transcultural Nursing, 20*(2), 227–223.

American Cancer Society. (2012). *Cancer Facts and Figures 2012*. Atlanta: American Cancer Society.

Arfken, C., Arnetz, B., Fakhouri, M., Ventimiglia, M., & Jamil, H. (2011). Alcohol use among Arab Americans: What is the prevalence. *Journal of Immigrant and Minority Health, 13*(4), 713–718. doi:10.1007/s10903-011-9447-8.

Aswad, M., & Hammad, A. (2001). *Health Survey of the Arab, Muslim and Chaldean Communities in Michigan* available at http://www.accesscommunity.org/site/DocServer/health_and_research_cente_19.pdf.

Australian Institute of Health and Welfare. (2000). *Australia's health 2000*. Canberra: Australian Institute of Health and Welfare.

Ayash, C., Axelrod, D., Nejmeh-Khoury, S., Aziz, A., Yusr, A., & Gany, F. M. (2011). A community intervention: AMBER: Arab American breast cancer education and referral program. *Journal of Immigrant and Minority Health, 13*(6), 1041–1047.

Barcenas, C., Wilkinson, A., Strom, S., Cao, Y., Saunders, K., Mahabir, S., et al. (2007). Birthplace, years of residence in the United States, and obesity among Mexican-American adults. *Obesity (Silver Spring), 15*(4), 1043–1052.

Baron-Epel, O., Haviv-Messika, A., Green, M., & Kalutzki, D. (2004). Ethnic differences in reported smoking behaviors in face-to-face and telephone interviews. *European Journal of Epidemiology, 19*, 679–686.

Centers for Disease Control and Prevention. (2012a). Cancer Screening—United States, 2010. *Morbidity and Mortality Weekly Report, 61*(3), 41–45.

Centers for Disease Control and Prevention. (2012b). *Prevalence and trends data*. Retrieved July 2010, from Centers for Disease Control and Prevention http://www.cdc.gov/brfss/index.htm

Daw, M. A., & Dau, A. A. (2012). Hepatitis C virus in Arab world: a state of concern. *Scientific World Journal*, 2012:719494. doi: 10.1100/2012/719494. Epub 2012 May 2.

de la Cruz, G. P., & Brittingham, A. (2003). The Arab population:2000. In U.S. Census Bureau (Ed.), *Census 2000 Brief* available at http//www.census.gov/prod/2003pubs/c2kbr-23.pdf.

Dey, A., & Lucas, J. (2004). Physical and mental health characteristics of U.S.-born and foreign-born adults 1997–2002. Retrieved from http://www.cdc.gov/nchs/ppt/duc2004/dey_lucas.ppt

El-Sayed, A. M., & Galea, S. (2009). The health of Arab-Americans living in the United States: A systematic review of the literature. *BMC Public Health, 9*, 272. doi:10.1186/1471-2458/9/272.

Ennis, S., Rios-Vargas, M., & Albert, N. (2011). The Hispanic Population: 2010. In U.S. Census Bureau (Ed.), *Census Brief 2010.* available at http://www.census.gov/prod/cen2010/briefs/c2010br-04.pdf

Fennelly, K. (2005). The 'healthy migrant' effect. *Minnesota Medicine, 5*(3), 1–4.

Ferley, J., Shin, H., Bray, F., Forman, D., Mathers, C., & Parkin, D. (2010). GLOBOCAN v1.2. Lyon France: International Agency for Research on Cancer. Retrieved from http://globocan.iarc.fr/

Hatahet, W., Khosla, P., & Fungwe, T. (2002). Prevalence of risk factors to coronary heart disease in an Arab-American population in southeast Michigan. *International Journal of Food Sciences and Nutrition, 53*(4), 325–335.

Hensley-Alford, S., Schwartz, K., Soliman, A., Cole-Johnson, C., Gruber, S., & Merajver, S. (2009). Breast cancer characteristics at diagnosis and survival among Arab-American women compared to European- and African-American women. *Breast Cancer Research and Treatment, 114*(2), 339–346.

Hunt, R., Xiao, S., Megraud, F., Leon-Barua, R., Bazzoli, F., van der Merwe, S., et al. (2011). *Helicobacter pylori* in develoing countries. World Gastroenterology Organisation Global Guideline. *Journal of Gastrointestinal and Liver Diseases, 20*(3), 299–304.

Hyman, I. (2001). *Immigration and health.* Ottawa: Health Canada.

Islam, S., & Johnson, C. (2003). Correlates of smoking behavior among Muslim Arab-American adolescents. *Ethnicity & Health, 8*(4), 319–337.

Jaber, L., Brown, M., Hammad, A., Zhu, Q., & Herman, W. (2004). The prevalence of the metabolic syndrome among Arab Americans. *Diabetes Care, 27*(1), 234–238.

Jamil, H., Templin, T., Fakhouri, M., Rice, V., Khouri, R., & Fakhouri, H. (2009). Comparison of personal characteristics, tobacco use, and health states in Chaldean, Arab American and non-Middle Eastern White adults. *Journal of Immigrant and Minority Health, 11*, 310–317.

John, E., Phipps, A., Davis, A., & Koo, J. (2005). Migration history, acculturation, and breast cance risk in Hispanic women. *Cancer Epidemiology, Biomarkers & Prevention, 14*(12), 2905–2913.

Kawar, L. (2009). Jordanian and Palestinian immigrant women's knowledge, affect, cultural attitudes, health habits, and participant in breast cancer screening. *Health Care for Women International, 30*(9), 768–782.

Lee, J., Demissie, K., Lu, S., & Rhoads, G. (2007). Cancer incidence among Korean-American immigrants in the United States and nataive Koreans in South Korea. *Cancer Control, 14*(1), 78–85.

Nanchahal, K., Mangtani, P., Alston, M., & Dos Santos Silva, I. (2001). Development and validation of computerized South Asian Names and Group Recognition Algorithm (SANGRA) for use in the British health-related studies. *Journal of Public Health Medicine, 23*(4), 278–285.

Nasseri, K. (2007). Construction and validation of a list of common Middle Eastern surnames for epidemiological research. *Cancer Detection and Prevention, 31*(5), 424–429.

Nasseri, K. (2009). Breast cancer in the MIddle Eastern population of California, 1988–2004. *The Breast Journal, 15*(2), 182–188.

Nasseri, K., Mills, P. K., & Allan, M. (2007). Cancer incidence in the Middle Eastern population of California, 1988–2004. *Asian Pacific Journal of Cancer Prevention, 8*(3), 405–411.

Passel, J. S., & Word, D. L. (1980). Construction of the list of Spanish surnames for the 1980 Census: An applicatin of Bayes' theorum.

Peterson, L., Soliman, A., Ruterbusch, J. J., Smith, N., & Schwartz, K. (2011). Comparison of exposures among Arab American and non-Hispanic White female thyroid cancer cases in metropolitan Detroit. *Journal of Immigrant Minority Health, 13*(6), 1033–1040.

Razum, O., Zeeb, H., & Rohrmann, S. (2000). The 'healthy migrant effect'—not merely a fallacy of inaccurate denominator figures. *International Journal of Epidemiology, 29*, 191–192.

Read, J. (2007). *Alternative definitions of Mexican and Arab identity: An examination across the top three census metropolitan standard areas of concentration*. Irvine: University of California.

Rice, V., & Kulwicki, A. (1992). Cigarette use among Arab Americans in the Detroit metropolitan area. *Public Health Reports, 107*, 589–594.

Rice, V., Weglicki, L., Templin, T., Hammad, A., Jamil, H., & Kulwicki, A. (2006). Predictors of Arab American adolescent tobacco use. *Merrill-Palmer Quarterly (Wayne State University Press), 52*(2), 327–342.

Schneider, K., Clark, M., Rakowski, W., & Lapane, K. (2009). Evaulating the impact of non-response bias in the Behavioral Risk Factor Surveillance System. *Journal of Epidemiology and Community Health, 66*(4), 290–295.

Schwartz, K., Fakhouri, M., Bartoces, M., Monsur, J., & Younis, A. (2008). Mammography screening among Arab American women in metropolitan Detroit. *Journal of Immigrant Minority Health, 10*(6), 541–549.

Schwartz, K., Kulwicki, A., Weiss, L. K., Fakhouri, H., Sakr, W., Kau, G., et al. (2004). Cancer among Arab Americans in the metropolitan Detroit area. *Ethnicity & Disease, 14*(141–146).

Shah, S. M., Ayash, C., Pharaon, N. A., & Gany, F. M. (2008). Arab American immigrants in New York: Health care and cancer knowledge, attitudes and beliefs. *Journal Immigrant Minority Health, 10*(5), 429–436.

Siegel, R., Desantis, C., Virgo, K., Stein, K., Mariotto, A., Smith, T., et al. (2012). Cancer treatment and survivorship statistics, 2012. *CA: A Cancer Journal for Clinicians, 62*(4), 220–241.

Singh, G., & Siahpush, M. (2001). All-cause and cause-specific mortality of immigrants and native born in the United States. *American Journal of Public Health, 91*, 392–399.

Sykes, L., Walker, R., Ngwakongnwi, E., & Quan, H. (2010). A systematic literature review on response rates across racial and ethnic populations. *Canadian Journal of Public Health, 101*(3), 213–219.

US Preventive Services Task Force. (2012). *Recommendations for Adults: Cancer*. Rockville: Agency for Healthcare Research and Policy.

Vicini, F., Shah, C., Wallace, M., Jones, P., Dykes, V., Tull, J., et al. (2011). Strategies for reducing cancer incidence and mortality in African American and Arab American and Chaldean communities in the Detroit metropolitan area. *American Journal of Clinical Oncology, 35*(4), 316–21.

Weglicki, L., Templin, T., Rice, V., Jamil, H., & Hammad, A. (2008). Comparison of cigarette and water pipe smoking by Arab and non-Arab-American youth. *American Journal of Preventive Medicine, 35*(4), 334–339. doi:10.1016/j.amepre.2008.06.037.

Williams, K., Mabiso, A., Todem, D., Hammad, A., Hill-Ashford, Y., Hamade, H., et al. (2011). Differences in knowledge of breast cancer screening among African American, Arab American, and Latina women. *Preventing Chronic Disease, 8*(1), A20.

Wiseman, M. (2008). The second World Cancer Research Fund/American Institute for Cancer Research expert report. Food, nutrition, physical activity, and the prevention of cancer: a global perspective. *Proceedings of the Nutrition Society, 67*(3), 253–256. doi:10.1017/S002966510800712X.

World Health Organization. (2009). *2008–2013 Action Plan for the Global Strategy for the Prevention and Control of Noncommunicable Diseases*. Geneva, Switzerland: World Health Organization.

World Health Organization. (2011). *WHO Report on the Global Epidemic, 2011: Warning about the Dangers of Tobacco*. Geneva, Switzerland: World Health Organization.

Yassine, M. W., & Galka, A. (2006). *Special cancer behavorial risk factor survey*. In Michigan Cancer Consortium: Michigan Public Health Institute (Ed.) available at http://www.mphi.org/pubs/MCCReports-SCBRFS.pdf.

Yassine, M. W., & Galka, A. (2010). Special Cancer Behavioral Risk Factor Survey, 2008

Chapter 17
Health Disparities and Advocacy Chapter

Adnan Hammad, Manal Said, and Cynthia L. Arfken

Definition of Health Disparities

In 1948, the World Health Organization defined *Health* as a state of complete physical, mental, and social well-being and not merely the absence of disease or infirmity (World Health Organization (WHO) 1979). The achievement of complete physical, mental and social well-being has generally been understood to be influenced by genetics, social and physical environment, behavior, and health care. However, in 2002 the Institute of Medicine report, *Unequal Treatment: Confronting Racial and Ethnic Disparities in Healthcare* called attention to *systematically worse* access to health care and worse health outcomes among certain racial and ethnic groups compared to the majority group (Smedley, Stith, & Nelson, 2002). This report was followed by analyses that showed at no time in US history has the overall health status of racial and ethnic minority populations equaled or even approximated that of the majority group (Liao et al., 2004; Ulmer, McFadden, & Nerenz, 2009). These systematic differences were reflected in the definition of *Health Disparities* by the Centers for Disease Control and Prevention (CDC, 2008):

> preventable differences in the burden of disease, injury and violence, or opportunities to achieve optimal health experienced by socially disadvantaged racial, ethnic, and other populations, groups, and communities. These disparities are unjust, unfair, and directly related to the historical and current unequal distribution of social, political, economic, and environmental factors.

A. Hammad (✉) • M. Said
ACCESS Community Health and Research Center, 6450 Maple Street,
Dearborn, MI 48126, USA
e-mail: ahammad@accesscommunity.org

C.L. Arfken
Department of Psychiatry and Behavioral Neuroscience, Wayne State University,
3901 Chrysler Drive, Detroit, MI 48201, USA
e-mail: carfken@med.wayne.edu

S.C. Nassar-McMillan et al. (eds.), *Biopsychosocial Perspectives on Arab Americans: Culture, Development, and Health*, DOI 10.1007/978-1-4614-8238-3_17,

Thus, health disparities was broaden to represent a systematic inequality adversely affecting groups independent of their legal classification as racial or ethnic minorities. To address the disparities requires advocacy for data, analysis and then action based upon these analysis. This advocacy represents a shift for the public health sector from concentrating on individual patient risk factors and education to broader political action in order to change social, political, economic and environmental conditions.

Determinants of Health Disparities

Health disparities result from many forces in society. Increasingly it is recognized as shaped by social determinants and cultural barriers. The social determinants range from broad societal issues such as poverty, racism, and hazardous environments, to health system factors such as lack of health care coverage/access and lack of workforce diversity. As such, disparities as summarized by the CDC and the IOM reflect discrimination within society and barriers to full participation in society.

Health disparities can be examined from a variety of theoretical perspectives. For immigrant groups which include Arab Americans, most frequently these approaches have included acculturation (Berry, 1997) and discrimination (Krieger, 1999). However, other approaches such as stress-coping and even traditional individual level exposure to risk factors such as environmental hazards and trauma for chronic diseases help inform approaches to eliminate disparities.

Social Determinants and Cultural Barriers

Social determinants of health and health care encompass socioeconomic status, education, health insurance, language, employment, transportation, housing, and geographic location of institutions where care could be received. However, it is difficult to disentangle the complex interaction between membership in a disempowered group and social determinants to understand direct determinants of health and treatment and how they may influence the receipt of optimal care (Guidry, Aday, Zhang, & Winn, 1997, 1998; Shavers & Brown, 2002). Common challenges associated with, for example, having low income such as limited transportation and affordability of office visits or prescriptions may negatively influence the ability to receive care. One frequently quoted example is that African Americans, a disempowered group in the USA, receive a lower quality of health care than the majority group even when social determinants, such as patients' insurance status and income are controlled (Saha, Arbelaez, & Cooper, 2003).

However, it is also important to examine more subtle cultural disparities. Findings from several studies suggest that cultural characteristics such as race, country of origin, and gender may influence a physician's perception of patients (Einbinder & Schulman, 2000; Rathore et al., 2000; Shavers & Brown, 2002; van Ryn & Burke, 2000).

These perceptions then are manifested in different referral patterns and treatment recommendations (Einbinder & Schulman, 2000; Rathore et al., 2000; Schulman et al., 1999; Shavers & Brown, 2002). One study (Schulman et al., 1999) tested specifically how race and gender influenced physicians' clinical decisions and recommendations using actors as patients with chest pain. The results suggested that a patient's race and gender influenced a physician's recommendation independent of the patient's clinical characteristics. Likewise, in a survey of eight New York State hospitals, physicians were more likely to have negative perceptions of disempowered groups (Shavers & Brown, 2002; van Ryn & Burke, 2000).

Other aspects of the patient and physician interaction influence health outcomes. For example, how patients perceive the physician, whether patients feel respected and listened to, and whether patients understand ongoing actions they need to take to care for chronic diseases (Michalopoulou, Falzarano, Arfken, & Rosenberg, 2009). Poor patient–physician communication can result from physicians' lack of familiarity with cultural norms and language barriers, coupled with time pressure during visits. Exacerbating the problem, poor patient–physician communication can lead to inefficient care and medical errors. Addressing these health care disparities requires special attention to cultural attitudes and perceptions that affect health behaviors and patterns of health care access and utilization (AHQR, 2008). One response has been that hospitals are now mandated to collect more detailed information on country of origin and preferred language of their patients and actively respond to disempowered group within their communities (The Joint Commission, 2011).

Health Disparities Between Arab Americans and Majority Group

Why Study Health Disparities Among Arab Americans?

Arab Americans trace their heritage to one of 22 countries with Arabic as one of the official languages. Arab Americans share common historical, cultural and social experiences in addition to a common linguistic heritage (Nydell, 2006). Important to the USA, they are a growing immigrant group (de la Cruz & Brittingham, 2003). Unfortunately, as a group they have been confused in published literature and in public discourse with "Middle Eastern," a group including Iranians, Turks, and other countries of origins in the Eastern Mediterranean area who may share religious or cultural values but who are not Arab Americans.

Although Arab Americans as a group enjoy a high median income relative to the majority group (de la Cruz & Brittingham, 2003), this statistic masks a large proportion of Arab Americans with low income who may be disempowered by economic forces. Moreover, disempowerment for a group may result from other factors. As documented by Shaheen (2001), Arabs and Arab Americans have been portrayed as evil and conniving since the advent of movies. After September 11, 2001, the negative depictions became more entrenched (Shaheen, 2008) even as it became politically incorrect to depict stereotypes of other racial or immigrant groups. Recent analysis of political speeches also documented overt negative public rhetoric (Merskin, 2004), contributing to a hostile environment for Arab Americans. Behavioral experiments confirmed that college students preferentially discriminated against Arab Americans compared to other minority groups (Bushman & Bonacci, 2004).

These depictions and rhetoric are also matched with government actions taken against Arab American and Muslim organizations and charities, including raids and freezing of assets. Ongoing racial profiling at airports, border crossings, and on the street similarly contributes to feelings of inequality within the larger US society. Lastly, the war in Iraq colored the perception of citizenship of Arab Americans by the rest of the society (Detroit Arab American Study Team, 2009).

Cultural factors affect the health disparities for Arab Americans, as well. One important cultural aspect is stigma. Chronic diseases such as cancer, diabetes, mental health, and substance abuse are traditionally viewed as highly stigmatizing with the result that Arab Americans may deny that there is a problem, leading to delayed diagnosis and lack of treatment. Infectious diseases requiring ongoing maintenance such as HIV are also traditionally viewed as highly stigmatizing. The stigma may be felt not only by the person with the disease but by the whole family. Two examples that the authors personally know include a woman diagnosed with breast cancer who refused to tell her family or seek treatment because she did not want to affect the chances of her daughter getting married. Another example was a young adult woman who was told by her mother that if she drank alcohol or used drugs that she and her sisters would not be able to marry. (Both of these examples demonstrate the strong Arab cultural values on family and personal behavior benefitting the family.) These examples are not presented to paint all Arab Americans as having these values; they are to remind the reader that they can exist. Having said that, stigma can be valuable as a prevention strategy, for example, to deter people from starting to smoke marijuana. However, once a problem behavior is initiated, the associated stigma may delay and complicate treatment.

Subgroups Within Arab Americans

The New York survey of physicians (Shavers & Brown, 2002) mentioned earlier also highlighted that negative perceptions towards patients were more likely to occur when the patients differed from the physicians. For Arab Americans, these differences from the majority group may encompass language skills (e.g., no or limited English proficiency or speaking English with an accent), skin color (e.g., darker skin for people with Sudanese and Yemeni heritage), rural versus urban background, religion, and religiosity (i.e., both observed behaviors and personal importance of religious beliefs). Other differences include gender roles, acceptable clothing (e.g., some countries of origin/subgroups believe men and women should dress modestly; other countries of origin/subgroups believe men and women should celebrate their beauty and emphasize their bodies), range of literacy, education and income, and health beliefs with a few traditional groups believing that health status is influenced by "evil eye" and demons. Equally important for immigrant groups are country or origin and generational differences between immigrant or first generation, second generation and third generations. These generational differences may not be predictable as Arab countries are experiencing rapid changes including Westernization of diet. Lastly, as Arab countries have and are experiencing conflict, exposure to conflict and trauma would constitute subgroups. Some of these differences may correlate with country of origin; others will not correlate well. It is important to keep in mind that the Arab countries vary dramatically from each and represent the full range from highly developed education and medical systems to countries struggling to provide basic services.

Mortality

The most dramatic health disparity is higher mortality rate. Until recently, little was known about mortality experiences among Arab Americans compared to the majority group in the USA as officially within OMB Arab Americans are classified as "White". The designation may be changing, as this chapter is being written, as the US Bureau of Census found improved accuracy when allowing a separate designation of Arab Americans. This impact on accuracy reflected similar improvements when the reporting of substance abuse treatment was expanded to include ethnicity of "Arab/Chaldean" and subsequently with the expansion of racial categories to include "Arab Americans".

The recent efforts of three groups of investigators to provide information on mortality data among Arab Americans reflect the difficulties in obtaining data. One group (Nasseri & Moulton, 2011) examined death certificates in selected Californian counties from 1997 to 2004. During this time period, California death certificates collected information on country of birth and country of birth of parents. The research group used countries from the Middle East (including Iran, Turkey, Afghanistan etc) and ignored countries from North Africa. The eligible Californian counties reflected where the majority of Iranian Americans live in the USA. Using proportional mortality measures, they found first generation Middle Easterners had higher odds for diabetes, colorectal cancers, and heart disease; they had lower odds for chronic obstructive pulmonary disease and suicide. Immigrant Middle Eastern men had higher odds for all cancers, lymphomas and pancreatic cancers. Immigrant Middle Eastern women had lower odds for lung cancer and dementia, but higher odds for breast cancer. The second generation Middle Eastern men had higher odds for all cancers and heart diseases, and second generation Middle Eastern women had lower odds for lung cancer and stroke. Second generation Middle Easterners overall had higher odds for colorectal cancers and lower odds for chronic obstructive pulmonary disease.

Another group (Dallo, Schwartz, Ruterbusch, Booza, & Williams, 2012) used a different methodology, time frame and geographic location. They examined death certificates for 1999–2001 in Michigan for persons 25 and older. To produce mortality rates, they used lists of Arab first names and surnames to identify deaths among Arab Americans. For the denominator, they used the number of Arab Americans living in Michigan from the 2000 Census. To obtain this number, they used self-reported Arab ancestry, birthplace in one of the 22 Arab countries or Arabic/Syriac language spoken at home. They found older Arab Americans (75 and above) had higher mortality rates than Whites or African Americans. Among men, all-cause mortality rates for Arab Americans did not differ substantially from that of Whites and African Americans. However, Arab American men had lower mortality rates from cancer and chronic lower respiratory disease compared to both Whites and African Americans. Among women, Arab Americans had lower mortality rates from heart disease, cancer, stroke, and diabetes than either Whites or African Americans.

El-Sayed, Tracy, Scarborough, and Galea (2011) used a methodology and time frame different from either the other two groups. Like Dallo and colleagues, they used Michigan as the geographic location. Combining Michigan death certificates for 1990–2007, they found life expectancies among Arab American men and women were 2.0 and 1.4 years lower than among White men and women. For men, the higher mortality rate was due to infectious diseases (septicemia and pneumonia/flu), chronic diseases (cancer, diabetes, heart diseases, strokes, and chronic respiratory disease), and homicide. For women the higher mortality rate was due to cancer, diabetes, heart diseases, and stroke. Most striking was the elevated mortality rates among the groups under 5 and 45 years and older for both males and females. For Arab Americans males, the elevated mortality rate was evident from birth through age 25, using their age groupings. To obtain these numbers, they used Arab ethnicity reported on the death certificates and self-reported ancestry from the 2000 census. Although they have 18 years of data, they did not examine temporal trends across this long period of time.

Finkton, El-Sayed, and Galea (2012) further examined infant mortality (death prior to 1 year of life), neonatal mortality (death prior to 28 days) and post-neonatal mortality (death between 28 days and 1 year) separately using records from all live singleton birth in Michigan between 1989 and 2005. They found Arab Americans had a lower infant mortality rate (4.7 per 1,000 live births) than non-Arab Whites (5.6 per 1,000 live births). However, when they adjusted for marital status, maternal tobacco consumption during pregnancy, and maternal birthplace there was no difference between the groups. Such lack of difference suggests that cultural protective factors may wane with acculturation but to date this has not been examined rigorously.

The Michigan Department of Community Health publishes online the infant mortality numbers by race and ethnicity (including Arab Americans). Infant mortality rate which had been lower than the White population in the early 2000s has steadily increased and since 2005 surpassed that of Whites (2008: 8.5 vs. 5.4 per 1,000 births). This consistent and disturbing trend is not attributed to maternal risk factors among Arab Americans as they appear similar in prevalence to that of other race/ethnic groups. However, Vital Statistics data showed that Arab American births in comparison to the major racial/ethnic groups had the highest proportion of precipitous labor, highest percentage of assisted ventilation immediately following delivery, and highest percentage of births with significant birth injury. These data suggest that access to health care or communication with providers may be a contributing problem. An alternative explanation is that, similar to the phenomena observed among Latinas, second-generation Arab American women who do not have resources/support are experiencing higher infant mortality rates than the first generation women. A third possibility is that the some of the Arab American women had been exposed to environmental hazards. Again rigorous research examining these hypotheses is needed.

The use of Arab ethnicity on the Michigan birth and death certificates is believed to underestimate the number of births and deaths identifying with the immigrant group (Michael Beebee, Michigan Department of Health, personal communication). When Michigan changed their birth and death certificates to the national standard by moving the physical location to designate Hispanic ethnicity, the number of births and deaths among Hispanics jumped with no corresponding increase among Arab Americans (personal communication). This bias would mean the actual mortality and number of births are even higher than reported.

Morbidity and Access to Care

Information on health disparities in morbidity experience among Arab Americans is also difficult to find. Although hospitals must now collect information on disempowered groups in their community, we have not seen hospitalization data on Arab Americans as of this writing. Thus, researchers have had to rely on national surveys with place of birth for immigrant Arab Americans, Michigan probability surveys with Arab ancestry questions, and convenience samples.

For national surveys, the National Health Interview Survey collects place of birth and in the public access datasets provides regions of birth. One such region is "Middle East" which encompasses Arab countries in the Levant as well as Iran, Turkey and other non-Arab countries. No analysis to date that we are aware of has accurately estimated the misclassification for Arab Americans.

Read, Amick and Donato (2005) used the 2000–2001 National Health Interview Surveys, to compared self-rated health and activity limitations of immigrant Middle Easterners to US-born white Americans. They found that immigrant Middle Easterners did not significantly differ from the majority group in their self-rated health but were less likely to report limitations in activity. Arguing against acculturation, length of time in the US had no effect on health. These results suggest that immigrant Middle Easterners enjoy superior health to the majority group.

Dallo and Borrell (2006) examined self-reported diabetes and hypertension among respondents to the 2002–2003 National Health Interview Surveys. They found a nonsignificant difference in diabetes prevalence of 4.8 % for immigrant Middle Easterners and 6.9 % for non-Hispanic Whites. Likewise the prevalence of hypertension was lower among immigrant Middle Easterners (13.4 % for immigrant Middle Easterners and 24.5 % for non-Hispanic Whites). From these analyses, it would also appear immigrant Middle Easterners enjoy superior health status to the majority group.

Other national databases with information on country of birth include the National Survey on Drug Use and Health. Country of birth is currently accessible under restricted use only. This annual survey has information on alcohol, tobacco, and other drug use as well as psychological distress and has been used to examine alcohol and drug use (Arfken, Arnetz, Fakhouri, Ventimiglia, & Jamil, 2011; Arfken, Jamil, & Arnetz, 2012). Although use of any substance was lower among immigrant Arab Americans, the prevalence of abuse or dependence showed no difference. Thus, immigrant Arab Americans who tried either alcohol or drugs were more likely to develop problems than US born Non-Hispanic Whites.

Michigan probability samples include the ongoing Behavioral Risk Factor Survey and specially funded survey on cancer control. In 2007, Michigan added a question: *Are you of Arabic or Chaldean origin?*. Using the expanded race data from 2007 to 2009 (Fussman, 2010), Arab Americans did not have significantly different prevalence of self-reported diabetes, heart disease, or asthma. Likewise, Arab Americans did not differ on cholesterol checked, HIV testing, leisure time activity, smoking cigarettes, or obesity from other racial and ethnic groups. Other tobacco delivery systems such as waterpipe were not included in the survey. From this source, it would appear that there are no disparities in burden of chronic diseases between Arab Americans and the majority group.

However, this same database showed clearly that Arab Americans had health disparities in access to health care. Arab Americans were significantly more likely to state that they had no health care access during past 12 months due to cost (21.7 vs. 10.8 % for non-Hispanic White Americans). This lack of access was highest among all race and ethnicities measured. This inequality was also supported by 16.8 % of the Arab Americans stating they have no health care coverage and 18.7 % stating they did not have a personal health care provider vs. 13.5 % and 11.9 % for non-Hispanic White Americans respectively.

Another difference found in the survey was a high level of binge drinking among Arab Americans who had drank alcohol in the previous month (Arfken et al., 2011). This later analysis shows the importance of contrasting findings from different sources of data when measuring disparity to gain insight into possible generational differences.

Specially funded government sponsored surveys also revealed data on Arab American health disparities. The Michigan Cancer Behavioral Risk Factor Survey was conducted in 2008. The phone-administered survey was conducted in English, Spanish, and Arabic. Self-identified Arab Americans were less likely to be asked by a physician about family history of cancer, a deficiency that may detract from monitoring patients and early detection. They were also less likely to use hospice care, a difference that might reflect cultural preference for family care. Finally, Arab Americans were more likely to state that if they smoked cigarettes they were trying to quit. There were no other behaviors in cancer control that showed disparities between Arab Americans and other groups.

Unfortunately, these state-level data are from Michigan only which limits the generalizability. Moreover, we have limited data to determine if the disparities are influenced by differences previously mentioned including acculturation, language fluency, exposure to trauma, or country of origin. Similarly, the surveys do not include measures of discrimination or other stresses to assess their impact on health disparities.

One stressor to the Arab American community and the country were the attacks of September 11, 2001. To measure the impact of this stressor, El-Sayed, Hadley and Galea (2008) analyzed Michigan birth certificated dating from September 11, 2000, to March 11, 2001, and from September 11, 2001, to March 11, 2002. The outcome measures were low birth weight, very low birth weight, and preterm birth. They found no association between birth before/after September 11 and risk of adverse birth outcomes among Arab Americans in Michigan by using either a name algorithm or self-reported ancestry to determine Arab American ethnicity. In fact, Arab name was significantly associated with lower risk of very low birth weight and preterm births in adjusted and unadjusted models. Additionally, Arab ethnicity was significantly associated with lower risk of very low birth weight and preterm births in adjusted and unadjusted models.

In contrast, Lauderdale found an impact of September 11, 2001 on birth outcomes (2006). She examined birth certificates in California for 2000–2002 using a name algorithm that identified a mother as Arab American if the surname included at least 20 % reporting an Arab country as birthplace. Lauderdale found increased preterm births and low birth weight among singletons in the 6 months after September 11, 2001 compared to the preceding 6 months. Moreover, there was no such trend for other racial and ethnic groups. The discrepancy between the study in California and the study in Michigan may reflect reporting problems or real differences between locations with differing social and institutional support systems.

The lack of agreement between these two studies was explored further when El-Sayed and Galea (2009b) examined all births in Michigan between 2000 and 2005. Arab ethnicity was again associated with lower preterm birth risk compared with non-Arab white subjects. In the final adjusted model, Arab ethnicity was no longer associated with preterm birth risk. The most important variables were immigrant versus later generations followed by marital status and tobacco use. Such findings suggest the importance of acculturation as well as traditional risk factors.

However, Arab Americans in Michigan are not immune from stressors. Abdulrahim and Baker (2009) analyzed the Detroit area Arab American study conducted soon after September 11, 2001 (Detroit Arab American Study Team, 2009). They found that immigrant Arabs were more likely to report worse self-rated health compared to US-born Arab Americans. Furthermore, Arabic-speaking immigrants were more likely to also report worse self-rated health compared to both US-born Arab Americans and to English-speaking immigrants.

Padela and Heisler (2010) reanalysis confirmed perceived post–September 11 abuse was associated with higher levels of psychological distress, lower levels of happiness, and worse health status, especially among Muslim Arab Americans and immigrant Arab Americans. Thus subgroups of Arab Americans, those who may be perceived as "different" may be more vulnerable to discrimination and stressors.

The above mentioned studies used secondary analysis of existing datasets. Samples collected prospectively, whether using probability sampling or convenience samples, have the opportunity to incorporate more measures, such as acculturation and generational status, into the protocol. Unfortunately, most of these studies have been conducted in southeastern Michigan and only recently have there been expansion to other places. For example, for asthma Johnson, Nriagu, Hammad, Savoie, and Jamil (2005) found that acculturation was associated with worse asthma severity. Jaber, Brown, Hammad, Zhu, and Herman (2003) in contrast found acculturation associated with lower diabetes prevalence, a finding that may reflect the growing diabetes epidemic in Arab countries (Badran & Laher, 2012). We refer the reader to the specific chapters to examine these and other issues in more detail.

A recent article explored in more detail the impact of discrimination on distress, including depressive, anxiety and behavioral symptoms among a convenience sample of 240 Arab American predominately Muslim adolescents from southeastern Michigan (Ahmed, Kia-Keating, & Tsai, 2011). They found that first generation Arab American adolescents had higher ethnic identity and a higher likelihood of reporting the use of religious coping. Adolescents who reported more perceived racism also had higher levels of acculturative stress, depression, anxiety, internalizing and externalizing symptoms, and less religious support. In the final structural model, the cultural resources of ethnic identity, religious coping and religious support were directly related to lower psychological distress. They, however, did not moderate the adverse effects of perceived racism and acculturative stress on psychological distress.

Challenges in Documenting Arab American Health Disparities

As has been reported repeatedly in this book, Arab American is not an OMB-defined ethnicity and thus data are scarce. The US Census has limited information on Arab ancestry with the most recent data from the 2000 Census. In that census, Michigan was the state identified as having the largest concentration of people with Arab ancestry. Fortunately, due to this concentration and the political strength of Arab Americans, Michigan has some data from Vital Statistics (birth and death records) and Behavior Risk Factor Survey data on Arab Americans. Unfortunately, it is the only state with these data. Other data on Arab Americans according to self-reported ancestry are available from the ongoing American Community Survey. This survey samples the US population, as opposed to the census which tries to reach everyone, to provide yearly information.

Arab American health disparities are thus incompletely documented due to following problems:

1. Lack of Arab American as an OMB-defined ethnicity.
2. Limited information on preferred language, generational status or other characteristics for Arab Americans when they are identified.
3. Limited information on health behaviors believed common in the Arab American community such as waterpipe use.

4. Limited information on strengths of the Arab American community, including family connection and religiosity.

The lack of Arab American as an OMB-defined ethnicity means that there is no federal requirement to collect the information. Thus, healthcare systems are not required to collect the data needed to identify healthcare access, needs and outcomes of Arab Americans. Healthcare systems were recently required to report on preferred language and ethnicities reflecting local community needs as part of accreditation and quality measure reporting. As of this date, we are unaware of their findings for Arab Americans.

The lack of information has stymied greater analyses of health problems among Arab Americans (El-Sayed & Galea, 2009a, 2009b, 2009c). However, more information continues to be reported. Thus, this chapter touches on some of the issues but is by no means an exhaustive review of the literature.

Advocacy

Advocacy to address these health disparities needs to take multiple forms. There are several community-based organizations working diligently to address health disparities. Nationally, there are other organizations advocating for the health equality with the most prominent ones being the American-Arab Anti-Discrimination Committee (ADC) and the Arab American Institute. In Michigan, these exemplary organizations include the Arab American and Chaldean Council (ACC), the Arab Heritage Center, and the Arab Community Center for Economic and Social Services (ACCESS), among others. In this section, we will discuss the approaches taken by one of these community-based organizations, namely, the Arab Community Center for Economic and Social Services (ACCESS).

ACCESS was formed in 1971 to address the lack of resources as well as presence of cultural barriers to work and health care for Arab Americans in the Detroit metropolitan area. Within ACCESS, the Community Health and Research Center has become the largest Arab community-based health center in North America, with over 50 programs in the areas of Medical Health, Public Health, Mental Health and Environment. It also serves as a role model for community-based health centers throughout the country.

Identification of Problems

For ACCESS, identification of problems and potential solutions starts with listening to the community. As an example of listening to the community, open discussion and targeted focus groups were hosted by ACCESS during the debate on health care reform. The results are then reviewed and disseminated internally at ACCESS and externally through newsletters, press releases and briefs for elected officials. For health care reform, the following points were made by the community:

- Improving access to quality healthcare services
- Addressing disease prevention with health education
- Increasing the number and improving the capacity of Arab American healthcare providers
- Improving the cultural sensitivity of healthcare personnel
- Increasing data collection and needs assessment research
- Developing and disseminating bilingual educational materials
- Advocating for increased funding opportunities to address health disparities
- Building community trust for health care providers

This information was then presented during a statewide Health Disparities Reduction Summit on September 9, 2009. It was incorporated into the Michigan Health Equity Roadmap 2009.

Partnering with Other Advocacy Groups

ACCESS has recognized the added value of partnering with other advocacy groups. It has national partnerships with organizations such as the National Health Policy Training Alliance for Communities of Color (The Alliance). The Alliance was created by Families USA Foundation, the Health Policy Institute at the Joint Center for Political and Economic Studies, the National Association of Latino Elected and Appointed Officials Education Fund, and the National Medical Association to strengthen the capacity of African American and Latino community leaders to become engaged in and address the health policies that affect their communities, and to train leaders to be a resource on minority health. ACCESS was invited to formally partner with the Alliance shortly after its creation to include a relevant Arab American perspective. From the very beginning of this partnership, The W.K. Kellogg Foundation's support allowed each partner organization to increase its organizational capacity to conduct Alliance-related activities and strengthen its health care work in minority communities and among its respective constituents. Partner organizations also learned how to more effectively work together by identifying their own individual niches and using that knowledge to determine how to move forward as a whole. These organizational partnerships have allowed the Alliance to engage a greater number of community leaders as well as build a foundation for broader collaboration on issues of disproportionate importance to communities of color.

Creating Specific Programs

ACCESS provides approximately 70 different programs to serve people from various ethnic and religious backgrounds. During the 2009–2010 fiscal year, ACCESS provided services to 442,721 individuals. Approximately 80–90 % of the contacts were with members of the Arab American community. These services included home visits which is an outreach health education strategy. To extend the reach of this care, ACCESS developed and disseminated culturally appropriate health education brochure in both Arabic and English. Below we will talk about specific programs of women's cancer prevention and treatment, and infant mortality reduction.

ACCESS has collaborated with the Wayne State University's Karmanos Cancer Institute's Breast Cancer Community Outreach and Education program since 1997. The Karmanos Cancer Institute (KCI) is a designated comprehensive Cancer Center by the National Cancer Institute. Other partners include the State of Michigan's Breast and Cervical Cancer Control Project (BCCCP) funded by CDC, American Cancer Society, Susan G. Komen Foundation, the Avon Foundation and the Michigan Cancer Consortium. The breast and cervical cancer control program trains lay community members to become health workers. They are then responsible for communicating with local women in their homes on the importance regular mammography. During these contacts, lay health workers reinforce the importance of healthy lifestyles, use of annual primary care check-up and designated screenings for early cancer detection. These contacts are followed with clinical cancer screening services, including translation, transportation and any follow-up services. Women may use a separate private entrance to the clinic for cancer screening if preferred.

ACCESS also actively collaborates with Michigan State University. The research conducted under the direction of Dr. Williams includes designing, testing and implementation of a multigenerational life-span breast and cervical cancer prevention and screening intervention focused on Black, Latina and Arab women—The Kin Keeper SM Cancer Prevention Intervention.

ACCESS is collaborating with the state of Michigan's Department on Community Health on efforts to reduce infant mortality. These efforts include serving on the Practices to Reduce Infant Mortality through Equity (PRIME) project taskforce. The project has three goals:

1. To develop a replicable workforce training and practice model that incorporates social justice and the elimination of racism in both organizational policy and practice. The model is to be used as a strategy for eliminating disparities in health outcomes and lower infant mortality in Michigan
2. To use a state/local partnership network identify and implement efforts to undo racism and improve infant health in Michigan.
3. To identify a sustainable quality assurance process that recognizes social determinants of health in policies, program models and practices, allocation formulas and/or program accreditation review.

As mentioned above, the infant mortality rates while initially low have been steadily rising over recent years in the Arab American community in Michigan. As partners in this project ACCESS is working to ensure the specific needs of the Arab American community are included within this process/model and the factors surrounding infant mortality are addressed.

ACCESS is the only community-based agency in the country to provide HIV/STD prevention, screening and treatment services among the Arab American community. Since 2008, the Ryan White Care program provides patients the opportunity to access HIV/AIDS treatment services. Outreach to Arab Americans who are at high risk for contracting HIV is also supported. Internally, ACCESS has provided containers of freely provided condoms for staff and visitors in the privacy of restrooms.

Other Advocacy Steps

ACCESS views that advocacy for Arab Americans includes fostering among the wider American society a greater understanding of Arab Culture as it exists both in the USA and in the Arab world. One example of this advocacy is the creation of the Arab American National Museum in Dearborn, Michigan. The museum is a part of the Smithsonian Affiliations.

Policy change to address social determinants and disparities is another advocacy step in which ACCESS is actively engaged. Most notable recent policy changes impacting the Michigan Arab American community were the passage of the state's Clean Air Act and increase in excise tax on cigarettes. ACCESS is working with businesses to inform and educate them on the Clean Air Act, especially as it relates to waterpipe smoke. Additionally ACCESS continues to work with the Michigan Department of Community Health and political leaders to increase the excise tax on other forms of tobacco and regulate waterpipe use.

ACCESS also originated and continues to support a biennial International Conference on Health Issues in Arab Communities. The conference offers various professionals and academia a forum to share their research and gain invaluable knowledge of the Arab American community and other immigrant Arabs (such as in Australia) and in Arab countries. Additionally, the conferences serve as a meeting site and network for researchers interested in health disparities affecting Arab communities.

Conclusions

To achieve health for all Americans, health disparities between disempowered groups and the majority group must be eliminated; these disempowered groups include Arab Americans. In this chapter we reviewed the definition of health and health disparities and social determinants of health disparities. Barriers to addressing the health disparities among Arab Americans begin with lack of data. Arab ethnicity is not an OBM-defined ethnicity (with accompanying requirement of data collection) so data on health status and health disparities are limited. There were some preliminary disparities identified in the state of Michigan including higher mortality rates, recent increases in infant mortality rates, and cost barriers to accessing health care. Findings on diabetes and cancer morbidity differ between sources and might reflect problems in detection and adequate treatment as well as vulnerability of subgroups. These subgroups within Arab Americans may be defined by generational status (in which case acculturation may change health status), economic, country of origin, religion, and other differences that may make Arab Americans less likely to blend into the majority culture. For these Arab Americans, discrimination, stressors, and quality of health care may result in disparities.

To advance the analysis of disparities, population-level prospective studies are needed which incorporates measures of acculturation and discrimination as well as demographic variables enabling the identification of relevant subgroups of Arab Americans. For Arab Americans who left countries in conflict, measures of trauma and exposure to environmental hazards are needed. When secondary data sources are used, construction of comparisons to illuminate the relative role of culture or acculturation may advance our understanding of identified disparities. Dr. Florence Dallo has examined immigrant Middle Easterners compared to immigrant Russians and immigrant Europeans to parcel out unique differences within this overall "White" race category of immigrants. Dr. Cynthia Arfken and colleagues have examined immigrant Arab Americans compared to immigrant Canadians and immigrant Iranians, Afghanstani, and Pakistani to parcel out the relative contribution of immigration versus culture (Arfken et al., 2012). Dr. Abdulrahman El-Sayed has also contrasted zipcodes for the impact of community context on health outcomes (El-Sayed & Galea, 2009a, 2009b, 2009c).

Addressing these health disparities requires sustained and multiple level efforts. One of these efforts is advocacy. In this chapter we reviewed the actions of one community-based agency, Arab Community Center for Economic and Social Services, and the advocacy work it does. The work includes identifying problems by listening to the community, partnering with other advocacy organizations, and creating targeted programs such as on breast cancer and infant mortality. Lastly, advocacy as we saw with the Arab Community Center for Economic and Social Services also entails educating the larger society about Arab Americans and supporting research dissemination on health disparities.

References

Abdulrahim, S., & Baker, W. (2009). Differences in self-rated health by immigrant status and language preference among Arab Americans in the Detroit Metropolitan Area. *Social Science & Medicine, 68*(12), 2097–2103.

Agency for Healthcare Research and Quality (AHRQ). (2008). *National healthcare disparities report 2008* (Publication No. 09–0002). Rockville, MD: U.S. Department of Health and Human Services AHRQ. Retrieved from www.ahrq.gov/qual/qrdr08.htm

Ahmed, S. R., Kia-Keating, M., & Tsai, K. H. (2011). A structural model of racial discrimination, acculturative stress, and cultural resources among Arab American adolescents. *American Journal of Community Psychology, 48*(3–4), 181–192.

Arfken, C. L., Arnetz, B. B., Fakhouri, M., Ventimiglia, M. J., & Jamil, H. (2011). Alcohol use among Arab Americans: What is the prevalence? *Journal of Immigrant and Minority Health, 13*(4), 713–718.

Arfken, C. L., Jamil, H., & Arnetz, B. B. (2012). Marijuana and non-medical prescription drug use among immigrant Arab Americans. *New Iraqi Journal of Medicine., 8*, 7–13.

Badran, M., & Laher, I. (2012). Type II diabetes mellitus in Arabic-speaking countries. *International Journal of Endocrinology, 2012*, 902873.

Berry, J. W. (1997). Immigration, acculturation, and adaptation. *Applied Psychology, 46*(1), 5–68.

Bushman, B. J., & Bonacci, A. M. (2004). You've got mail: Using e-mail to examine the effect of prejudiced attitudes on discrimination against Arabs. *Journal of Experimental Social Psychology, 40*, 753–759.

Centers for Disease Control and Prevention (CDC). (2008). *Health Disparities among Racial/Ethnic Populations*. Community Health and Program Services. Centers for Disease Control and Prevention. Retrieved from http://www.cdc.gov/NCCDPHP/DACH/chaps/disparities/index.htm

Dallo, F. J., & Borrell, L. N. (2006). Self-reported diabetes and hypertension among Arab Americans in the United States. *Ethnicity & Disease, 16*(3), 699–705.

Dallo, F. J., Schwartz, K., Ruterbusch, J. J., Booza, J., & Williams, D. R. (2012). Mortality rates among Arab Americans in Michigan. *Journal of Immigrant and Minority Health, 14*(2), 236–241.

de la Cruz, G. P., & Brittingham, A. (2003). The Arab population. U.S. Census Bureau C2KBR-23.

Detroit Arab American Study Team. (2009). *Citizenship and crisis*. New York, NY: Russell Sage.

Einbinder, L. C., & Schulman, K. A. (2000). The effect of race on the referral process for invasive cardiac procedures. *Medical Care Research and Review, 57*(suppl. 1), 162–180.

El-Sayed, A. M., & Galea, S. (2009a). Community context, acculturation, and low birth weight risk among Arab-Americans: Evidence from the Arab-American Birth Outcomes study. *Journal of Epidemiology and Community Health, 64*(2), 155–160.

El-Sayed, A. M., & Galea, S. (2009b). Explaining the low risk of preterm birth among Arab Americans in the US: An analysis of 617,471 births. *Pediatrics, 123*(3), e438–e445.

El-Sayed, A. M., & Galea, S. (2009c). The health of Arab-Americans living in the United States: A systematic review of the literature. *BMC Public Health, 9*(1), 272.

El-Sayed, A. M., Hadley, C., & Galea, S. (2008). Birth outcomes among Arab-Americans in Michigan before and after the terrorist attacks of September 11, 2001. *Ethnicity & Disease, 18*(3), 348–356.

El-Sayed, A. M., Tracy, M., Scarborough, P., & Galea, S. (2011). Ethnic inequalities in mortality: The case of Arab-Americans. *PLoSOne, 6*(12), e29185.

Finkton, D. W., El-Sayed, A. M., & Galea, S. (2012). Infant mortality among Arab-Americans: Findings from the Arab-American birth outcomes study. *Maternal and Child Health Journal, 17*(4), 732–745.

Fussman, C. (2010). *Estimates for chronic health conditions, risk factors, health indicators, and preventive health practices by race/ethnicity state of Michigan behavioral risk factor survey 2007–2009*. Retrieved October 20, 2012 from http://www.michigan.gov/documents/mdch/2007-2009_Expanded_Race_Tables_FINAL_321428_7.pdf

Guidry, J. J., Aday, L. A., Zhang, D., & Winn, R. J. (1997). Transportation as a barrier to cancer treatment. *Cancer Practice, 5*(6), 361–366.

Guidry, J. J., Aday, L. A., Zhang, D., & Winn, R. J. (1998). Cost considerations as potential barriers to cancer treatment. *Cancer Practice, 6*(3), 182–187.

Jaber, L. A., Brown, M. S., Hammad, A., Zhu, A., & Herman, W. H. (2003). Lack of acculturation is a risk factor for diabetes in Arab immigrants in the US. *Diabetes Care, 26*(7), 2010–2014.

Johnson, M., Nriagu, J., Hammad, A., Savoie, K., & Jamil, H. (2005). Asthma prevalence and severity in Arab American communities in the Detroit Area, Michigan. *Journal of Immigrant Health, 7*(3), 165–173.

Krieger, N. (1999). Embodying inequality: A review of concepts, measures, and methods for studying health consequences of discrimination. *International Journal of Health Services, 29*(2), 295–352.

Lauderdale, D. S. (2006). Birth outcomes for Arabic-named women in California before and after September 11. *Demography, 43*, 185–201.

Liao, Y., Tucker, P., Okoro, C. A., Giles, W. H., Mokdad, A. H., & Harris, V. B. (2004). REACH 2010 Surveillance for health status in minority communities: United States, 2001–2002. *Morbidity and Mortality Weekly Report. Surveillance Summaries, 53*(SS06), 1–36.

Merskin, D. (2004). The construction of Arabs as enemies: Post-September 11 discourse of George W. *Bush. Mass Communication and Society, 7*(2), 157–175.

Michalopoulou, G., Falzarano, P., Arfken, C., & Rosenberg, D. (2009). Physicians' cultural competency as perceived by African American patients. *Journal of the National Medical Association, 101*(9), 893–899.

Nasseri, K., & Moulton, L. H. (2011). Patterns of death in the first and second generation immigrants from selected Middle Eastern countries in California. *Journal of Immigrant and Minority Health, 13*(2), 361–370.

Nydell, M. K. (2006). *Understanding Arabs: A guide for modern times* (4th ed.). Boston: Intercultural Press.

Padela, A., & Heisler, M. (2010). The association of perceived abuse and discrimination after September 11, 2001, with psychological distress, level of happiness, and health status among Arab Americans. *American Journal of Public Health, 100*, 284–291.

Rathore, S. S., Lenert, L. A., Weinfurt, K. P., Tinoco, A., Taleghani, C. K., Harless, W., et al. (2000). The effects of patient sex and race on medical students' ratings of quality of life. *American Journal of Medicine, 108*(7), 561–566.

Read, J. G., Amick, B., & Donato, K. M. (2005). Arab immigrants: A new case for ethnicity and health? *Social Science & Medicine, 61*(1), 77–82.

Saha, S., Arbelaez, J. J., & Cooper, L. A. (2003). Patient-Physician relationships and racial disparities in the quality of health care. *American Journal of Public Health, 93*(10), 1713–1719.

Schulman, K. A., Berlin, J. A., Harless, W., Kerner, J. F., Sistrunk, S., Gersh, B. J., et al. (1999). The effect of race and sex on physicians' recommendations for cardiac catheterization. *The New England Journal of Medicine, 340*(8), 618–626.

Shaheen, J. G. (2001). *Reel bad Arabs: How Hollywood vilifies a people*. Northampton, MA: Olive Branch Press.

Shaheen, J. G. (2008). *Guilty: Hollywood's verdict on Arabs after 9/11*. Northampton, MA: Olive Branch Press.

Shavers, V. L., & Brown, M. L. (2002). Racial and ethnic disparities in the receipt of cancer treatment. *Journal of the National Cancer Institute, 94*(5), 334–357.

Smedley, B. D., Stith, A. Y., & Nelson, A. R. (2002). *Unequal treatment: Confronting racial and ethnic disparities in health care. Institute of Medicine*. Washington, DC: National Academy Press.

The Joint Commission. (2011, February 9). *R3. Report requirement, rationale, reference*. A complimentary publication of The Joint Commission, Issue 1.

Ulmer, C., McFadden, B., & Nerenz, D. R. (2009). *Race, ethnicity, and language data: Standardization for health care quality improvement*. Washington, DC: National Academies Press.

van Ryn, M., & Burke, J. (2000). The effect of patient race and socio-economic status on physicians' perceptions of patients. *Social Science & Medicine, 50*(6), 813–828.

World Health Organization (WHO). (1979). *Health for all.* Paper presented at the International Conference on Primary Health Care. Retrieved from http://www.who.int/about/definition/en/print.html

Chapter 18
Health and Well-Being in Arab Americans: Prevention Strategies Using a Biopsychosocial Approach

Julie Hakim-Larson, Sylvia C. Nassar-McMillan, and Kristine J. Ajrouch

Immigration from the Arab world has resulted in settlements over a wide expanse of the globe both within and outside of North America, including other destinations within the Arab region. Thus, contemporary Arab Americans or their ancestors may have been displaced successively more than once before finally settling in the United States and many may currently have familial connections in other parts of the world, including but not restricted to the Middle East. Recent estimates of the Arab Diaspora or number of such Arab refugees, immigrants, and their offspring by the United Nations are tentative due to classification disparities by the destination countries as compared to the data provided by the countries-of-origin (Fargues, 2006, May); nonetheless, for the early 2000s, the United Nations estimated over 4 million Arab immigrants from eight Arab countries (i.e., Morocco, Algeria, Tunisia, Egypt, Palestine, Jordan, Syria, and Lebanon), not including Iraq, to other parts of the world. In 2007, the United Nations High Commissioner for Refugees reported that there were an estimated 4 million displaced Iraqis worldwide, with approximately 1.9 million internally displaced within Iraq, 2 million resettled in other Middle Eastern countries, and the remaining thousands dispersed throughout Europe, the Americas, and other regions of the world (UNHCR, April 2007). More recently, as of November 2012, the United Nations Refugee Agency reported that

J. Hakim-Larson (✉)
Department of Psychology, University of Windsor, Windsor, ON, Canada, N9B 3P4
e-mail: hakim@uwindsor.ca

S.C. Nassar-McMillan
Department of Curriculum, Instruction, and Counselor Education, North Carolina State University, 2310 Stinson Dr., Poe 520, Campus Box 7801, Raleigh, NC 27695-7801, USA
e-mail: snassar@ncsu.edu

K.J. Ajrouch
Department of Sociology, Anthropology, Criminology, Eastern Michigan University, 712 Pray-Harrold, Ypsilanti, MI 48197, USA
e-mail: kajrouch@emich.edu

S.C. Nassar-McMillan et al. (eds.), *Biopsychosocial Perspectives on Arab Americans: Culture, Development, and Health*, DOI 10.1007/978-1-4614-8238-3_18,

there were an estimated 400,000 refugees that had left Syria due to civil war and who were attempting to resettle in the neighboring countries of Turkey, Lebanon, Jordan, and Iraq (UNHCR, 2012, November). The long-term settlement destinations of these refugees are yet to be determined. The many socio-cultural, psychological, and health issues addressed in this book are ones that likely have implications for Arab immigrants and refugees dispersed globally, even though we do not know as yet which research findings can be generalized and which cannot. Future research strategies that address the biological, psychological, and social needs of Arab Americans will need to take a broad, comprehensive approach that includes attention to historical events as well as both proximal and distal contexts in their efforts to prevent disorder and disease and promote well-being and optimal health. Longitudinal as well as epidemiological studies are needed.

The conflicts and wars of the last half of the twentieth century into the first decade of the twenty-first century and the ongoing regional conflicts into the second decade of the twenty-first century—especially in Iraq, Syria, Lebanon, and the Palestinian territories, as well as the dozen or more countries involved in the Arab Spring that began late in December of 2011 that has resulted in protests ranging from civil uprisings to governmental overthrows—have significant implications for the current health and well-being of Arab Americans of all ages. Many Arab Americans still have family ties to these regions and visit their relatives routinely or at least on occasion. With the virtually instant relaying of news events via the media, and the advances in communication, it is possible for those within the Arab Diaspora internationally to maintain and foster social connections and generate information and personal opinions about events whether they are of immediate proximal relevance or not (Joseph, 2011). In addition, organizations such as the Arab American Institute in Washington, DC (http://www.aaiusa.org) recognize the importance of events in the Arab world for the health and well-being of Arab Americans and thus maintain an active involvement in generating and disseminating information and trying to help inform American policies relevant to Middle East affairs.

Interdisciplinary research and practice are increasingly being encouraged in academic and community settings alike. Taking a biopsychosocial approach to Arab health and well-being is promising because it incorporates ecological models that have emerged from a variety of disciplines in the social and medical sciences, all of which have their own unique stakes in mental and physical health promotion (Richard, Gauvin, & Raine, 2011). As described in various chapters throughout this book, ecological models are appropriate in structuring our understanding of the complexity of factors involved socially, psychologically, and biologically across multiple cultural contexts and across generations of time. Psychologists, sociologists, and other social scientists have become increasingly aware of the important influences of the larger social-political-economic and cultural contexts on individual health and well-being; likewise, medical epidemiologists focusing on individual risk factors for diseases have also noted their limitations in not sufficiently accounting for the broader ecological context in their statistical models (Richard et al., 2011). Thus, taking an ecological systems approach is widely acknowledged as one way that a complex array of potentially important biological, psychological, and socio-cultural factors can be addressed in health promotion and illness/disease prevention efforts.

There are many reasons that we need to better understand the Arab segment of the global population. For one, it is especially noteworthy that the greatest population growth of people in the world who are younger than 25 years of age is in Arab countries, with the proportion of such youth expected to rise even further in the coming decades (United Nations Development Programme, 2006). It appears to be this growing voice of youth who are initiating contemporary political changes in the Middle East. There is some international recognition that this new "baby boom" in Arab countries is resulting in the growth of a youth population in search of their identities and a sense of meaningful purpose to their lives (e.g., Joseph, 2011). In 2009, for example, the UNICEF Middle East and North Africa Regional Office, and the Issam Fares Institute for Public Policy and International Affairs (2011) at the American University of Beirut in Lebanon began an initiative to better understand the needs, identities, and state of mind of Arab youth within the changing socio-political contexts in which they live. There is increasing recognition of the lack of knowledge concerning the consequences for youth of unresolved regional, social, and political conflicts arising out of longstanding emotional strife, grudges, and the need for vengeance, and territorial disputes that sometimes extend for generations backward. This bulge of Arab youth internationally will have an effect worldwide. The economic impact of such a young labor force in the Middle East and North Africa has not escaped attention, and with a new global economy, there are a whole range of possibilities both positive and negative (Joseph, 2011).

In the following sections, we summarize the various ways in which taking a biopsychosocial approach to Arab health and well-being can potentially inform our understanding of social relationships and socio-cultural factors, psychosocial development and psychological factors, and medical interventions within the Arab Diaspora. In each case our focus is on future preventative intervention strategies.

Social Relationships and Socio-cultural Factors

Social relationships and socio-cultural factors are increasingly recognized as key factors to more completely understand health and well-being. A focus on the social context also requires attention to the cultural contexts that both shape as well as are formed through relationships on both the micro and macro-levels. In the section below, we consider the ways in which cultural contexts inform social relations and their potential links to health.

The first section of this edited volume illustrated the multiple ways in which social relationships stimulate a more systematic account of cultural context. A cultural framework for Arab American life was established through the elaboration of socio-political history, inter-ethnic diversity, family, gender, aging, and forgiveness. At the macro level, the socio-political history of Arab Americans as well as the identity issues that surface via multiple ethnic and religious affiliations provided critical background as to the heterogeneity that marks the Arab American experience. Yet, together these assessments also contribute to a deeper appreciation of the ways in which relations with American society facilitated a need to recognize a unique Arab American experience. Issues of incorporation and discrimination emerge from these macro-level social relations, each having implications for health. At the micro level, interactions within family, the role of gender, and the aging process drew attention to cultural assumptions that influence interactions between and among Arab Americans. As such, the cultural expressions of interpersonal relationships and whether or not those relations serve as a resource or a stressor also hold value for better addressing health issues among Arab Americans. The cultural account of forgiveness within an Arab American context highlighted social relations at both the macro and micro levels, showing how cultural frames of forgiveness hold promise for attending to hurtful situations, and hence potentially become a protective resource. A focus on forgiveness speaks to the multiple levels of social relations. Below we elaborate on the ways in which the multiple levels of social relations have implications for health and well-being.

Relationships between individuals, such as within the family or between co-workers, are affected by a number of socio-cultural factors including but not limited to socio-political history and recent events, religion, demographic status, and cultural traditions. Such socio-cultural factors interact with the ongoing social exchanges that occur among various generations of family members (e.g., Antonucci, Birditt, Sherman, & Trinh, 2011). For example, Arab ethnic groups who uphold collectivistic values place an emphasis on intrafamilial family obligations. As a consequence, there are likely to be more frequent intergenerational social exchanges among Arab American ethnic group family members than between the generations of many members of the European American public. Various forms of tangible (e.g., financial) and intangible (e.g., emotional) support are likely to be part of these social interactions and are affected by community resources and the changing social context that fluctuates over time (e.g., Antonucci et al., 2011). Consider an Arab American family in which there is a breadwinner who provided support for decades to both the older and younger generations. If such a breadwinner experiences a job loss due to the downsizing of a corporate employer, his or her family will have a significant loss of financial support within the family network. In addition, the underlying tension and stresses may have the secondary effect of emotional support losses within the family context. Preventative interventions for Arab Americans include at a minimum the same economic and community supports that promote well-being in the general American public.

While the immediate family environment plays a strong proximal supportive role, an area of particular importance is the underlying emotional climate of the nation. After the tragedy of 9/11, there was a recognized and understandable increase in fear among the general American public, including Arab Americans (see Bakalian & Bozorgmehr, 2009; Marvasti & McKinney, 2004). Unfortunately, however, there is evidence that this fear may have translated into a backlash of prejudicial attitudes and discriminatory practices with effects on the mental health of some Arab Americans (e.g., Aprahamian, Kaplan, Windham, Suter, & Visser, 2011;

Nassar-McMillan, Lambert, & Hakim-Larson, 2011). Arab Americans incur a kind of double consciousness in that as Americans they mourn the horror, death, and destruction brought on by this terrible event, yet because of their ethnic membership, they come under scrutiny as affiliated with those who carried out this heinous act. Though negative opinions about Arab Americans are not new, after 9/11 damaging encounters are no longer isolated and occur in a more sweeping and patterned manner. Arab Americans now more than ever before are asked to explain their political, religious, and personal beliefs, altering their daily lives in multiple ways. Prevention of prejudice and discrimination of Arab Americans is the mission of agencies and organizations such as the American-Arab Anti-Discrimination Committee (http://www.adc.org). Yet, difficulty in fighting discrimination is heightened due to fact that Arab Americans are not a legal minority (considered White by the US government), and therefore do not benefit from resources in place to combat discrimination that occurs because of ethnicity (Cainkar, 2009).

One means of preventing future societal trends that discriminate against Arab Americans is to be proactive in promoting attitudes that are incompatible with defensive reactions to feelings of fear. According to deMause (2002), the emotional climates of cultures within the various nations of the world are represented in the accepted childrearing practices of parents within the society. These can range from empathy, forgiveness, compassion, secure attachments, and love to abusive actions leading to fear, revenge, hatred of others, and further interpersonal violence. In the first case, the collective memories of individuals are likely to lead to peaceful coexistence with others, while in the latter case they are likely to promote ongoing wars and unresolved intransigent conflicts. In particular, some community groups and non-profit organizations (e.g., Asseily, 2007) advocate the idea that societal healing can occur through the use of narratives and the promotion of feelings of forgiveness. Beyond the family unit, however, is the role played by other societal institutions including the government and the media. Categorization of groups based on factors such as national origin characteristics, religion, or language provides an important means for understanding cultural world views (as well as ways in which culture impacts health and well-being). Such processes are encouraged by government and media as a means to simplify the world, and thereby serve a functional goal. Yet, using such differences to claim inferiority, backwardness, and/or to show that a culture is simply lacking in basic human qualities endangers not only the group targeted, but the entire nation. Such processes risk a homogenization process where the actions of a few come to represent an entire, diverse group of peoples. This risk runs extremely high when members of a society have little opportunity to interact and connect with members of the defined group. Because Arab Americans have historically constituted a small proportion of the overall US population and have generally integrated into dominant White society (Gualtieri, 2009), the demonization of Arabs, especially in a post 9/11 world, becomes easier to achieve. A main goal in the United States should be to recognize differences without attributing value judgments. A common value of human dignity, in all the diversity of the world, has been the hallmark of American society. As Blumer (1958) advanced, social group positions are what encourage prejudiced attitudes and the willingness to discriminate. Engendering a more inclusive ideal of what it means to be American will ensure the promotion of inter-ethnic relations that result in coexistence, understanding, and national strength.

In sum, social relationships that occur among Arab Americans as well as between Arab Americans and others provide key pathways for promoting cultural understanding and well-being. Societies within the Middle East and social agencies addressing Arab issues within North America can assist in prevention efforts by providing resources and programs to help individuals and groups of Arab descent (e.g., youth groups, senior groups, English as a second language/ESL classes) learn skills that will help them navigate emotionally as well as socially. Moreover, they can serve as catalysts for promoting intra-cultural understanding within the broader society.

Psychosocial Development and Psychological Factors

Psychologists and other social scientists remain quite Western and Eurocentric in their focus in spite of the attempts over the last 40 years to be more inclusive in their understanding of the psychosocial development of different racial and ethnic groups (e.g., Hall & Breland-Noble, 2011). Given the globalization of knowledge across the many domains of the social and natural sciences, the need is greater than ever for understanding just what dimensions of psychological functioning are unique to the experiences of Arab Americans and which are similar to that of other ethnic groups. Both are worthy of our attention.

Many normative developmental experiences are similar and are shared by Arab Americans and the mainstream given that Christianity is the dominant religion in the United States, and that the earliest immigrants to the United States were primarily Christian with descendants in the third, fourth, and fifth generation sometimes among those who consider themselves Arab American (Suleiman, 1999). Over the last 100 years or so, there are normative experiences of adolescents and young adults as they encounter the developmental tasks of achieving career, religious, and political identities, as well as finding an intimate life partner. Like other Americans, Arab Americans over the past century have also faced the Great Depression, two World Wars, the civil rights, and women's movements of the 1960s and 1970s, among the other significant wars and changes affecting the United States and others around the world.

Like their Christian Arab American counterparts, Muslim Arab Americans face the same normative experiences and developmental tasks as other Americans. However, some issues faced by Arab Americans may not necessarily fall into the normative mainstream pattern of experiences given their beliefs in the Islamic religion or their traditional ethnic traditions. Hall and Breland-Noble (2011) suggest that therapists need to embrace the new global paradigm by attaining a well-informed understanding of Islam and by taking into account the spirituality of

Muslim Arab Americans; in doing so, they will be in a better position to promote their well-being and prevent the avoidance of help-seeking behavior due to feelings of stigma when mental health services are needed. As noted below, addressing stigma and the effects of trauma from war and political strife are two noteworthy areas of interest in addressing the psychosocial health of Arab Americans.

Prevention of Stigma

Counteracting the stigma of mental health help-seeking, assessment, diagnosis, and intervention is a crucial issue among those interested in the psychosocial issues affecting Arab Americans. As is often common in collectivistic cultures, shame or dishonor in Arab families involves disgracing the family name, and likewise pride in accomplishments reflects favorably upon the whole family and extended family system of relatives (e.g., Simon, 1996). Family stigma involves the feelings of prejudice or discrimination encountered by people who have a relative with mental illness, and this is not restricted to the Arab American population (e.g., Larson & Corrigan, 2008).

However, given the collectivistic values of Arab Americans, the family repercussions of stigma may be exacerbated and amplified as is noted by Dalky (2012) in a study comparing family stigma in various Arab countries; a number of negative emotional reactions were reported by family members of a person with mental illness. Dalky (2012) also reviews literature highlighting the fact that Arab families are more likely to shoulder the responsibility for caring for their ill extended family members rather than rely on social services, and to keep mental illness secret given that it may affect a female family member's chances for marriage. Thus, it is particularly important that destigmatizing mental health issues be included among the prevention efforts for Arab Americans.

Larson and Corrigan (2008) suggest a dual approach to tackling stigma. First, public stigma must be addressed through comprehensive educational programs and outreach publicity campaigns that help to neutralize public attitudes that are stigmatizing. Second, self-stigma is problematic given that individuals may have already internalized stigma and have low self-esteem. In this case, group self-esteem enhancement programs that address an individual's feelings of competence and worthiness may be one way to combat self-stigma whether it is for the person with a mental illness or for a family member who has felt stigmatized. Empowering both individuals and family members is an important preventive measure.

Mruk (1995, 2006) reviews the literature on self-esteem enhancement and describes how group treatment approaches can be effectively utilized to realistically improve feelings of competence (e.g., at work and in daily life) and feelings of worthiness (e.g., lovability among family members, and likability among peers). Such preventive intervention programs hold promise for working with Arab Americans.

Preventive Strategies in Traumatized Societies and Traumatized Individuals

The emotional and social lives of Arab Americans are affected by the various wars and conflicts between groups in the Middle East. Prevention of the effects of trauma resulting from such conflicts takes place at two levels: societal and individual. At the societal level, wars and traumatic societal conflicts inflict pain and suffering on many individuals who are members of large social groups, and the consequences often have collective implications for the groups for many generations after the initial trauma (e.g., Volkan, 2000, 2011). For Arab Americans, the groups and subgroups vary and may be religious (e.g., Christian Egyptian Copts, Druze, Lebanese Maronite Catholics, Sunni Muslims, Iraqi Chaldean Catholics, Orthodox, Shiite Muslims) or based on ethnicity (e.g., Saudi Arabian, Kuwaiti, Iraqi, Palestinian, Jordanian) or on regional or political affiliation. Thus, generations after a traumatic event, prejudicial feelings and discriminatory attitudes may prevail. According to Volkan, coping with trauma and mourning the inevitable losses is not an easy task, and unfortunately when it is ineffective or unfinished mourning, the work is transmitted to yet another generation to handle. The collective identity of members of a large group, whether political, regional, or religious, has implications for the unresolved traumatic memories that are stored and transmitted, and the dormant old issues can get reignited periodically in the service of political action (Volkan, 2011). Prevention of the cyclical effects of trauma and warfare (e.g., vengeance) involves the facilitation of a process of healthy mourning, where what is lost isn't forgotten but it does not preoccupy the group either; the group is freed from feelings of helplessness and humiliation and can effectively assert itself to accomplish new goals (Volkan, 2011). In addition, dialogues between the leaders of opposing groups can facilitate this healing with one result being more business and social collaborations among opposing group members as part of the healing process. For Arab immigrants to North America, relationships between the various groups and subgroups in the Middle East continue to be noteworthy at times and are followed closely via access to television and internet news from the Arab world.

While Volkan's approach considers the broader societal level, Kira's approach highlights the more direct impact of trauma psychologically on individuals (e.g., Kira et al., 2008). Kira et al. note that the various forms of trauma may vary by the age and background of the person involved. A person may either directly or vicariously experience trauma, and the trauma may occur once or more than once. The frequency, duration, and variety of events are important considerations, as are the ages at which the traumas were experienced. A careful assessment of a person's trauma history can be instrumental in considering prevention measures. To assist in providing such an assessment, Kira et al. (2008) present a questionnaire and a taxonomy of trauma based on developmental and contextual considerations such as attachment, identity, personal and collective traumas, interdependence, indirect or secondary traumas, self-actualization, and physical survival traumas. This taxonomy also includes another dimension that represents additional features to consider:

cumulative stresses including internal medical pain, and nature-made, person-made, and socially made traumas. These may be simple single-episode traumas or ones that are more complex and have occurred multiple times. The importance of Kira et al.'s taxonomy is that it allows for the classification of traumas by individual and by group so that trauma profiles can be created for use in intervention planning.

One promising area of study with individuals who have experienced trauma involves the study of posttraumatic growth. Kira and his colleagues (2006) found that Arab American immigrant survivors of torture were more resilient, had better adaptation and greater religiosity, and were more tolerant of others than their non-tortured refugee counterparts in spite of having poorer physical health. Preventive interventions among those who are tortured include addressing the secondary traumatization of the spouses and children of survivors in addition to members of their communities (Kira et al., 2006). According to Kira et al. (2006), positive health benefits ensue to survivors and their families when there is retributive and restorative justice regarding the perpetrators of torture, and when survivors are able to experience forgiveness and reconciliation with respect to those who may have been ambivalent or unwilling collaborators with the perpetrators.

Resilience and Protective Factors in Preventive Health Interventions

The process of resilience within the field of developmental psychopathology involves unexpected adaptive outcomes in the face of adversity; that is, even though a person has significant risk factors that outweigh protective factors, the person nonetheless performs well in adaptive life tasks (e.g., Masten, 2007). According to Masten, the process of resilience takes place within multiple systems and resilience science has now advanced to where there are ten hot spots that researchers know to have beneficial effects on the life trajectories of individuals. These resilience factors help to buffer individuals and families from risks and stressors that could potentially derail them. Each of these will be considered in turn as part of a multilevel analysis and discussed in the context of the Arab American experience.

According to Masten (2007), the most basic levels of analysis of resilience include: (1) the health and stress system of the individual where there is normal immune and hormonal functioning, (2) the information processing and problem-solving systems where there is normal cognitive and intellectual functioning, and (3) secure attachment systems with parents, friends, and others who provide competent age-appropriate care and supports. For Arab Americans, promoting environmental health seems to be of critical importance in preventing disruptions to the immune, hormonal, cognitive, and attachment systems of developing children. Smoking cessation and prevention especially during pregnancy and preventing lead poisoning by increasing awareness about the problem are both issues addressed by community agencies such as the Arab Community Center for Economic and Social

Services (ACCESS) and the Arab American and Chaldean Council (ACC) in their respective work with Arab American families.

In addition, Masten (2007) describes how the underlying temperamental characteristics of the individual affects two additional systems: (4) self-regulation, self-direction, and response inhibition, and (5) mastery over the environment and rewards involving having a positive outlook, sense of self-efficacy, and achievement motivation. For Arab immigrant families, overcoming the barriers to their full participation in American society includes learning and using the English language, obtaining an education, and attaining employment that makes use of one's full potential to succeed and feel mastery over the environment.

Finally, Masten (2007) discusses five broader social systems that are hot spots for the multilevel integration of resilience ideas and research. These are: (6) spirituality and religion, (7) family, (8) peers, (9) school and teachers, and (10) community and culture. Ecological models focus on prevention and early intervention at the group level rather than on merely remediation of individuals after a problem has been identified (Gutkin, 2012). To take such an approach within Arab communities would involve prevention programs designed with the input of spiritual and religious leaders (e.g., priests, imams), schoolteachers, religious organizations and groups, extended families, peer networks and youth groups, community programs and school systems, and personnel including university level academic faculty members with a vested interest in the community. In taking such a broad approach to prevention, it would be possible to make full use of Bronfenbrenner's (1994) ecological model where even small changes in one level of a micro-meso-, exo-, or macro-system environment can have a significant interaction with another level and reverberate throughout (Gutkin, 2012).

In this book, taking a biopsychosocial perspective to the study of Arab Americans highlights the idea that these three levels of analyses work together, and ultimately a comprehensive understanding to prevention science cannot be reduced to any one level of analysis whether socio-cultural, psychological, or biobehavioral and medical.

Biological Factors and Medical Preventive Interventions

To complete the comprehensive biopsychosocial perspective adopted throughout this book, we now turn to role of biological factors and medical preventive interventions with Arab Americans. Because of the stigma associated with disability in general within the Middle East and among the many and varied traditional cultures of Arab American immigrants, some Arab Americans may somaticize their emotional issues, whether or not they are specifically linked to traumas (e.g., Hakim-Larson, Kamoo, Nassar-McMillan, & Porcerelli, 2007; Nassar-McMillan, 2010). Thus, medical doctors and other medical staff may be the first to encounter Arab Americans in distress. In addition, the medical profession in the Middle East has a long, venerable history harking back to the physicians of the pharaohs and still is held in high esteem in the Arab world where the opinions of medical doctors are highly respected.

It would therefore seem that medical preventive interventions hold great promise for outreach efforts with Arab Americans. The domains of interest for medical preventive interventions include mental health, environmental health, nicotine and other substance abuse prevention, diabetes prevention, prevention of maternal and child health risks, cancer prevention, and cardiovascular health promotion through improvements in diet and exercise. As many medical hospitals and clinics are increasingly acknowledging, mental health issues permeate nearly every facet of medical intervention, and thus cannot be considered solely as a separate domain of intervention.

Public Health Issues and Health Care Disparities

The many public health environmental problems in the Middle East have led to some rudimentary and still-developing advocacy and intervention efforts there as noted by Jamil in Chap. 12; for immigrants to the United States, environmental problems continue especially for those of lower socioeconomic status. There are consequently negative effects of exposure to lead poisoning in poor Arab children and adults, as well as exposure to other toxic substances more prevalent in industrial regions in the US where there are more dense Arab enclaves (Nriagu, Senthamarai-Kannan, Jamil, Fakhori, & Korponic, 2011). From a biopsychosocial perspective, not only is medical intervention needed to assess and remediate the toxic exposures, but also psychological interventions to promote adequate cognitive functioning and learning skills, as well as social interventions to assist with issues such as relocation and housing.

There are a number of health disparities when Arab Americans are compared to other ethnic groups and the mainstream American population, as noted in the chapters from Part III of this volume. Contributing factors to these disparities are access to health care, fear among immigrants of communicating with government systems given their traumatic histories, and actual and perceived prejudice and discrimination.

With respect to substance abuse, the statistics indicate a lower prevalence of drinking but a higher prevalence of smoking, corresponding to Arab cultural and religious values. There are higher risks of diabetes due to lifestyle factors, acculturation, and the precipitous shift for some immigrants who have come from nonindustrialized societies to an industrialized one upon entering the United States. Arab American mothers and children who come from lower socioeconomic groups or who may have an illegal immigrant status are at higher risk due to their limited access to health care and the various barriers to their utilization of the help that is available to them. Cancer and cardiovascular risks for Arab Americans vary by lifestyle adaptations and environmental exposures, in many cases relative to their country of origin and socioeconomic status.

To address these public health issues that seem particularly important for working with Arab Americans, public education of prevention strategies and increased provider awareness are key strategic goals. Medical databases need to more clearly specify which clients have an Arab ethnic background so that better comparative epidemiological data can be garnered. This issue is one that needs to be undertaken globally as advances are made in integrating culturally relevant diagnoses into the DSM-V and ICD-10 diagnostic classification schemes, and improvements are made in facilitating international communication about diagnoses (e.g., American Psychological Association, 2012). International partnerships, as well as national, regional, and local collaborations, are needed to optimize the development of such a research database on diagnostic classifications and treatment. Ultimately, the goal is to have an impact on advocacy, public policy, and service delivery.

Biopsychosocial Perspectives on Arab Americans: Concluding Recommendations

In summary, stakeholders with an interest in the health and well-being of individuals within the Arab Diaspora would do well to prioritize the implementation of preventative intervention measures. Consistent with the ecological approach to preventive medicine, more will be gained in the long run by not merely focusing on remediation of already identified problems. Towards that end, we recommend that consideration be given to the following preventive courses of action:

1. Early preventative interventions are needed for Arab Americans representing particularly vulnerable groups such as youth, elderly, and other potentially underresourced groups. At the micro-level, continued efforts are needed to identify and ameliorate the various environmental toxic risks (e.g., lead, air pollution; exposures to nicotine smoke both prenatally and postnatally). Improving the air quality and physical environment, especially of children, is known to have long-term neurological positive benefits for cognitive, emotional, and behavioral functioning. Public education about the sources of lead poisoning, particularly about the gains in children's development when they are not exposed to toxins such as lead and smoke, would be beneficial.
2. For those Arab Americans who are recent immigrants, preventive measures at micro- and macro-levels include facilitation of the grieving process within the private domain of one's own individual experiences as well as in a public forum. At the private or individual level, the feeling of forgiveness for actual or perceived enemies, coupled with the feeling that there has been justice for perpetrators of crimes, can also assist in promoting well-being. Therapeutic interventions need to take into account the full impacts of the immigration experience, particularly those associated with trauma, and incorporate this aspect of healing into the counseling process. The more public aspect of grieving would need to take place at a macro-level of analysis within the broader collective community. One way that this might be accomplished is for religious and community leaders and event organizers, artists, writers, and musicians to help in placing memories of what has been lost in adaptive perspectives about the past.

3. Public health campaigns are needed to promote better nutrition for Arab Americans consistent with the traditional Mediterranean diet of whole grains, fresh fruits and vegetables, and healthy fats. While one primary focus of this intervention would be preventing obesity, concomitant foci are ameliorating major health risks for cancer, diabetes, and child maternal health burdens and improving mortality rates for Arab Americans locally and nationally. Moreover, public health campaigns can be effective at preventing and combating stigmas about a variety of health issues that may still be held by Arab Americans, particularly among those who are less acculturated.
4. At public policy levels locally and nationally, Arab Americans need to be regarded as a unique population. Continued efforts and resources need to be directed at determining culturally appropriate ways to count Arab Americans within governmental (e.g., Census, Centers for Disease Control) and other data gathering initiatives. More accurate data will promote more culturally competent research and practice, thereby ensuring more effective preventive and clinical intervention measures.
5. At the macro-level nationally, organizations such as the Arab American Institute (http://www.aaiusa.org) and American-Arab Anti-Discrimination Committee (http://www.adc.org) have taken as their mission the task of promoting the well-being of Americans of Arab ethnicity. Support for these organizations and disseminating the information that they provide will be helpful in preventing anti-Arab attitudes within the general American public.
6. Lastly, but perhaps most importantly, cultural competence training needs to occur that includes a portrayal of Arab Americans as both humanistic and adaptive. This training needs to occur at all levels—both micro and macro—locally, nationally, and globally. It is incumbent upon professionals spanning the biopsychosocial disciplines to recognize and act upon the need for this type of training, and in some cases, to themselves provide relevant consultation and training. Organizations such as AAI and ADC, along with others such as Arab World and Islamic Resources (AWAIR, http://www.awaironline.org/) and America-Mideast Educational and Training Services (AMIDEAST, http://amideast.org/), can and do provide referrals and other training resources for various groups.

References

American Psychological Association (2012). Practice update—February 9, 2012. *Transition to the ICD-10-CM: What does it mean for psychologists*? Retrieved from http://www.apapracticecentral.org/update/2012/02-09/transition.aspx

Antonucci, T. C., Birditt, K. S., Sherman, C. W., & Trinh, S. (2011). Stability and change in the intergenerational family: A convoy approach. *Ageing & Society, 31*(7), 1084–1106. doi:10.1017/S0144686X1000098X.

Aprahamian, M., Kaplan, D.M., Windham, A.M., Sutter, J. A., & Visser, J. (2011). The relationship between acculturation and mental health of Arab Americans. *Journal of Mental Health Counseling, 33*, 80–92.

Asseily, A. (2007). *Breaking the cycles of violence in Lebanon - and beyond.* Great Britain: Guerrand-Hermes Foundation for peace publishing. Retrieved from http://www.ghfp.org/publications.aspx

Bakalian, A., & Bozorgmehr, M. (2009). *Backlash 9/11: Middle Eastern and Muslim Americans respond.* Berkeley, CA: University of California Press.

Blumer, H. (1958). Race prejudice as a sense of group position. *The Pacific Sociological Review, 1*(1), 3–7.

Bronfenbrenner, U. (1994). Ecological models of human development. International Encyclopedia of Education (2nd ed., Vol. 3, pp. 1643–1647). Oxford: Elsevier. In M. Gauvain & M. Cole (Eds.), *Readings in the development of children* (2nd ed., 1993, pp. 37–43). NY: Freeman.

Cainkar, L. (2009). *Homeland Insecurity: The Arab American and Muslim American Experience After 9/11.* New York, NY: Russell Sage Foundation Press.

Dalky, H. F. (2012). Perception and coping with stigma of mental illness: Arab families' perspectives. *Issues in Mental Health Nursing, 33,* 486–491. doi:10.3109/01612840.2012.676720.

deMause, L. (2002). The emotional life of nations. New York: Karnac.

Fargues, P. (2006, May). *International migration in the Arab region: Trends and policies.* Beirut, Lebanon: United Nations Expert Group Meeting on International Migration and Development in the Arab Region. Retrieved from http://www.un.org/esa/population/migration/turin/Symposium_Turin_files/P09_Fargues.pdf

Gualtieri, S. (2009). *Between Arab and White: Race and ethnicity in the early syrian American Diaspora.* Berkeley: University of California Press.

Gutkin, T. B. (2012). Ecological psychology: Replacing the medical model paradigm for school-based psychological and psychoeducational services. *Journal of Educational and Psychological Consultation, 22*(1–2), 1–20. doi:10.1080/10474412.2011.649652.

Hakim-Larson, J., Kamoo, R., Nassar-McMillan, S., & Porcerelli, J. H. (2007). Counseling Arab and Chaldean American families. *Journal of Mental Health Counseling, 29,* 301–321.

Hall, R. E. & Breland-Noble, A. (2011). Spirituality vis-a-vis Islam as prerequisite to Arab American well being: The implications of Eurocentrism for mainstream psychology. *American Journal of Psychotherapy, 65,* 151–162.

Issam Fares Institute for Public Policy and International Affairs-American University of Beirut. (2011). *A generation on the move: Insights into the conditions, aspirations and activism of Arab youth – Executive summary.* Beirut, Lebanon: Author. Retrieved from http://www.aub.edu.lb/ifi/public_policy/arab_youth/Documents/20111118ifi_unicef_youth_report/20120126ifi_unicef_menaro_youth_report_agotm_english.pdf

Joseph, S. (2011). *The future today: Youth and adolescents of the Middle East and North Africa/ Situation analysis on adolescents and youth in MENA.* Beirut, Lebanon: Issam Centre for Public Policy and International Affairs-American University of Beirut.

Kira, I. A., Lewandowski, L., Templin, T., Ramaswamy, V., Ozkan, B., & Mohanesh, J. (2008). Measuring cumulative trauma dose, types, and profiles using a development-based taxonomy of traumas. *Traumatology, 14,* 62–87. doi:10.1177/1534765608319324.

Kira, I. A., Templin, T., Lewandowski, L., Clifford, D., Wiencek, P., Hammad, A., et al. (2006). The effects of torture: Two community studies. *Peace and Conflict: Journal of Peace Psychology, 12,* 205–228. doi:10.1207/s15327949pac1203_1.

Larson, J. E., & Corrigan, P. (2008). The stigma of families with mental illness. *Academic Psychiatry, 32,* 87–91.

Marvasti, A., & McKinney, K. D. (2004). *Middle Eastern lives in America.* Lanham, MD: Rowman & Littlefield.

Masten, A. S. (2007). Resilience in developing systems: Progress and promise as the fourth wave rises. *Development and Psychopathology, 19,* 921–930.

Mruk, C. J. (1995). *Self-esteem: Research, theory, and practice.* New York, NY: Springer.

Mruk, C. J. (2006). *Self-esteem research, theory, and practice: Toward a positive psychology of self-esteem* (3rd ed.). New York, NY: Springer.

Nassar-McMillan, S. C. (2010). *Counseling Arab Americans*. Pacific Grove, CA: Brooks-Cole/Cengage.

Nassar-McMillan, S. C., Lambert, R. G., & Hakim-Larson, J. (2011). Discrimination history, backlash fear, and ethnic identity among Arab Americans: Post 9–11 snapshots. *Journal of Multicultural Counseling and Development, 39*(1), 38–47.

Nriagu, J., Senthamarai-Kannan, R., Jamil, H., Fakhori, M., & Korponic, S. (2011). Lead poisoning among Arab American and African American children in the Detroit metropolitan area, Michigan. *Bulletin of Environmental Contamination and Toxicology, 87*, 238–244. doi:10.1007/s00128-011-0346-4.

Richard, L., Gauvin, L., & Raine, K. (2011). Ecological models revisited: Their uses and evolution in health promotion over two decades. *Annual Review of Public Health, 32*, 307–326. doi:10.1146/annurev-publhealth-031210-101141.

Simon, J. P. (1996). Lebanese families. In M. McGoldrick, J. Giordano, & J. K. Pearce (Eds.), *Ethnicity and family therapy* (2nd ed.). New York: Guilford Press.

Suleiman, M. (1999). *Arabs in America: Building a new future*. Philadelphia, PA: Temple University Press.

The United Nations Refugee Agency. (UNHCR, 2007, April). Statistics on displaced Iraqis around the World –UNHCR. Retrieved April, 2007, from http://www.unhcr.org/461f7cb92.pdf.

The United Nations Refugee Agency. (UNHCR, 2012, November). Syria regional refugee response: Information sharing portal. Retrieved from http://data.unhcr.org/syrianrefugees/regional.php.

United Nations Development Programme. (2006). Arab youth strategizing for the Millennium Development Goals (MDGs). Retrieved from http://www.arab-hdr.org/mdg/regional.aspx.

Volkan, V. D. (2000). Traumatized societies and psychological care: Expanding the concept of preventive medicine. *Mind and Human Interaction, 11*, 177–194.

Volkan, V. D. (2011). Shared trauma, transgenerational transmission and societal well-being. Invited paper presentation at the International Conference on Healing the Wounds of History: Addressing the Roots of History, November 11-13, 2011, Byblos, Lebanon.

Index

S.C. Nassar-McMillan et al. (eds.), *Biopsychosocial Perspectives on Arab Americans: Culture, Development, and Health*, DOI 10.1007/978-1-4614-8238-3,

W

Y